INFANT PERCEPTION: FROM SENSATION TO COGNITION

volume I   Basic Visual Processes

THE CHILD PSYCHOLOGY SERIES
EXPERIMENTAL AND THEORETICAL ANALYSES OF CHILD BEHAVIOR

EDITOR
DAVID S. PALERMO
DEPARTMENT OF PSYCHOLOGY
THE PENNSYLVANIA STATE UNIVERSITY
UNIVERSITY PARK, PENNSYLVANIA

INFANT PERCEPTION: FROM SENSATION TO COGNITION

volume I Basic Visual Processes

Edited by

Leslie B. Cohen

Department of Psychology and
Institute for Child Behavior and Development
University of Illinois
Champaign, Illinois

Philip Salapatek

Institute of Child Development
University of Minnesota
Minneapolis, Minnesota

ACADEMIC PRESS New York San Francisco London

A Subsidiary of Harcourt Brace Jovanovich, Publishers

7137-7529

OPTOMETRY

*BF723
I6I53l v. 1 Repl
v. 1*

ACADEMIC PRESS, INC.
111 Fifth Avenue, New York, New York 10003

United Kingdom Edition published by
ACADEMIC PRESS, INC. (LONDON) LTD.
24/28 Oval Road, London NW1

Library of Congress Cataloging in Publication Data
Main entry under title:

Infant perception.

        (Child psychology)
        Includes bibliographies and index.
        CONTENTS: v. 1.   Basic visual processes.
        1.   Infant psychology.   2.   Visual perception.
3.   Auditory perception.   I.   Cohen, Leslie B.
II.   Salapatek, Philip.   [DNLM: 1.   Cognition—In
infancy and childhood.   2.   Perception—In infancy
and childhood.   3.   Sensation—In infancy and
childhood.   WS105 I41]
BF723.I6153   155.4'22   75-3582
ISBN 0-12-178601-3

PRINTED IN THE UNITED STATES OF AMERICA

Acknowledgment is made for the following excerpts:
Page 144: From Hochberg, J. Attention, organization, and consciousness. In D.
Mostofsky (Ed.), *Attention: Contemporary theory and analysis,* © 1970. By permission of Prentice-Hall, Inc., Englewood Cliffs, New Jersey.
Page 206: From Humphrey, N. K. Seeing and nothingness. *New Scientist,* 1972, 30
March, 682–684. This extract first appeared in *New Scientist,* London. The weekly review of science and technology.

Contents

chapter 3: Pattern Perception in Early Infancy

PHILIP SALAPATEK

chapter 4: Early Visual Selectivity

ROBERT L. FANTZ, JOSEPH F. FAGAN, III,
AND SIMÓN B. MIRANDA

chapter 5: Infant Visual Memory

LESLIE B. COHEN AND ERIC R. GELBER

List of Contributors

Numbers in parentheses indicate the pages on which the authors' contributions begin.

Leslie B. Cohen (347), Department of Psychology, Institute for Child Behavior and Development, University of Illinois, Urbana–Champaign, Illinois

Joseph F. Fagan, III (249), Department of Psychology, Case Western Reserve University, Cleveland, Ohio

Robert L. Fantz (249), Department of Psychology, Case Western Reserve University, Cleveland, Ohio

Eric R. Gelber (347), Department of Psychology, University of Arizona, Tucson, Arizona

Bernard L. Karmel (77), Department of Psychology, University of Connecticut, Storrs, Connecticut

Eileen B. Maisel (77), Department of Psychology, University of Connecticut, Storrs, Connecticut

Daphne Maurer (1), Department of Psychology, McMaster University, Hamilton, Ontario, Canada

Simón B. Miranda (249), Department of Psychology, Case Western Reserve University, Cleveland, Ohio

Philip Salapatek (133), Institute of Child Development, University of Minnesota, Minneapolis, Minnesota

Preface

Perceptual development has been one of the most rapidly expanding areas of investigation over the past two decades. A number of
factors have converged to make this expansion possible: the
dissemination of Piagetian theory and data, the application of
ethology to human behavior, the redemonstration by Fantz (originally demonstrated by the German psychophysicists) that even the
newborn can be cajoled into answering interesting research questions, improvements in both technology and methodology, and
finally, striking recent advances in developmental neurophysiology.

The study of infant perception has experienced a particularly
fruitful proliferation during this period. Although isolated reports of
the infant's ability to see and hear date back to the nineteenth
century, it has only been within the last few years that investigators
have begun comprehensive programmatic examinations of early
sensory, perceptual, and cognitive systems. The present volumes,
which constitute the first synthesis of recent research and theorizing on infant perception, reflect this trend. The contributors do
more than list what the infant is capable of perceiving; their
approach is to organize the material in a cohesive, systematic
framework. Several authors outdid themselves, summarizing large
bodies of existing research, reporting in some detail previously

unpublished data, and integrating the two into an original theoretical system. What has emerged is a view of the infant as a curious blend of neural–behavioral systems—reflex and voluntary, sensory and perceptual, sensorimotor and representational—who provides a likely bridge between advances in ethology, neurophysiology, and sensory systems on one hand, and the cognitive linguistic mature human on the other.

We did not feel compelled to include systematically all areas or modalities of infant perception in these two volumes. Our constant goal was to represent and analyze the flow of programmatic investigations, rather than isolated studies or pockets of research. The amount of research has been most pronounced in infant vision, and to a lesser extent in infant audition. For this reason the organization of the volumes reflects that emphasis with the first volume and most of the second devoted to infant visual perception. Although a search was made, we were unable to fulfill our goal in the "other" sensory systems, e.g., taste, smell, touch, the vestibular and kinesthetic senses. However, given the continuing proliferation of research in all areas of early perceptual development, we expect such chapters to be feasible in the very near future.

Volume I begins with a chapter by Maurer in which most of the major physiological and behavioral techniques used to measure infant vision are assessed. Each technique is critically evaluated in terms of the method employed, the type of data which can be obtained, and the anatomy of the visual system. In Chapter 2, Karmel and Maisel show how one of these techniques (measurement of visually evoked responses) can be used to assess infant visual preferences for patterns varying in amount of contour. They also propose a neuronal model to explain developmental changes in these preferences.

The value of the corneal reflection technique for the study of infant attention and visual scanning patterns is amply demonstrated by Salapatek in Chapter 3. Integrating considerable evidence from his own work as well as data from other laboratories, he provides answers to basic questions about the innate organization of perception, focal versus peripheral processing, and oculomotor involvement in perceptual learning. The evidence is also used as a basis for evaluating a variety of existing theories of perceptual development.

In Chapter 4, Fantz, Fagan, and Miranda examine both developmental changes and individual differences in early pattern perception. The authors present a large body of data, accumulated over a number of years, in order to trace the development of visual preferences for variations in form, pattern arrangement, size versus number of elements, and novelty versus familiarity. They show that most of these changes are a function of gestational age rather than age since birth, and that their techniques are also sensitive to differences between retarded and normal infants.

The final chapter in Volume I could be considered a continuation of the preceding one. Cohen and Gelber concentrate on evidence of infant visual preferences for novelty and on the implications of such evidence for models of early recognition memory. The pros and cons of habituation versus paired comparison techniques are discussed, and evidence from both is shown to be remarkably consistent on such issues as the type of visual information infants can remember, how long they can remember, and the conditions most likely to produce interference with that memory.

Volume II begins where Volume I leaves off. The chapters in Volume I are arranged along a continuum from basic sensory and neurophysiological functioning to information processing and memory. All of the chapters deal primarily with two-dimensional pattern perception. In Volume II the third dimension, depth, is added. The first chapter by Yonas and Pick discusses the difficulties prior research has had in assessing infant perception of depth or space. Two research strategies are proposed which would provide more powerful evidence of early space perception, and several specific experiments are suggested which employ these new strategies. The second chapter by Bower provides a link between infants' perception of space and their perception of objects. In the first half of the chapter he argues that occlusion information is critical to an infant's perception of depth, and in the second half he argues that the development of object permanence seems to require both an infant's perception of three-dimensional boundedness and his understanding of the transformation involved when one object goes inside another.

The development of object permanence is discussed further in the next chapter, by Gratch. After a brief description of Piaget's sensorimotor stages, Gratch critically evaluates both psychometric studies of object concept development and studies focusing specifically on Piaget's theory. The chapter closes with a comparison of "constructivist" (Piaget) versus "realist" (Gibson) theories, and the conclusion is reached that neither can provide a completely adequate account of all the data.

"Constructivist" versus "realist" theories are also compared in the chapter by Lewis and Brooks, but this time in reference to social perception. The authors reject the notion that theories constructed to explain infant nonsocial perception are also sufficient for social perception. Considerable emphasis is placed on the infant's development of the concept of self, and that concept is used to explain the infant's perception of other persons.

The theme changes in the final two chapters of Volume II, from infant vision to infant audition. Nevertheless, the organization of the chapters reflects the same continuum from basic sensory and neurophysiological functioning to information processing and social–linguistic ability. In Chapter 5 Hecox describes in detail the developmental anatomy of the auditory pathway. Major anatomical structures from the middle ear to the cortex are discussed in terms of both function and development. Next comes an examination of electrophysiological functioning, followed by the description of experiments in which one electrophysiological measure (the brainstem evoked response) is effectively used to assess infant auditory capacity.

In the concluding chapter of Volume II Eimas describes a series of studies on the infant's receptiveness for the segmental units of speech, his ability to perceive phonemic feature contrasts, and the manner in which this perception occurs. A theoretical mechanism for infant speech perception is also proposed, and an attempt is made to relate the findings on early speech perception to the development of the full linguistic competence.

The task of editing these two volumes was somewhat more difficult than we had anticipated but also considerably more rewarding. We became more and more pleased as one chapter after another appeared with original theoretical and methodological statements as well as reviews of research. We would like to express our appreciation to the authors for their obvious expenditure of time, effort, and thought on their contributions. We would also like to thank our students and colleagues for their help in editing manuscripts, and, in particular, Richard Aslin, Martin Banks, Ruth Pearl, Elliot Saltzman, and Robert Schwartz for preparation of the subject index.

Contents of Volume II

INFANT PERCEPTION: FROM SENSATION TO COGNITION

volume I   Basic Visual Processes

chapter 1:   Infant Visual Perception: Methods of Study

DAPHNE MAURER
McMaster University

I. INTRODUCTION

It is hard to study visual perception in human infants. Direct methods do not work—one cannot ask a neonate what he sees—and indirect methods, such as recording the visually evoked potential (VEP), can become horrendously involved and time consuming.

Furthermore, indirect methods often produce data that are difficult to interpret. Take the visually evoked potential, for instance. Its amplitude depends, at least in adults, on all these factors: the location of the electrodes; the size, intensity, wavelength, and patterning of the stimulus; the location of the stimulus on the retina; and the subject's visual acuity and state of alertness. Only after we understand all these influences can we ask what the data show about perception—and even then there will be complications. If the amplitude of the infant's response is less than the amplitude of the adult's, that may be because the infant's acuity is poorer—or because his macula is less developed.

This chapter is a guide to reading studies which have used indirect methods to study the visual perception of infants. It outlines the methods, examines their advantages and shortcomings,

1

points out any peculiar pitfalls, summarizes the studies with infants, and suggests appropriate interpretations. The methods include anatomical analysis, electroretinography, electrooculography, corneal reflection, and the studies of optokinetic nystagmus and the visually evoked potential. Each one is treated separately and in three parts: (1) general methodological considerations, (2) summary of the studies done with infants, and (3) interpretation.

II. ANATOMY

A. General Methodological Considerations

Psychologists have examined the anatomy of the infant's visual system to find out if the infant has all the physiological bases for vision. They have studied the dimensions of his eye to find out how well it should be able to deal optically with light (Figure 1.1 shows these dimensions in an adult's eye), and they have studied all parts of his visual pathway to find out how well it should be able to translate light into nervous impulses and then transmit and process those impulses. Most of these studies have by necessity been done on dead organisms—which presents a serious problem, for the eye changes after death.[1]

For one thing, several structures change in size, some increasing and others decreasing. Studies of the adult show that the disk (Last, 1968) and some other parts of the eye (Kestenbaum, 1963) may swell, including the cornea if it is not kept with intact epithelium and endothelium and at 31°C, the normal temperature of aqueous humor (Davson, 1972). Studies of the infant show that other parts of the visual system shrink: the cortex of the brain, because it contains so much water (Conel, 1939), and probably the eyeball itself (Todd, Beecher, Williams, & Todd, 1940).

Death also causes changes of pressure, which in turn cause more changes of size and also of shape. In adults, intraocular tension is reduced; so the volume of the eye decreases, the length of all diameters is reduced by 5%, and the outer coats of the eye (the sclera and the cornea) become thicker (Kestenbaum, 1963). Moreover, in the living adult's eye, but not in the dead eye, the lens is

---

[1] These changes can probably be minimized by freeze-drying the eye immediately after death, but no one who has studied the anatomy of the infant's visual system has done this.

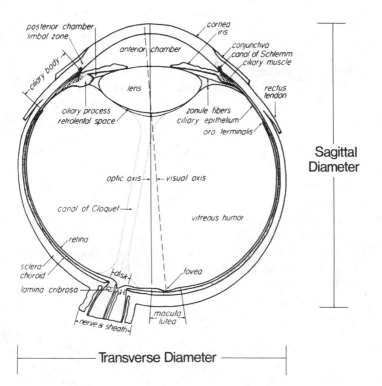

posterior chamber
limbal zone
anterior chamber
cornea
iris
conjunctiva
canal of Schlemm
ciliary muscle
ciliary body
lens
rectus tendon
ciliary process
retrolental space
zonule fibers
ciliary epithelium
ora terminalis
optic axis
visual axis
canal of Cloquet
vitreous humor
retina
sclera
choroid
disk
fovea
lamina cribrosa
nerve & sheath
macula lutea

Sagittal Diameter

Transverse Diameter

Figure 1.1   Horizontal section of the right human eyeball. [Adapted from Walls, 1942, p. 7.]

displaced forward because of a difference in osmotic pressure between the vitreous and acqueous humors (Kestenbaum, 1963).

These changes as they occur in adults have been confirmed by Kestenbaum (1963), who compared measurements of living eyes made by optical techniques with direct measurements of dead eyes. But not all studies of infants' eyes have found such striking differences. Sorsby and Sheridan (1960) note a close agreement of their measurements of dead corneas with both measurements made on dead eyes (by Schneller) and estimates made on living eyes (by Kaiser and by Hymes). And they claim the newborn's eyes do not change even a long time after death, since they found no difference between measurements made sometime within the first week after death and measurements made 6 weeks later. However, they did not take any measurements soon enough after death to catch immediate changes.

In addition to changes in the dimensions of the visual system, death also causes changes in its chemical composition—at least in the adult. The chloride content of the lens increases a few hours after death; the concentration of lactic acid increases within 40 hr in even the best of artificial media; and cooling causes the potassium content to drop and the sodium content to rise (Davson, 1972).

The typical anatomical preparation is not only dead, it is also in a fixative, which causes more disruption. Ehlers, Matthiessen, and Anderson (1968) studied the effects of fixatives on 107 fetuses and found they caused changes in all dimensions of the eye. Fixation in 4% neutral buffered formaldehyde caused a 2% reduction in the weight of the eye and in its sagittal diameter, plus a 4% reduction in its corneal diameter and a 10% reduction in the lens's weight (yet it had no effect on the transverse diameter or on the lens's diameters). Preservation in a mixture of ethanol, formaldehyde, and acetic acid had more serious consequences: The weight of the eye decreased 22%, the sagittal diameter decreased 5%, the transverse diameter decreased 2%, the corneal diameter decreased 10%, and the lens's weight and diameter decreased 30% and 10% respectively. Note the serious problem here: Most dimensions change, but they do not change to the same extent. Moreover, greater reductions occur in smaller fetuses.[2]

Death and fixation also affect the body's weight and size, so the age of a specimen cannot be gauged using norms determined from living infants. And since the amount of shrinkage depends on the type of fixation, norms determined from dead infants will be unreliable. As a result, eyes from babies born prematurely are often confused with eyes from babies born at term.

For histological studies, the tissue is not only dead and fixed, it is also stained, usually, if from infants, with Cresyl violet, Golgi-Cox impregnation, Weigert's method, or Cajal silver impregnation. And staining also disrupts preparations: The paraffin-embedding of

---

[2] Scammon and Armstrong (1925) also studied eyes from fetuses preserved with formaldehyde, but note no effect on sagittal diameter when comparing their measurements to those made by others on unpreserved eyes; and Todd *et al.* (1940), who studied eyes from infants of all ages as well as from adults, conclude that preservation with formaldehyde will not change the eyeball's weight if the eyeball is distended with water to its maximum size in a reasonable period of time. But note that Ehlers *et al.* (1968) found the eyeball's weight and sagittal diameter are two of the parameters least affected by formaldehyde. Fixatives certainly have effects on other dimensions.

Weigert's procedure, for example, causes from 25% to 35% shrinkage in cortical tissue, with the amount of shrinkage dependent on the amount of myelin present (the more myelin, the less shrinkage) (Rabinowicz, 1967a). Moreover, a stain can color one structure within a preparation more deeply than another similar structure, even if they are the same size (Scheibel & Scheibel, 1971).

Partial and uneven staining makes the study of myelinization difficult, because myelinization is usually gauged by the density of stained fibers and the intensity of their coloration. Moreover, these criteria do not indicate the maturity of myelinization since some fibers remain light gray while others pass through many gradations of intensity.

The standard counting technique can also lead to errors. The procedure is first to count the number of cells in a section 25μ thick and then to multiply the outcome by 4, thereby estimating the number of cells in a unit 100μ thick. A slice 25μ thick at birth represents a greater proportion of the total retina or the total cortex than it will later. Moreover, at any age the count will vary with the magnification of the microscope, the exact thickness of the section, the darkness of the stain, the experimenter's criteria, and other highly variable factors (Rabinowicz, 1967b). Even more serious is a developmental change affecting the detectability of cells: The larger neurons grow, the more they are underestimated (Rabinowicz, 1967b).

A few recent studies using ultrasound to measure living subjects have avoided the problems of using dead, fixed, and stained preparations. When high frequency sound waves are beamed into the eye, they reflect off the various surfaces in the eye. These reflections can be converted into an electrical signal by a transducer and then displayed on an oscilloscope. By noting the time lag between the reflections of the beam off two surfaces, it is possible to calculate the distance between them—if it is known how fast the medium between them transmits ultrasound, and if the beam is directed straight into the eye along the optic axis. Agreement between measurements made by ultrasound and by optical techniques is generally good (Jansson, 1963; Larsen, 1971b).

But ultrasound has its own set of methodological problems: Its resolving power is only about .8 mm, so the posterior wall of the cornea cannot be measured (Jansson, 1963); the velocities of its transmission through some media in the eye can only be estimated; and errors will occur if the path of the beam is off the optic axis. With adults, this last error seems to be small: Ten measurements of the depth of one eye's anterior chamber produced a mean of 3.9037 mm with a standard deviation of .033 mm (Larsen, 1971a), while a similar test on the lens produced a mean of 3.65 mm with a standard deviation of .066 mm (Larsen, 1971b). But in newborns this error is greater: Five measurements on each of three placid infants yielded a deviation around the first measurement of .1 mm.

Also, ultrasound may be hazardous: It may harm the eye through thermal absorption, local accelerations as high as 140,000 g, and variations in pressure as great as 3.7 atm (Jansson, 1963). But Jansson notes that the average local displacement is only .04μ, and that animals exposed to ultrasound of low intensity or for a short period of time show no signs of damage.

B.   Summary of the Data from Infants

Anatomical studies must be read cautiously: Measurements of weight are suspect because of the problems from death and fixation; size estimates also suffer from these problems, or from the problems of ultrasound; and measurements of myelinization and of the number and density of cells are, in addition, affected by staining and counting. For reliable information one must compare a great number of studies carried out under a variety of procedures and hope the results give a consistent picture—which, in general, they do.

1.   DIMENSIONS OF THE BULBUS

Many investigators have measured the diameters (Barber, 1955; Duke-Elder & Cook, 1963; Larsen, 1971a, b, c, d; Scammon & Armstrong, 1925; Sorsby & Sheridan, 1960; Wilmer & Scammon, 1950) and the volume (Scammon & Armstrong, 1925; Wilmer & Scammon, 1950) of the newborn's eye. Typical measurements are 17.5 mm for the sagittal diameter, 17.1 mm for the transverse diameter, 16.5 mm for the vertical diameter and 3.25 ml for the volume. Comparable figures for the adult are 24 mm, 24 mm, 23 mm, and 6.6 ml.

At birth the sagittal diameter is longer than the vertical diameter, but the vertical diameter grows faster, allowing the eye to become more nearly spherical (Barber, 1955; Knighton, 1939; Last, 1968; Sorsby & Sheridan, 1960). Growth of all the diameters is rapid during the first two postnatal years and continues through the middle of childhood (Duke-Elder & Cook, 1963; Knighton, 1939;

Larsen, 1971a, d). But compared to the rest of the body the eye grows relatively little: It only doubles in size while the body increases 20 times (Mann, 1964; Scammon & Armstrong, 1925). In this respect the eye resembles the rest of the central nervous system, which increases by a factor of 3.5.

2. THE ORBIT

During fetal development the eyeballs rotate forward in the head: The angle of the optic nerves at the optic chiasm decreases from 105° to 71°, with the most extensive change during the formation of the face in the second and third months (Zimmerman, Armstrong, & Scammon, 1934). A further reduction to 68° occurs sometime before adulthood, probably because of ossification and the union of different bony parts of the orbit.

3. THE CORNEA

The cornea grows less than the rest of the eye, and faster: The transverse diameter at birth is about 10 mm, and by 1 year the diameter nears the adult's value of 12 mm (Barber, 1955; Hymes, 1929; Parks, 1966; Scammon & Armstrong, 1925; Sorsby & Sheridan, 1961; Wilmer & Scammon, 1950). The shape of the newborn's cornea is similar to the adult's with two exceptions: The radius of curvature is about 1 mm less (Walton, 1970), and the cornea is more curved at the periphery, so it is more spherical (Duke-Elder & Cook, 1963; Last, 1968; Parks, 1966; Sorsby & Sheridan, 1961). The cornea is also thinner (Mann, 1964), and refracts more than the adult's (50.5 D versus 43.0 D).

4. THE LENS

Many studies of the lens's dimensions have been done (Larsen, 1971b; Mann, 1964; Scammon & Hesdorffer, 1937; Sorsby & Sheridan, 1961; Wilmer & Scammon, 1950). Typical figures are 4 mm for thickness, 6 mm for diameter, 4 mm for anterior radius, and 66 mg for weight. The lens of the newborn is more spherical than the lens of the adult (Duke-Elder & Cook, 1963; Knighton, 1939; Last, 1968; Mann, 1964; Parks, 1966; Walton, 1970), and as it grows flatter it becomes less refractive. Unlike other parts of the eye, the lens grows throughout life, albeit very little (Duke-Elder & Cook, 1963; Knighton, 1939; Scammon & Hesdorffer, 1937).

5. THE RETINA

By 5½ months after conception the retina has all its layers present in their final arrangement (Mann, 1964). By 7 months after conception the retina has substantially the adult's proportions, and the visual pathway is anatomically complete and capable of functioning. Even the fovea has begun to form.

As early as 23 weeks after conception, rods and cones can be distinguished. The beginnings of the cones' synapses can also be observed: A few processes, probably from bipolar and horizontal cells, end near primitive pedicles, which contain a few synaptic vesicles and tubules (Yamada & Ishikawa, 1965). Before term, rods, cones, and the cones' synapses become structurally indistinguishable from those in the adult's retina: the rods and cones at 36 weeks, and the cones' synapses at 27 weeks.

Even so, at birth the macula is less mature than the rest of the retina (Duke-Elder & Cook, 1963; Last, 1968; Mann, 1964; Peiper, 1963). The cones in the macula are shorter, stumpier, and less numerous than they will be later; and there are many layers of ganglion, amacrine, and bipolar cells present which will eventually move to the periphery. By 4 months after birth most of the ganglion, bipolar, and amacrine cells have disappeared from the macula, and the cones are longer and more densely packed.

6. THE OPTIC NERVE

The optic nerve in the newborn's eye is both thinner and shorter than that in the adult's: The diameter of its anterior end is about 1 mm as opposed to about 1.5 mm in the adult's; the diameter of its posterior end is about 2 mm as opposed to about 3 mm in the adult's; and its length is about 1.2 mm as opposed to 1.4 mm (Mann, 1964; Scammon & Armstrong, 1925; Wilmer & Scammon, 1950). Growth precedes from the region of the optic chiasm toward the retina (Bembridge, 1956; Duke-Elder & Cook, 1963; Larroche, 1966; Parks, 1966; Walton, 1970), and axons originating in the macula tend to myelinate first (Bembridge, 1956; Nakayama, 1968; Walton, 1970).

Myelin is first detectable on the optic nerve during the sixth fetal month (Bembridge, 1956; Nakayama, 1968), although Langworthy (1933) did not detect it until the eighth fetal month. Subsequent progress is rapid: Various investigators have found the completion of myelinization at 3 weeks (Last, 1968), 1 month (Nakayama, 1968), 10 weeks (Keibel, 1912; Knighton, 1939; Mann, 1964), 3 months (Yakovlev & Lecours, 1967), and 4 months (Duke-Elder & Cook, 1963; Parks, 1966; Walton, 1970). Whichever is the case, the optic nerve has one of the quickest rates of myelinization in the nervous system.

Some studies have shown that exposure of the eye to light accelerates myelinization (Langworthy, 1933; Last, 1968), but not all studies have supported this idea (Nakayama, 1968).

7. THE VISUAL CORTEX

Differentiation of the visual cortex is marked after the twenty-eighth week of fetal life (Larroche, 1966). There is no longer evidence of mitosis by the eighth fetal month (Rabinowicz, 1964), but at birth many neurons are not in their proper layers (Conel, 1939) and there are no Nissl bodies or neurofibrils (Conel, 1939; Larroche, 1966). Differentiation continues into early childhood at a steady pace: The density of cells decreases and cells are more likely to be in their proper layers; dendrites get larger, end in layers farther away from the cell's body, and develop more pedunculated bulbs; axons and their branches get longer; chromophil becomes more plentiful and more differentiated; and neurofibrils appear (Conel, 1941, 1947, 1951, 1955, 1959). Areas differ in when they first show evidence of myelin, and there is a general increase in myelin with development. In general, vertical fibers myelinate before horizontal fibers, which in turn myelinate before tangential fibers.

C. Interpretation of Results

The problem with using anatomical data to make inferences about infants' visual perception is that the correlation between physiology and behavior is as yet very poorly understood. For example, consider this datum about the newborn's retina: The macula is less developed than the rest of the retina, with fewer and stumpier cones. Now, macular cones are involved in visual acuity, so one can safely say newborns have relatively poor acuity. But since the contribution of any one cone or the effect of its particular size and shape is not known, we cannot make any more specific predictions.

The easiest data to correlate with visual behavior would be discontinuous data, data showing a sudden anatomical change that coincides with a change in visual behavior. Unfortunately, most anatomical development is continuous: Myelinization gradually increases, cones gradually change their shape and number, dendrites gradually elaborate, etc. And when there are discontinuous anatomical changes (like the first detection of myelin on a certain type of fiber, the first appearance of neurofibrils, or the first appearance of Nissl bodies), they are rarely correlated with behavioral changes.

Nevertheless, one can infer the effect of myelinization on the functioning of the nervous system: Myelin speeds neural transmission, so increased myelinization of the optic tract and the visual cortex should aid visual perception. Still, myelinization is not *necessary* for neural functioning since there are many examples of functioning without it: The fetal rat moves many days before its brain is myelinated; the newborn opossum can locate its mother's pouch and nipples even though there is no sign of myelin on its central nervous system; and the human optic nerve can function after 28 weeks' gestation when myelinization has only just begun (Gottlieb, 1971; Langworthy, 1933; Robinson, 1969).

More helpful data are the shape and dimensions of the cornea and lens. The high refractivity of the cornea and lens should compensate for the shortness of the newborn's eyeball. And spherical aberration and hence peripheral acuity should be worse in the newborn's eye than in the adult's, since the adult's flatter peripheral cornea compensates for spherical aberration at least to some extent.[3]

The simple fact that the infant's eye is smaller than the adult's also has an implication for the infant's vision. Since stimuli subtending equal visual angles will fall on a smaller area of retina in the infant than in the adult, therefore fewer receptors will be stimulated in the infant and he should have poorer acuity.

III. THE ELECTRORETINOGRAM

A. General Methodological Considerations

An electroretinogram (ERG) is a record of slow changes of electrical potential produced by the retina when it is exposed to light. In humans the potential is usually recorded by two electrodes, an active electrode embedded in a contact lens placed against the anterior surface of the eye, and a reference electrode placed on the forehead. The eyelid is held open, and often the eye is anesthetized and the pupil is dilated.

Diffuse light is almost always used as the stimulus. In the human adult, the ERG produced in response to it consists of a negative a-wave followed by a large, positive b-wave, a slowly rising, positive c-wave, and finally a small, positive d-wave occurring after the end of the stimulus (see Figure 1.2). When the stimulus is red light, a positive x-wave precedes the b-wave. This wave has also been called the photopic b-wave.

The signal is small—only about 50 μV—so random noise may obscure it, especially when weak stimuli are used. The ratio of signal to noise can be increased by averaging the signal, presenting the stimulus repeatedly and then combining the several responses into an average response.

The more light that reaches the retina, the stronger the response; so, for example, when the pupil dilates, the b-wave increases (Karpe, 1945). And as the intensity of the stimulus increases, so usually does the amplitude of the response, with the exact effect dependent on the organism. In the cat the a-wave is present only with high intensities (Brown, 1968; Granit, 1933). In the frog, cat, and adult human, if the intensity of the stimulus increases, so does the amplitude of the b-wave, while the latency—and duration— decrease (Karpe, 1945), at least over a middle range of intensities (Armington, 1968; Riggs & Wooten, 1972). Also, in the adult human the a- and x-waves increase in amplitude with increases in intensity (Armington, 1968; Riggs & Wooten, 1972).

The duration of the stimulus and its wavelength are also impor-

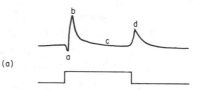

Figure 1.2   (a) The electroretinogram of a light-adapted human to a 1-sec light. (b) The electroretinogram of a light-adapted human to a flash of red light.

tant. In the adult human both the amplitude and latency of the b-wave vary greatly with different wavelengths, and an x-wave appears only with wavelengths over 600 mμ (Armington, 1966).[4] The amplitude of the b-wave increases with the duration of the stimulus, up to a duration of 1 sec (Riggs & Wooten, 1972).

Another parameter is the location of the stimulus on the retina. In the human adult, the b-wave is more prominent when the stimulus is directed toward the peripheral retina than when it is directed toward the central retina (Davson, 1972), while the x-wave (in response to red light) is largest when the fovea is stimulated (Armington, 1966). These findings have serious methodological implications: The responses recorded to two stimuli may differ simply because they happen to fall on different parts of the retina. Two safeguards are to distribute the stimulus over the entire retina by placing a diffusing sphere over the eye (Brunette, 1973), or to locate the stimulus precisely on just one part of the retina. But it is difficult to locate the stimulus precisely because light scatters: Recordings made when light is directed at the blind spot are similar to recordings made when the light is directed at adjacent regions (Davson, 1972).[5]

The size of the stimulus also affects the response, although part of that effect may be caused by different stimuli's falling on different parts of the retina or creating different amounts of stray light. In the cat, a stimulus 1° wide produces no trace of the a-, c-, and d-waves found with a stimulus 5° wide (Granit, 1933); and the latency of the b-wave decreases as the width of the stimulus increases (Karpe, 1945). In adult humans, the amplitudes of both the a- and b-waves decrease with reductions in the size of the stimulus until there is almost no response to a stimulus of less that 2° (Armington, 1968).

Dark adaption also changes the response, with components affected differently in different organisms. Adaptation increases the amplitude of the b-wave in the cynomolgus monkey and pigeon; abolishes the a-wave in the cat; has no effect on the x-wave in any organism; and in organisms like man with both rods and cones, it increases the amplitudes of both the b- and the c-waves while diminishing the d-wave (Adrian, 1946; Brown, 1968; Davson, 1972; Karpe, 1945; Riggs, 1954; Riggs & Wooten, 1972).

---

[4] Some of the effects, however, may be caused only by differences in luminance between wavelengths (Riggs & Wooten, 1972).

[5] See Riggs and Wooten (1972) for a summary of methods devised to overcome this problem.

Finally, recordings from adults are made when the subjects are awake, but recordings from infants are usually made when the subjects are asleep. This may make a difference, since when an adult shuts his eyes the amplitude of his ERG decreases (Barnet, Lodge, & Armington, 1965). Unfortunately, the only relevant study (Lodge, Armington, Barnet, Shanks, & Newcomb, 1969) in infants compared just two different states of sleep: It compared the ERG during stage 1 and stage 2 sleep (as defined by the voltage of the electroencephalogram, the presence of spindling, and the presence of eye and muscle movements), and found unsystematic variation. But this might have been caused by the position of the pupil: In stage 1 sleep the pupil is aligned with the stimulus, while in stage 2 sleep it sometimes moves under the eyelid.

B. Summary of the Data from Infants

Table 1.1 summarizes the data on ERG that have been gathered from newborn infants. It shows that with intense stimuli and/or dark adaptation and/or averaging, the a-wave and the b-wave can be found in the newborn. Moreover, with red light an x-wave is obtained. No investigator has used a long enough stimulus to test for the c-wave. The latency of the b-wave is usually longer than that in the adult, and its amplitude is lower.

When responding to changes of intensity, the newborn's ERG behaves in most respects like the adult's. As the stimulus gets more intense, the amplitudes of the a-, b-, and x-waves increase, and the latency of the b-wave decreases (Barnet *et al.*, 1965; Horsten & Winkelman, 1962; Lodge *et al.*, 1969).

Another similarity of the infant's and adult's ERG is its critical flicker fusion frequency (CFF), the slowest rate at which the stimulus can be flashed on and off that will elicit not a discrete response to each flash, but a continuous response beginning with the first flash and continuing till the last. Dark-adapted newborns and even prematures show the adult's CFF of 72 flashes per second (Horsten & Winkelman, 1962, 1964) (although non-dark-adapted newborns show a lower CFF—Zetterstrom, 1955; Heck & Zetterstrom, 1958a). And like the adult's, the newborn's CFF increases with an increase in the intensity of the stimulus (Horsten & Winkelman, 1962, 1964).

Surprisingly, the "refractory period" of the infant's ERG is

TABLE 1.1 SUMMARY OF STUDIES OF THE ELECTRORETINOGRAM IN NEWBORNS

Study	Subjects					Stimuli					Results		
	Number	State	Local anesthesia	Pupil dilation	Dark adaptation	Intensity	Size	Flash rate (no. per min)	Color	Averaging	Components present	Amplitude b-wave (mV)[a]	Latency b-wave (msec)[b]
Algvere & Zetterstrom, 1967	15	asleep by the end	yes	yes	5 min	33,000 lux	90°	1	white	no	a,b, wavelets on b	.10	longer[c]
Barnet, Lodge, & Armington, 1965	12	often asleep	yes	yes	15 min	various, including 64.9 lux	8°	180	white	yes	a,b	less[d]	96
Barnet, Lodge, & Armington, 1965	12	often asleep	yes	yes	15 min	various, including 64.9 lux	8°	180	orange	yes	a,b,x	—	longer[c]
Heck & Zetterstrom, 1958a	18	asleep	yes	yes	—	700 lux	—	60	white	yes	b, off	less[d]	75

Study													
Horsten & Winkelman, 1962	10	asleep	yes	yes	5 min	1.5, 6, 25, 60 lux at 25 cm from eyes	—	—	white	no	a,b	less[d]	—
Horsten & Winkelman, 1962	10	asleep	yes	yes	15 min	1.5, 6, 25, 60 lux at 25 cm from eyes	?	?	white	no	a,b	less[d]	—
Lodge, Armington, Barnet, Shanks, & Newcomb, 1969	12	often asleep	yes	yes	15 min	various	8°	24	blue-white	yes	a,b	21.2	76
	9	often asleep	yes	yes	5 min–15 min	various	8°	24	orange	yes	a,b,x	7.9	58
Shipley & Anton, 1964	10	often asleep	yes	yes	1 hr	650,000 lux at 6 inches from lamp	53°	2	white	no	a,b	91	—
Zetterstrom 1951	35	—	no	yes	—	20, 80, 1600 lux	—	—	white	no	none	—	—

[a] Measured from the trough of the a-wave to the peak of the b-wave.
[b] Measured from the onset of the stimulus to the peak of the b-wave.
[c] Slightly longer than in the adult.
[d] Less than in the adult.

shorter than the adult's: An infant (1 to 12 months) will give a second b-wave that is at least 70% of the first one after an interval of only 300 msec, while an adult requires an interval of 500 msec (Francois & de Rouck, 1964).

There is evidence that both physical maturity and experience affect the development of the ERG. Studying premature children, Zetterstrom (1952) found a positive correlation between the weight of the child at birth and the age at which the ERG was first detected.[6] But the prematures that weighed the most developed an ERG within 2 weeks of birth, just as full-term babies did (when she measured them without averaging).

C. Interpretation of Results

To compare one study of the ERG with another, all these factors must be identical: the intensity, wavelength, duration, and retinal size of the stimulus; its location on the retina; and the subject's states of sleep and of dark adaptation. But these parameters differ across studies and probably cannot be held constant across ages: The effects of any given intensity or wavelength, and the requirements for dark adaptation, are likely to change with age.

One approach to interpreting the ERG is to present scotopic and photopic conditions to enable identifying different scotopic and photopic components. A scotopic component is one that occurs to stimuli weaker than about 5 lux, increases after dark adaptation, and appears in organisms with all-rod retinas. A photopic component occurs to intense stimuli (10–100 lux) and to red light, decreases with reductions in the stimulus' intensity and with dark adaptation, and appears in cone-dominated retinas. Table 1.2 shows how various aspects of the ERG can be divided.

This information is useful in assessing how well the receptors are functioning: The presence of scotopic components indicates good rod function; the presence of photopic components, good cone function. Some clinical cases illustrate the correlation: Patients with normal central vision and good color perception but no vision after dark adaptation show normal photopic components but reduced or no scotopic components; patients with poor acuity and color vision but normal vision after dark adaptation show only scotopic components (Brunette, 1973; Gouras, 1970).

---

[6] Shipley and Anton (1964) could find no relation between birth weight and ERG amplitude, but their sample included only a narrow range of weights.

TABLE 1.2   THE DIVISION OF THE ELECTRORETINOGRAM INTO PHOTOPIC AND SCOTOPIC COMPONENTS

Component	Photopic	Scotopic	Response in all-rod retinas	Response in cone-dominated retinas	Response after dark adaptation	Response to red light	Response to weak light	Response to intense light	Response to light in fovea
a-wave	yes	no[a]	no	yes	no	yes	no	increases	?
b-wave	no[a]	yes	yes	?	increases	decreases	?	increases	decreases
d-wave	yes	no	no	yes	no	?	no	increases	increases
x-wave	yes	no	no	yes	yes	yes	yes	yes	increases
CFF[b] below 30 sec	no	yes	yes	?	?	?	yes	no	?
CFF[b] above 30 sec	yes	no	no	yes	?	?	no	yes	?

[a] With high intensity stimuli, the a-wave and the b-wave in the human have both photopic and scotopic components (Riggs, 1965).
[b] Critical flicker–fusion frequency.

17

However, other clinical cases show the inadequacies of this approach. A normal ERG with a normal CFF can be recorded in people with macular degeneration, subnormal visual acuity, partial color blindness, or central scotoma (Francois, 1968; Riggs, 1954; Riggs & Wooten, 1972; Zetterstrom, 1956), and sometimes a normal ERG cannot be recorded in patients whose vision is nearly normal (Riggs, 1954; Riggs & Wooten, 1972).

These cases are not surprising since the presence of a component of the ERG proves that a certain type of receptor is functioning, but not how well it is functioning. Analyses of the amplitude and latency of the response and its relation to parameters like intensity and size may provide better information (see Gouras, 1970, for such analyses). But even so, information about the ERG cannot be translated into predictions about perception: Functioning cones do not guarantee good visual acuity; production of an x-wave to orange light does not prove that the subject perceives color; and the CFF does not indicate the frequency at which the subject *sees* the flashes as fused together, since in adults these two frequencies resemble each other only with high luminance (Davson, 1972).

Note that all the photopic components have been found in the newborn by one or another investigator, except for the d-wave which has never been looked for. This indicates that the vision of the newborn resembles in some respects that of the adult, but it does not indicate what the baby sees, how good his acuity is, whether he perceives color, etc.—especially since there are differences in the amplitude, duration, and latency of the responses. And again, the CFF does not indicate whether he sees the flashes as fused together.

Another tack is to watch changes in the ERG as the eye is affected by anoxia or drugs. Granit (1933) did the classic study: He examined the ERG when the eye was exposed to various periods of anoxia (caused by clamping the retinal blood vessels) or of etherization. Different parts of the response survived for different lengths of time. He concluded that no single part of the retina produces an entire wave; rather, many parts produce components which, measured together, form the ERG. Figure 1.3 shows Granit's analysis of the ERG into components: P_1 was obliterated most quickly, P_2 was affected next, and P_3 was the most resilient.

Researchers after Granit found that component P_2 actually consists of two components (Brown, 1968; Davson, 1972; Kawasaki, Tsuchida, & Jacobson, 1972). The two components, the b-wave component and the d.c. component (so named because it

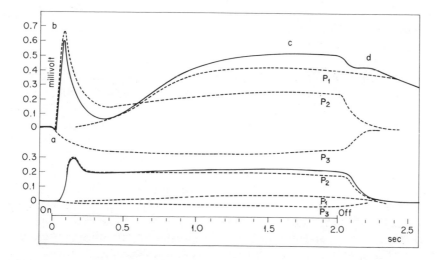

Figure 1.3   Analysis of the ERG to stimuli of two intensities, 14 mL and .14 mL. Components are shown by broken lines. The a-wave is broadened slightly out of scale to show its derivation more clearly. [Adapted from Granit, 1933, p. 221.]

looks like a d.c. potential), are probably generated by different parts of the retina, at least in some nonhuman organisms (Kawasaki *et al.*, 1972).

But two cautions are in order. First, Granit's study and much of the subsequent work was done on the cat, an organism that has many fewer cones than the human. And second, Granit and most other researchers assume that the several parts of the retina are affected sequentially by anoxia or ether, without overlapping in time. That is, they assume the drug first affects whatever generates P_1, and only after P_1 is knocked out does it begin to affect whatever generates P_2. Yet it is more likely all parts of the retina are affected simultaneously, with the rate of decay varying from part to part;[7] and allowing this alternative assumption, interpretations multiply.

Nonetheless, this approach does imply that an understanding of the newborn's ERG will require analyzing its underlying components, not just detecting the waves. One cannot use anoxia or ether on a human newborn, but one could analyze his ERG to find out what combinations of amplitudes and latencies of various components would produce it.

A third approach to interpreting the ERG is to try to pinpoint

[7] See Rodieck (1972) for this type of analysis.

which parts of the retina generate each wave. The simplest way to do this would be to correlate histological changes of the retina with changes in the waves, but this method has been unsuccessful: There is no particular histological change that corresponds to the first appearance of any aspect of the ERG in either the dog or the human (Horsten & Winkelman, 1960; Winkelman & Horsten, 1962).

But three more involved methods have shown some success. The first is inserting a microelectrode into the eye and noting the depth at which a maximum response occurs for each wave, plus any reversals in polarity. The second uses organisms, like the cat and cynomolgus monkey, whose retinal circulation does not support all parts of the retina: Their retinal circulation is cut off, and the changes in the ERG are noted. And finally, the last method is examining the ERG in eyes lacking some part of the retina because it never exists at all (like the cone-free retina of the night monkey or the rod-free retina of the squirrel monkey), because it never exists in some part of the eye (like the absent layer of ganglion cells in the center of the cynomolgus monkey's retina), or because it was removed or destroyed.

Results from these three methods can be summarized as follows.

1. THE a-WAVE

The a-wave is measured at maximum amplitude when the microelectrode is on the retinal side of the pigment epithelium, about at the level of the receptors (Brown, 1968; Davson, 1972). It is induced partly by cones: It can be recorded only if the eye has cones and has not adapted to the dark; and a part of it can be recorded from the fovea. But only part of it can be recorded from the fovea; the full wave requires input from the periphery of the retina. So, clearly, the a-wave is also caused by rods (Davson, 1972).

2. THE b-WAVE

The b-wave is measured at maximum amplitude when the microelectrode is approximately halfway through the retina, about at the inner nuclear layer (Brown, 1968; Davson, 1972). This means it could be generated by bipolar cells, horizontal cells, amacrine cells, or glial cells of Muller. Miller and Dowling (1970) suggest it reflects depolarization of Muller cells: The timing is appropriate, the polarity is correct, and the two are affected similarly by changes in intensity.

3. THE c-WAVE

Most evidence indicates the c-wave is generated by the pigment epithelium. Sodium iodate, which destroys the pigment epithelium, obliterates the c-wave without affecting the rest of the ERG (Noell, 1954). Sodium azide increases the amplitude of the c-wave—if the pigment epithelium is present (Noell, 1954). The c-wave is measured maximally on the retinal side of the pigment epithelium (Brown, 1968). It cannot be produced in retinas isolated from cold-blooded animals and thus lacking pigment epithelium. And in the cat, the response is not obliterated by clamping the retinal circulation, a manipulation which would not affect the pigment epithelium (Brown, 1968).

4. THE d-WAVE

The generation of the d-wave is probably related to the generation of the a-wave: Their maximum amplitudes are measured at the same depth; their magnitudes co-vary across species; and potentials from cones seem to be involved in the onset of both (Brown, 1968; Granit, 1933). In addition, the falling phase of the d-wave reflects activity in the inner nuclear layer (Brown, 1968).

5. THE x-WAVE

The x-wave must be induced by the cones because it occurs only to red light; because it is found only in species whose retinas contain a high proportion of cones; and because in humans it is most distinct when produced to foveal stimuli (Adrian, 1946; Armington, 1966; Brown, 1968).

Data on the ERG suggest certain parts of the newborn's retina are functioning. Both rods and cones are probably working: The a-wave reflects both, while the x-wave is attributed to cones. The presence of the b-wave suggests that Muller cells are depolarizing.

Still, the newborn's ERG is different from the adult's in latency and amplitude. These differences may mean either fewer cells are functioning or each cell is functioning less efficiently. More parametric studies could help sort out these alternatives by comparing the functions relating the amplitude (or latency) of a component to intensity (or duration or size) in both infants and adults. Differences in the shapes of the functions would indicate the cells responsible for that component do not behave in the same way in the two eyes.

Differences in the locations of the functions would indicate that fewer cells are operating in one eye. But even with this added information the ERG would not indicate what the infant is seeing.

IV. VISUALLY EVOKED POTENTIAL

A. General Methodological Considerations

A visually evoked potential (VEP) is a change in the electrical potential produced by the brain in response to a visual stimulus. It is usually recorded from electrodes on the scalp. It can be recorded bipolarly from two electrodes placed over the same part of the cortex, or monopolarly with one "active" electrode over the cortex and a second "reference" electrode on some other part of the head.

The type of response depends on the nature of the stimulus, on whether it is diffuse light, a pattern, or a small spot of light. The typical VEP in response to diffuse light consists of four positive and four negative deflections. The deflections have been labeled in so many different ways that to determine which deflection a given investigator is describing one must examine its latency, position, and polarity. This chapter will use the labeling by Ellingson (1970) of a response measured monopolarly from the occiput of an adult (see Figure 1.4 and Table 1.3).

The VEP in response to a patterned stimulus is similar, but two additional "pattern-caused" effects often appear, a negative deflection at about 100 msec and a positive deflection at about 200 msec. However, when the stimulus is a small spot of light, the VEP is entirely different; then it is a sinusoidal wave of 8 to 12 Hz.

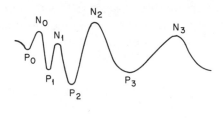

Figure 1.4   The VEP of an adult to a flash of diffuse light as recorded monopolarly from the occiput.

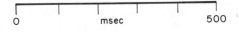

The type of response also depends on the rate of presentation of the stimulus. If the stimulus is flashed on and off at a slow enough rate, a separate VEP will occur after each flash. If it is flashed very frequently, the first flash will elicit a VEP (called the "on-response") but the signal will not return to the baseline until after the last flash (the return to baseline is called the "off-response"). And at intermediate rates of presentation, a phenomenon called photic driving will occur: single deflections after every flash combining to make the response look sinusoidal.

The signal is little stronger than background electroencephalographic (EEG) activity, so placement of the electrodes is critical. In the adult, some VEP can be recorded from many parts of the scalp, but the response reaches its greatest complexity, maximum amplitude, and minimum latency when it is measured over the occiput; in particular, before the inion (1.5 to 4 cm) and on either side of the midline (Rietveld, Tordoir, Hagenouw, Lubbers, & Spoor, 1967; Spehlmann, 1965; Vanzulli, Bogacz, Handler, & García-Ausst, 1960). In the infant the response, at least to diffuse light, can be picked up well only over the occiput (Ellingson, 1958a; Hrbek, Hrbkova, & Lenard, 1969; Hrbek, Karlberg, & Olsson, 1973; Hrbek & Mares, 1964; Lodge *et al.*, 1969; Umezaki & Morrell, 1970; Vanzulli, Wilson, & García-Ausst, 1964; Vitova & Hrbek, 1970b); and responses recorded from different parts of the infant's occiput do not correlate perfectly with each other. The correlations average .68 to .70, as opposed to .85 to .90 in the adult (Ellingson, Lathrop,

TABLE 1.3 LATENCY OF VARIOUS COMPONENTS OF THE VEP IN HUMAN ADULTS (MSEC)

Component	Ellingson, 1970	Kooi & Bagschi, 1964	Rietveld et al., 1967	Spehlmann, 1965	Armington, 1966
P_0	20–25	—	—	—	—
N_0	40–45	—	—	—	—
P_1	50–60	60–80	—	—	—
N_1	60–80	80–120	60	—	70–95
P_2	100–110	90–120	100	80–120	105–150
N_2	130–140	120–170	170–210	—	—
P_3	170–180	—	200–235	120–200	—
N_3	220–240	—	—	—	—

Danahy, & Nelson, 1973; Ellingson, Lathrop, Nelson, & Danahy, 1972).

Ellingson (1967a) recommends placing an active electrode on midline slightly above the inion with a reference electrode toward the back of the head or on an earlobe. The reference electrode can be closer to the active electrode on an infant than on an adult, but to avoid recording eye movements or potential changes not related to the visual processing of the stimulus, it should not be placed on the forehead or over the vertex.

Because the signal is so weak there is also a lot of noise. This should be reduced by averaging the recording—presenting the stimulus repeatedly and combining a number of responses into an average response. Averaging also eliminates the large and obfuscating variability of the individual responses. In the infant, to be certain of including all the information available, at least 500 msec of each response should be averaged. Unfortunately, averaging also destroys any information about the variability of the response, and it may destroy the response itself if the response varies sufficiently in latency. (See Chapter 2 by Karmel and Maisel for a more comprehensive discussion of these and other aspects.)

The number of responses averaged need not be large, since noise decreases as a function of the square root of the number of trials (Ellingson, 1967a). Ellingson claims that 10 responses is about right, since 20 or 30 give no better reliability, and since averages based on 100 responses do not differ significantly from averages based on 32 responses (Ellingson, 1967a; Ellingson et al., 1973). He also cautions that some EEG activity in the background may not average out, but instead may lock to the rhythm of the flashes. For this reason he suggests using irregular intervals between the stimuli.

One difficulty with using the VEP is its large variability among individuals. Its amplitude interacts with parameters like the size of the pupil and the rate of the stimuli's presentation—and that interaction varies from subject to subject (Fleming, Wilson, & Merrill, 1972). Even the shape of the response differs: Some subjects do not show some components (Vanzulli et al., 1960).

Infants are still more variable. Responses at a given age differ in waveform (Ellingson, 1958a, b; Vanzulli et al., 1964), in amplitude (Ellingson, 1958a, b; Vanzulli et al., 1964; Watanabe, Iwase, & Hara, 1972, 1973), and in latency (Engel & Benson, 1968; Watanabe et al., 1973). An interaction with state of arousal varies from infant to infant (Hrbek, 1969; Hrbek *et al.*, 1969). And all this variability is great even within a pair of monozygotic twins (Umezaki & Morrell, 1970).

Within an infant, visually evoked potentials may or may not be consistent in amplitude and latency: Some studies (Engel & Benson, 1968; Ellingson, 1958a, b, 1960, 1964a, b; and Umezaki & Morrell, 1970) have found consistency, but others have shown that any aspect of the VEP may vary within the same session. The response may disappear for a while or be present only in one hemisphere (Engel, 1964; Engel & Butler, 1963). The small waves preceding P_2 may disappear (Hrbek *et al.*, 1969). The latencies of N_1, N_2, and P_3 may vary, especially during the first 3 months (Ellingson, 1970). And the amplitudes of the peaks may vary within a session (Ellingson, 1970; Groth, Weled, & Batkin, 1970; Heck & Zetterstrom, 1958b) even when the infant is in the same sleep state (Watanabe *et al.*, 1972). On top of all this, there are individual differences in variability: Some infants are more stable than others. By 12 months the variability has decreased, but even at 20 months it is greater than in the adult (Ellingson *et al.*, 1972). At all ages P_2 is the most stable deflection (Ellingson, 1970; Ellingson *et al.*, 1972).

The nature of the VEP depends on the properties of the stimulus, its intensity, wavelength, rate of presentation, patterning, clarity, and position on the retina.

In adults, as the intensity of a diffuse stimulus is increased, the response becomes more complex (Vanzulli *et al.*, 1960), different components become most prominent (Armington, 1966), the latency decreases (Riggs & Wooten, 1972; Vanzulli *et al.*, 1960), and the amplitude increases (although when the stimulus is directed only at the fovea, the amplitude eventually reaches a maximum and then drops off again with further increases in the stimulus' intensity) (Armington, 1966; Vanzulli *et al.*, 1960). In infants, as the intensity of a diffuse stimulus is increased, the response becomes more complex (Ellingson, 1967a; Vanzulli *et al.*, 1964), its amplitude increases (although it may decrease again at very high intensities) (Ellingson, 1964a; Lodge *et al.*, 1969; Vanzulli *et al.*, 1964), and its latency decreases (Ellingson, 1964a, 1966, 1967a; Lodge *et al.*, 1969; Vanzulli *et al.*, 1964).

The VEP also varies with the wavelength of the stimulus. In adults, the amplitude is greater to red stimuli than to blue (Armington, 1966).[8] In infants (and older children), the latency changes. It decreases as the wavelength increases, though it is shortest in response to white light (Fichsel, 1969).

The amplitude of the VEP to diffuse light is reduced by increasing the rate of presentation of the stimulus, both in adults (Fleming *et al.*, 1972; Kooi & Bagchi, 1964) and in infants. In the newborn the response may disappear if the rate is greater than one flash per second (Ellingson, 1958b; Hrbek & Mares, 1964).

Another variable affecting the VEP is the design of the stimulus. When the stimulus is patterned the VEP in adults often includes the pattern-caused components, the negative component at about 100 msec and the positive component at about 200 msec. Whether these pattern-caused components occur, and their amplitudes, depends on the type of patterning. Rietveld *et al.* (1967) found that black-and-white patterns made of contiguous acute—or right-angled elements seemed to maximize the response: Stripes evoked no pattern-caused components at all, but only the VEP that occurs to diffuse light; isosceles right triangles evoked the strongest pattern-caused components, while diamonds with similar angles evoked similar components regardless of the length of the sides. But angles are not the only cause: Polka dots will evoke the pattern-caused components too (Harter, 1971). And John, Herrington, and Sutton (1967) tried diamonds, circles, and squares and found that different shapes containing the same area caused different responses, while similar shapes containing different areas caused responses similar in components and amplitudes.

In adults the patterned-caused components will reach a maximum amplitude when the stimulus contains some particular size or number of elements. Thus, for example, the positive pattern-caused component reaches a maximum amplitude when the stimulus contains a certain number of borders between black and white (Spehlmann, 1965); or if the stimulus is checkered, when the checks are a certain size (Harter & White, 1970; Rietveld *et al.*, 1967); or if the stimulus is dotted, when the dots have a certain size and spacing (Harter, 1971).

In infants, the only patterns tested have been made of checks. These do not add any components to the response, but the number of checks does affect the amplitude of P_2. The determining variable

---

[8] The subjects in these studies might be responding to brightness, not color, since the apparent brightness of a given intensity varies with its wavelength in adults, and apparently in infants (Peiper, 1963; J. M. Smith, 1936; Trincker & Trincker, 1967).

could be either the checks' size (Harter & Suitt, 1970) or how many inches of edge there are per square inch of stimulus at the retina (Karmel, Hoffman, & Fegy, 1974). In any case, the arrangement of the checks has no effect (Karmel, White, Cleaves, & Steinsiek, 1970; Karmel *et al.*, 1974).

The optimal size of pattern is also related to visual acuity, at least in adults. If the pattern is degraded by its being placed behind a screen or by the subjects' viewing it through a lens, both pattern-caused components decrease (Harter & White, 1968, 1970), and a larger check is necessary to produce the largest possible positive component. If the pattern is sufficiently degraded (IO D), the pattern-caused components disappear and the VEP becomes the same as the response to diffuse light (Rietveld *et al.*, 1967; Spehlmann, 1965). But degradation has no effect on the response to large checks (greater than 40 min) or to diffuse light.

Any refractive error of the subject's eye can be determined by noting the effect on the patterned-caused response of lenses of different powers. The refractive error corresponds to the power of the lens with whose aid he produces either *(1)* the largest pattern-caused components (Harter & White, 1968) or *(2)* the response to a patterned stimulus which differs maximally from his response to diffuse light (Duffy & Rengstorff, 1971). The error of these methods ranges from .0 to -1.0 D for spherical acuity and is usually less than $\pm.50$ D for axis determination (Duffy & Rengstorff, 1971; Ludlam & Meyers, 1972).[9]

The amplitude of the pattern-caused components in adults depends on where the stimulus falls on the eye: the closer to the fovea, the greater the response (Harter, 1970; Rietveld *et al.*, 1967). As the stimulus becomes more peripheral, larger checks are needed to maximize the response, and in general, variations in size of check have less effect (Harter, 1970). If the stimulus is sufficiently peripheral (4° 4'), the pattern-caused components disappear altogether (Rietveld *et al.*, 1967).

Eason *et al.* (Eason, Oden, & White, 1967) mapped the effects of the stimulus' location on the sinusoidal waves evoked by a spot of light. They aimed a light at the fovea and then moved it along the horizontal meridian of the eye. The farther out was the light, the

[9] Note that the size of check which elicits the maximum pattern-caused response is not a measure of visual acuity threshold: Checks subtending 20 min of arc commonly elicit the maximum VEP, but most adults can perceive checks subtending a mere 2 min of arc (Rietveld *et al.*, 1967).

smaller were the earlier deflections of each response, and the larger the later deflections. The latency of each response also decreased as the light was moved outward; but after the light reached 20°, the latency began to increase.

Eason *et al.* (Eason, White, & Oden, 1967) found similar effects when they moved the light away from the fovea along the vertical meridian. The farther out was the light, the shorter was the amplitude of the response and the longer its latency. The amplitude was also greater when the light was in the lower half of the field, as was the latency of the fourth deflection.

Eason, White, and Bartlett (1970) confirmed these findings with checkered stimuli: The latencies of two components were shorter when the stimulus was in the upper visual field than when it was in the lower, and the amplitude of an early positive component was larger in the lower field. Moreover, the amplitude of that component was related to the checks' size in different ways in the upper and lower fields: In the lower field the relation looked like an inverted U with medium-sized checks eliciting the maximum amplitude, while in the upper field the relation was linear (although the curve looks as though it might have decreased again if the experiment had been continued with smaller checks).

Finally, the response to diffuse light varies with the location of the stimulus on the retina. The amplitude of the response is larger when the stimulus is presented to the fovea than when it is presented elsewhere, with the greatest disparity when the light is red (Armington, 1966). And the shape of the spectral sensitivity curves (wavelength plotted against VEP) varies for different parts of the retina: It resembles the inverted U photopic luminosity function for the fovea and is lower and flatter for the temporal retina and the blind spot.

Not only do stimulus variables affect the VEP, but so does at least one subject variable: state of arousal.

In adults, the waveform, amplitude, and latency of the response to diffuse light vary with the state of sleep or wakefulness of the subject. When an adult goes to sleep, the positive deflections become larger (Vanzulli *et al.*, 1960), N_1 decreases (Vanzulli *et al.*, 1960), N_3 increases (Ellingson *et al.*, 1972, 1973), and the latencies of late deflections (N_2, P_2, N_3, and P_3) increase (Ellingson *et al.*, 1972, 1973; Lodge *et al.*, 1969; Vanzulli *et al.*, 1960). While a subject is awake, amplitudes are slightly greater with his eyes shut than with his eyes open (Vanzulli *et al.*, 1960). Some of these effects may be caused by changes in the intensity of the stimulus reaching the retina; and some of them may be caused by dark adaptation, the first 10 min of which cause a dramatic increase in the amplitude of the response (Riggs & Wooten, 1972). Manipulations of attention also affect the response: If the subject is told to release a button at the onset of a stimulus in one part of the visual field, then a stimulus in that part of the field elicits a greater VEP than a stimulus in a different part, which may even elicit no VEP at all (Eason, Harter, & White, 1969). The VEP also decreases during eye movements (Riggs & Wooten, 1972).

Most studies of the infant have found no relationship between phase of the sleep–wake cycle and the waveform, amplitude, or latency of the VEP (Ellingson, 1958a, 1970; Ellingson *et al.*, 1972, 1973; Ferriss *et al.*, 1967; Vanzulli *et al.*, 1964; Watanabe *et al.*, 1972). However, there are four exceptions. In newborns, Hrbek *et al.* (1969, 1973) found that the amplitude of various components of the VEP to diffuse light varied with state of sleep or wakefulness, but though the variation within any subject was consistent, the variation among subjects was inconsistent. In premature infants, Watanabe *et al.* (1973) found that the amplitudes of three components (N_1, P_2, and N_2) were larger after the infants had been awake with their eyes open for more than 1 min than when they were asleep. Moreover, the latencies of all components were shorter when the infants were awake. And Lodge *et al.* (1969) note that the latency of the response to orange light is shorter when a newborn is awake than when he is in most sleep states.

The amplitude and latency of the infant's VEP also differ with states of sleep: The amplitudes of some responses (P_2, N_1, and N_2) to white light are higher in REM sleep (rapid eye movements, occasional gross body movements, continuous slow wave EEG) than in quiet sleep (no rapid eye movements, no body movements, episodic EEG), at least at some conceptional ages (Lodge *et al.*, 1969; Watanabe *et al.*, 1973). And the latency of the response is longer during REM sleep than during other sleep states (Lodge *et al.*, 1969).

In older infants, the response to flickering light is clearly related to state (Vitova & Hrbek, 1970a, b). When a baby from 1 week to 6 months is awake, the VEP is driven in rhythm with a flashing light, unless the light flashes too quickly. But when the baby is asleep, low rates of flashing (3 to 5 Hz) elicit only a single on-response, and higher rates elicit no response. After 6 months, photic driving occurs even when the baby is sleeping, but the maximum rate of flashing is always much lower than when he is awake.

Fleming *et al.* (1972) found that the amplitude of the VEP also depended on the size of the subject's pupils: It was greater with dilated pupils (produced by 10% neosynephrine) than with naturally mobile pupils. However, three other investigators could find no relation between the size of the subject's pupils and the amplitude or latency of his response (Kooi & Bagchi, 1964; John *et al.*, 1967; Spehlmann, 1965).

So then, to maximize the VEP in infants one should use intense stimuli which cover the fovea and occur at random intervals exceeding 1 sec; and one should record over the occiput, average at least 500 msec of the signal, and try to keep the babies awake. To make comparisons across studies of infants, all of these variables should be matched: the placement of electrodes, the intensity and wavelength of the stimulus, the patterning of the stimulus, its position on the retina, the frequency of its presentation, the state of the subjects' arousal and the sizes of their pupils. To make comparisons across ages is even more difficult, since the fovea matures, accommodation and refraction change, and infants of different ages look longest at different amounts of brightness and patterning.

B.   Summary of the Data from Infants

If the signals are averaged, some VEP can be obtained from almost all newborns and most prematures (Ellingson, 1970; Engel, 1965, 1967; Ferriss *et al.*, 1967; Hrbek, 1969; Hrbek & Mares, 1964; Umezaki & Morrell, 1970). Even in his early studies done without averaging, Ellingson (1958a, b, 1960, 1964b) obtained it from more than half of the newborns he tested (though in no case did a subject respond to every flash).

The typical newborn's response to diffuse light usually consists of a positive deflection (P_2) followed by a negative deflection (N_2), but some newborns show only one of these deflections. Ferriss *et al.* (1967) always found at least the negative peak; Ellingson (1970) and Hrbek and Mares (1964) always found the positive peak. Some newborns show additional components: P_1 (which may be present at birth or may differentiate from P_2 during the first week of life) (Ferriss *et al.*, 1967); several small waves preceding P_2 (Hrbek *et al.*,

1969; Hrbek & Mares, 1964); or an assortment of up to eight different waves (Ellingson, 1970; Vanzulli *et al.*, 1964). By 2 months the form of the infant's VEP is similar to the adult's (Ferriss *et al.*, 1967).

The latency of the infant's VEP is always longer than the adult's (Ellingson, 1958a, b, 1960, 1964a, b, 1966; Engel, 1964, 1967: Engel & Butler, 1963; Ferriss *et al.*, 1967; Harter & Suitt, 1970; Lodge *et al.*, 1969; Umezaki & Morrell, 1970). But if newborns are awake, the latency is not so much longer (Lodge *et al.*, 1969).

Latencies are generally longer in male infants than in female infants (Ellingson, 1967b; Engel, 1965, 1967; Engel & Benson, 1968; Engel, Crowell, & Nishijima, 1968). But in both sexes the latencies of all components decrease during the first 3 months of life, particularly during the first 2 weeks and at about 4 weeks (Ellingson, 1964b, 1966; Ellingson *et al.*, 1973; Ferriss *et al.*, 1967; Harter & Suitt, 1970; Jensen & Engel, 1971). After 3 months, latencies decrease more slowly until they reach the adult level at 18 to 24 months (Ellingson *et al.*, 1973). Latencies in response to all wavelengths of light decrease at about the same rate (Fichsel, 1969). But all these changes are less evident in any individual's data than in a group's data.

The amplitude of the newborn's VEP has frequently been reported to be higher than the adult's (Ellingson, 1958a, b, 1964b; Umezaki & Morrell, 1970), and to increase during the first 2 months of life (Ferriss *et al.*, 1967; Harter & Suitt, 1970). However, Barnet *et al.* (Barnet, Lodge, Armington, Shanks, & Newcomb, 1968) report identical amplitudes for infants and adults. And Ellingson (1966, 1967b) discovered that the amplitude of averaged responses is no greater in infants than in older children or adults. One reason why high amplitudes are often found in infants may be that they are usually sleeping: In adults, the amplitude of the positive components is greater during sleep or with the eyes closed.

When the stimulus is a checkerboard, the amplitude of P_2 depends on the size of check. The size that produces the maximum response at a given age is similar to the size of check that other infants of the same age stare at longest (Harter & Suitt, 1970; Karmel, 1973; Karmel *et al.*, 1974)—even though that size changes systematically with age, becoming smaller and smaller as the infants get older. Moreover, infants who look "advanced" because unusually small checks evoke the maximum response also tend to look advanced because P_2 occurs with a short latency (Karmel *et al.*, 1974).

For most newborns the flashes must be at least 1 sec apart if the second flash is to evoke a response, and in some infants they must be 3 sec apart (Ellingson, 1958a, b, 1960, 1964b), while in adults the flashes need to be separated by only 100 msec. At high flash rates the first flash elicits an on-response, the last flash an off-response.

At some intermediate flash rates driving can be obtained. With averaging and/or intense stimuli and/or alert subjects, it is possible to obtain photic driving in almost all newborn infants (Ellingson, 1967b; Vitova & Hrbek, 1970a, b, 1972). The optimal flash rates during the first 2 months are between only 3 and 5 Hz. The optimal rate changes to 8 to 10 Hz during the third month, and photic driving can sometimes be obtained to flashes as high as 12 Hz. At 6 months, 15 Hz also works. During the first few months photic driving lasts only for a few seconds and the response is of very small amplitude. By 4 months, photic driving of a higher amplitude occurs the whole time the stimulus is flashing. Mirzoyants (1961) reports the interesting observation that priming sometimes works; that is, a high frequency sometimes elicits driving if—but only if—the driving was first started by a lower frequency.

The VEP and photic driving can be obtained as easily in premature babies as in full-term babies (Ellingson, 1960; Engel, 1964; Engel & Butler, 1963; Vitova & Hrbek, 1970a, b, 1972). However, prematures frequently show a negative deflection (N_2) without the preceding positive deflection (P_2), especially if their conceptual ages are 32 weeks or less (Ellingson, 1960; Hrbek et al., 1973; Hrbek & Mares, 1964; Umezaki & Morrell, 1970). The amplitudes of all deflections are greater in the premature (Engel, 1964; Hrbek et al., 1973; Umezaki & Morrell, 1970), and prematures have longer latencies than full-term babies even at the conceptional ages of 38 to 42 weeks, latencies being inversely correlated with conceptional age until about 50 weeks (Ellingson, 1960, 1964a, 1967b, 1968; Engel, 1965, 1967; Engel et al., 1968; Engel & Benson, 1968; Hrbek et al., 1973; Watanabe et al., 1972, 1973). The correlations run about −.50 to −.74 (Ellingson, 1968; Engel, 1964, 1968; Engel & Benson, 1968; Engel & Butler, 1963; Umezaki & Morrell, 1970). Interestingly, postnatal age does not correlate with latency (Umezaki & Morrell, 1970).

In newborns and also in older infants, the latency also correlates inversely with body weight at about −.80 (Ellingson, 1960, 1968). Ellingson, in an early study (1964b) done without averaging, postulated that the curve relating latency and weight leveled off and then dropped again at 8 or 9 pounds. However, in later studies

(Ellingson, 1966, 1967b, 1968) done with averaging he found instead that the correlation is significant up to about 13 pounds, and then declines toward zero.

These correlations with conceptional age and with body weight indicate that the latency of the VEP is related to maturity. It is not surprising that latency correlates with both conceptional age and body weight, since these two variables correlate even more highly (about .90) with each other (Ellingson, 1968). In fact, if weight is held constant, then the partial correlation between conceptional age and latency is only either −.34 (if based on the obstetrician's estimate of conceptional age) or −.16 (if based on the mother's estimate) (Engel & Benson, 1968). Interestingly, Engel and Benson (1968) found that twins do not differ significantly from each other in latency, even when they differ in weight. Also, babies who had had short latencies at birth scored higher on a test of mental abilities at 8 months than babies (matched for conceptional age) who had had longer latencies (Engel, 1964); they were more likely to be walking unaided at 1 year (Jensen & Engel, 1971); and they articulated consonants better at 3 years (Engel & Fay, 1972). However, the latency of the VEP at birth (adjusted for conceptional age) does not correlate with performance at 3 years on a test of verbal comprehension (Engel & Fay, 1972), at 4 years on an IQ test (Engel & Fay, 1972), or at 7 years on IQ tests, achievement tests or perceptual–motor tests (Henderson & Engel, 1974).

C. Interpretation of Results

Interpreting the VEP is even more difficult than interpreting the electroretinogram since the VEP is recorded farther from the visual input, and since it can be affected by nonvisual factors.

At least the VEP does seem to be related to visual input and processing: It is strongest and most detailed over the occipital cortex; its amplitude and latency vary with the intensity, wavelength, and patterning of the stimulus; it differs with the acuity of the subject and the proximity of the stimulus to the fovea; it disappears when the subject can no longer see the stimulus because he is making an eye movement; and the curve relating the sensitivity of the VEP to the wavelength of the stimulus resembles the photopic luminosity function.

However, a subject can have a VEP without seeing the stimulus at all: There is no change in the VEP as a stabilized retinal image fades

(Riggs & Wooten, 1972); subjects with severe visual deficits may show an apparently normal VEP (Ellingson, 1968; Engel, 1964); and nearly every other conceivable relationship between VEP and clinical condition has been found (Ellingson, 1964b). Nor does a VEP indicate generally good neurological functioning: In one study (Watanabe *et al.,* 1972) all 11 small-for-dates infants (i.e., undersized for their conceptional age) produced normal VEPs even though two had abnormal neurological symptoms (hyperexcitability and convulsions).

Which part of the brain is responsible for the VEP is disputed. One camp attributes components to particular types of synapses: Rose (1971) and Hrbek and Mares (1964) associate changes in P_2 and N_2 with changes in axosomatic connections, basilar dendrites, and axodendritic synapses; and Umezaki and Morrell (1970) and Purpura (cited in Scheibel & Scheibel, 1971) attribute P_2 more specifically to the basilar dendrite system of deep-lying pyramidal cells. Another camp attributes P_2 to axonal and dendritic neuropil, especially in stellate cells, because all these develop at the same time (Scheibel & Scheibel, 1971). While a third camp, e.g., Eason *et al.* (1970), Harter (1971), and Karmel (Karmel, 1973; Karmel *et al.,* 1974; see also Chapter 2), relates the optimal check size to the sizes of the receptive field centers of cells somewhere in the visual pathway.

In infants, so many aspects of the visual system and cortex are changing simultaneously, one can only speculate about the anatomical bases of developmental changes in the VEP. Ellingson (1960) attributes the decrease in latency to an increase in the conduction velocity of afferent fibers, but Karmel *et al.* (1974) point out that the decrease could also be caused by foveal development, or by increases in myelinization, in dendritic branching, or in the number of dendritic spines. Ellingson (1967b) suggests the response in the newborn can occur no faster than once per second because of one or more of these factors: long refractory periods of immature axons, large cortical postexcitatory depression, and an inhibitory influence on sensory end organs. Vitova and Hrbek (1970b, 1972) assume the improvement in driving between birth and 6 months is caused by an increase in exogenous fibers in the cortex (especially thalamocortico fibers), by an increase in dendritic branching in the cortex, by increases in myelin on the optic nerve and on cortical fibers, and by the development of neuropil in layer I of the cortex. But they also admit that the improvement could be related to changes in membrane properties, in synaptic transmitters, or in the inhibition of synaptic connections.

However, there is one clear anatomical relationship: Both the occipital cortex and the VEP of the infant are immature, and more immature than some other parts of the cortex and some other potentials. Thus, the occipital cortex is less mature than the somatosensory cortex; and the VEP is less mature than the somatosensory evoked potential, which more closely resembles the adult form at birth and which becomes apparent earlier (Hrbek *et al.*, 1973).

Several relationships have been suggested between the development of the VEP and the development of vision. All of these things develop coincidentally in rabbits (there are no data for humans): the mature form of the VEP, optokinetic nystagmus, visual control of the placement of the limbs, avoidance of the visual cliff, and the final level of amino acids in the occipital cortex, retina, and superior colliculus (Riesen, 1971). And in humans, the latencies of the VEPs to red, blue, and white light all decrease with age at the same rate, so those decreases must depend on some development affecting all wavelengths equally (Fichsel, 1969).

Harter and Suitt (1970) deduced another relationship between the infant's VEP and his visual development. First, they found that after their subject was 70 days old, the function relating amplitude of VEP to size of check had the same inverted U-shape which has been found in adults (though in adults the curve relates size of check to the pattern-caused components). Now in adults, the size of check producing the maximum pattern-caused components depends *(1)* on the visual acuity of the subject and *(2)* on whether the stimulus is located on the macula. That "optimal" size of check when their subject was 3 months old was the same as the optimal size for an adult with a 3 D degradation (about 20/250 acuity). Since infants are known to have better visual acuity than this, Harter and Suitt (1970) conclude that the changes in optimal size of check are probably related to macular development.

But there are two weaknesses with this argument. First, Harter and Suitt (1970) studied only one infant but used others' estimates of visual acuity—even though there are large individual differences. And second, the amplitude of P_2 in adults varies not only with acuity and location of the stimulus, but also with the intensity and form of the stimulus and the placement of electrodes. Two of these variables (placement of electrodes and intensity of stimulus) are known to be important in infants and others might be. Moreover, any one of them might have a different effect on an infant's immature visual system than it has on an adult's.

In general, it seems dangerous to make comparisons of the VEP across ages because so many parameters affect it and most of these parameters change developmentally. What is possible and valuable is to see how each of these parameters affects the response at every age.

V. ELECTROOCULOGRAPHY

A. General Methodological Considerations

Electrooculography (EOG) is the recording of electrical potentials produced in the eye and picked up by electrodes placed on the skin nearby. The potential probably arises from the retina (and not from ocular muscles): It can be recorded from an isolated retina, it changes at the ora serrata, and drugs that damage the pigment epithelium will alter it (Arden & Kelsey, 1962). It probably arises because a membrane (either the external limiting membrane, the membrane of Bruch, or the pigment epithelium) separates the negatively charged choroid from the positively charged retina (Alpern, 1962b). In a human eye looking straight ahead it is about 10 to 30 mV.

Changes of potential indicate eye movements: As the eye moves closer to an electrode the potential increases; as it moves farther from an electrode the potential decreases. The relationship, about 25 μV per degree (Larson, 1970; Shackel, 1961), is linear over the central part of the visual field: Alpern (1962b) claims linearity to at least 15° from the center, and Shackel (1960, 1961) to 30°, with the relationship fairly linear to 40°.[10]

Electrooculography is very sensitive. It can detect a movement of only .5° (Larson, 1970; Shackel, 1960, 1961; Young, 1963) out to at least 40° or 50° from the center of the field (Shackel, 1961; Young, 1963), and the technique has been used out to 70° (Kris, 1960) and even 90° (Young, 1963).

Calibration is necessary to translate changes of potential into

[10] Other investigators recommend relating the change of potential to the sine of the angle through which the eye rotated, but make similar claims about linearity (Marg, 1951; Miles, 1939).

degrees of eye movement. For best results the entire visual field should be calibrated for each subject, since the relationship is not linear in all regions or all subjects (Alpern, 1971; Byford, 1963). Such extensive calibration will also reveal whether the subject is one of the rare people in whom a change of potential sometimes occurs without any eye movement, or an eye movement occurs without any change of potential (Byford, 1963).

An additional reason for calibrating each subject exhaustively is to check for cross talk between the electrodes recording horizontal movements and the electrodes recording vertical movements (Gaboresk, 1968, 1969). Some of this cross talk happens when the axes of the vertical and horizontal electrodes are not perpendicular to each other (Shackel, 1961). The electrodes can be adjusted to minimize the problem, but some cross talk will still remain in some subjects. This residual cross talk may be caused by shifts of the axis around which the eye rotates (Alpern, 1962b, 1971).

It is also necessary to calibrate each subject repeatedly, because the resting potential (the potential measured while the eye is stationary) drifts. It fluctuates considerably in some people (Aantaa, 1970; Arden & Kelsey, 1962; Larson, 1970; Shackel, 1961), often rhythmically (Arden & Kelsey, 1962).

Some systematic changes of the resting potential are caused by changes of illumination. When a subject is placed in the dark or closes his eyes, the potential decreases about 30% during the first 10 to 12 min, then it increases until about the twenty-fifth minute, and finally it slowly declines to the original value (Aantaa, 1970; Arden & Kelsey, 1962; Kris, 1958). Re-exposing the subject to light leads to an increase of potential within 8 or 9 min, with the amount of increase dependent on the light's intensity and on the length of the preceding time in the dark (Arden & Barrada, 1962; Arden & Kelsey, 1962; Aserinsky, 1955; Kelsey, 1967a, b; Kris, 1958). Later the potential falls to the same trough it reached in the dark, but it may rise again at about the thirty-sixth minute (Arden & Kelsey, 1962; Kris, 1958).

The timing of all these changes varies from subject to subject and may be very slow. Changes in the dark occur in some people for 50 min (Gonshor & Malcolm, 1971), and a new steady state in the light (presumably necessary for most psychological experiments) may not happen until after 60 (Kris, 1958) or 120 min (Gonshor & Malcolm, 1971). And—most importantly—if the illumination changes and then returns to the original level, the resting potential will *not* return immediately to its original level (Arden & Kelsey,

1962). So if the control trial or intertrial interval is dark, or if the subject closes his eyes as babies are wont to do, the resting potential will change, continue to change after the subject opens his eyes or the new trial starts, and require continual calibration.

The resting potential also fluctuates with time of day: The amplitude is highest early in the morning (Aantaa, 1970; Aantaa & Elenius, 1968), and is higher when people first wake up than during a period of darkness just before they go to sleep (Aserinsky, 1955). Also, the potential varies with galvanic skin response (Alpern, 1971), fatigue (Kris, 1960), metabolic cycle (Kris, 1960), exercise (Kris, 1960), and time since the last meal (Kris, 1960).

To record vertical eye movements, electrodes should be above and below one eye. To record horizontal eye movements they can be placed either on the external and internal canthi of one eye or on the external canthi of the two eyes. The placement of the electrodes determines the strength of the signal. When the electrode on the external canthus is moved 1 cm farther from the eye, the change of potential for a 30° eye movement decreases to 93% of the original level. Displacements of 2, 3, and 4 cm cause reductions to 83%, 72%, and 60% of the original level, respectively (Aantaa, 1970).

To get a strong signal, the electrical resistance of the skin must be reduced by careful preparation. The skin should be cleaned with alcohol and then abraded by either rubbing with an abrasive jelly or rasping with a burr. But in the infant this process is less critical because his thinner skin has lower resistance (Dayton, Jones, & Dizon, 1963).

When EOG is used to determine where a subject is fixating, his head must remain steady. If the subject rotates his head while maintaining his fixation, a change of potential is registered because the front of the cornea has changed its position with respect to the electrodes.

Other precautions are necessary to minimize the possibility of artifacts from muscle-action potentials and galvanic skin potentials. Muscle-action potentials should be filtered out: Twenty Hz and 100 Hz cutoffs eliminate most of them (Larson, 1970), though artifacts may still occur from clenched jaws (Shackel, 1961). Skin potentials, which can be stronger than EOG potentials and are in the same frequencies, should be reduced by anesthetizing the skin, abrading it, using aluminum salts to minimize sweating, and maintaining a low temperature in the room (Shackel, 1961).

With problems of linearity, cross talk, drift, and head movement,

EOG is not particularly accurate when used to measure fixation. Shackel (1961) found a maximum error of 1.35° on 95% of the fixations on stimuli within 30° of the center of the field. Yarbus (1967) concluded that EOG is an appropriate technique only if error may exceed 1°. Edwards (1971) found that EOG, photographed corneal reflection, or an unaided observer were equally accurate in judging the initial direction of eye movements exceeding 5°, but EOG picked up the fewest small movements, particularly if they were vertical.[11] And Byford (1963) found that EOG does not accurately show the duration or velocity of saccades.

But for many studies of infants, an error of 1° or 2° is quite tolerable. And for studies of the direction or latency of *long* eye movements, or of the simultaneity of the two eyes' movements, it may not even be necessary to calibrate. On the other hand, calibration is essential for studies of the amplitude of eye movements, and for any study of short eye movements. But a perfect calibration is impossible with an infant since one cannot tell him what to look at. One can only present an interesting target and hope he will look directly at it and not, say, to its side.[12]

In every case, head movements must be eliminated from the data. An infant's head movements can be restricted by some sort of swaddling (e.g., ear pads, a padded helmet, or a harness attached to a board) and/or by placing an immobile nipple in the baby's mouth. But none of these methods will eliminate head movements completely. So a better approach with infants is to monitor head movements and subtract them from the data (see, for example, Trevarthen and Tursky, 1969, and Tronick and Clanton, 1971).

Finally, infants' EOGs should be measured across one eye rather than both, because infants' eyes may not always move in the same direction at the same time (i.e., they may not be conjugate), and because both eyes may not always converge on the same point.

B. Summary of the Data from Infants

Infants move their eyes differently when they are doing different things. When newborns are lying quietly awake their eye move-

---

[11] Note that Edwards does not mention any calibration procedure for the EOG.

[12] This is a real problem (see p. 58 for a detailed discussion). The best tack is first to present the target centrally and then to move it slowly toward the side (Dayton & Jones, 1964). But in very young infants this procedure should work only some of the time, and then for only the central parts of the visual field (Dayton *et al.*, 1963).

ments are more frequent, more regular, and shorter than when they are sleeping (Prechtl & Lenard, 1967; Schulman, 1973). When newborns are crying their eye movements seem less organized than when they are quiet (Schulman, 1973). Bruner (1973) found that while 3-month-olds are watching movies, the frequency of long, horizontal eye movements is lower when the babies are holding pacifiers in their mouths than when they are not, and lower still when they are sucking on them. And in the same study, Bruner found that while 3-month-olds watch an "unconventional" movie (achromatic and variously textured stripes and geometric shapes moving around, appearing, and disappearing without the appropriate perspectival or size transformations), they make as many large horizontal eye movements as while watching a "conventional" movie (an Eskimo mother playing with her child)—unless they do not have pacifiers. Then they saccade more often while watching the unconventional film.[13]

The eye movements of newborns are frequently conjugate (Dayton & Jones, 1964; Dayton, Jones, Aiu, Rawson, Steele, & Rose, 1964; Dayton, Jones, Steele, & Rose, 1964; Kris, 1967; Prechtl & Lenard, 1967) to at least some extent, but to just what extent is not known. The figures from all five studies are somewhat suspect: Only Dayton and Jones (1964) mention calibration, and their procedure detected eye movements only if they were longer than 2° and occurred within 20° of midline.

Among newborns who are awake, about half will fixate and track a target presented centrally and then moved to the right or left at about 15° per second (Dayton *et al.*, 1963; Dayton & Jones, 1964; Dayton, Jones, Steele, & Rose, 1964). Compared to adults and older infants, the newborns pursue the target for a shorter distance, and make more and longer saccades.

Finally, Tronick and Clanton (1971) identified four patterns of looking at and following brightly colored cubes that are variously stationary and moving. At any age between 4 and 15 weeks an infant might show one of these patterns: a "shift pattern" in which both eyes and head move rapidly; a "search pattern" involving a series of saccades and fixations occurring with slow head movements; a "focal pattern" in which the head is steady and only small saccades occur; and a "compensation pattern" in which head and

---

[13] Unfortunately, Bruner neither controlled nor measured head movements, and in this study head movements might not be just artifacts; they may themselves vary with sucking.

eyes movements compensate for each other. The authors also noted saccades as speedy as 200° to 400° per second, and an increase with age in the amplitude of saccades. Unfortunately, their method of calibration did not allow the distance of a head movement or of an eye movement to be determined, so the last two observations plus the "focal pattern" must be considered suspect.[14]

C. Interpretation of Results

The presence of any EOG indicates functioning receptors, an intact pigment epithelium, and adequate choroidal and retinal blood supplies (Aantaa, 1970; Kelsey, 1967a). But further interpretations are problematical because of artifacts. Head movements are indistinguishable from eye movements and may themselves change developmentally. Inadequate calibration leads to misestimates of position, amplitude, velocity, etc. And if adequacy of calibration changes with age, then the error will change with age too.

The effect of sucking on visual scanning is difficult to interpret without data on where the infants are fixating, how organized their scanning is, the nature of their smaller saccades, etc. Only then we will be able to evaluate Bruner's (1973) claim that sucking is a form of buffering which protects the infant from his great receptivity. Alternatively, sucking may reduce the infant's state of arousal so that he scans less, or it may simply distract him.

VI. OPTOKINETIC NYSTAGMUS

A. General Methodological Considerations

When a subject watches a repetitive pattern move in front of him at a constant speed he will (1) fixate some part of the pattern and follow it for a short time, then (2) saccade back to fixate some succeeding part. This response, which occurs repeatedly and rhyth-

---

[14] Tronick and Clanton measured both head and eye movements but they calibrated neither. They also combined the two signals and then balanced them by presenting a target to the infant and, while he seemed to be fixating it, rotating his head and adjusting the summed signal until it registered no change. The result was an excellent indicator of the sheer presence of fixation: If the subject changed his fixation point by moving either his head or his eyes, a change was registered. But the signal could not indicate magnitude.

mically, is called optokinetic nystagmus (OKN). It happens in nature when a person watches telephone poles from a moving train, and it happens in the laboratory when he looks at a rotating field of stripes. It can be recorded by electrooculography (see Figure 1.5), or it can be directly observed.

During the tracking or "slow" phase, the eyes usually move about 20% or 40% slower than the stimulus, depending on whether the stimulus is moving vertically or horizontally (Collins, 1972). But if the field moves too fast, 30° or 40° to 60° per second (Stark, 1971; Young, 1971), then the eyes lag farther behind, and their movement is no longer controlled by the speed of the stimulus.

To a certain extent OKN appears to be involuntary. When the field is filled entirely with stripes and the subject is awake with his eyes open, he cannot avoid the response (Davson, 1972; Gardner & Weitzman, 1967)—though he can delay it up to 30 sec by not fixating on any part of the stimulus and instead looking "through" it (Davson, 1972; Gardner & Weitzman, 1967; Walsh & Hoyt, 1969). Then the magnitudes of the slow phases are decreased (Gardner & Weitzman, 1967; Stark, 1971); the magnitudes of both the slow and the saccadic, "fast" phases become irregular (Stark, 1971); and the velocity of tracking is no longer a function of the stimulus' velocity (Stark, 1971).

Several effects seem to show OKN is influenced by changes in attention. It cannot be obtained when a subject is sleeping, even when his pupil is directed toward the stimulus (Gardner & Weitzman, 1967; Walsh & Hoyt, 1969). The probability of a response is decreased by drowsiness, intoxication (Duke-Elder & Scott, 1971), barbiturates, tranquilizers, and many sedatives and narcotics (J. L.

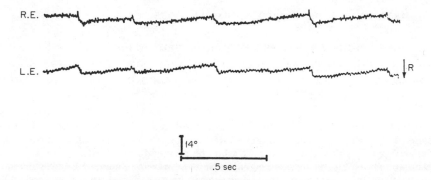

Figure 1.5　Optokinetic nystagmus. Eye movements in response to a drum of vertical stripes rotating to the left. [Reprinted from Alpern, 1962, p. 82.]

Smith, 1963). And as the stimulus decreases in size below 40°, the magnitude of OKN declines (Young, 1971). Yet experiments dealing with length of trial are not so clear-cut: Collins (1972) could find no changes during trials lasting up to 120 sec, and Dix and Hood (1971) report only that the velocity of the first slow phase is less than the velocity of any succeeding slow phase.

OKN is usually conjugate (Shackel, 1960) and is not affected by inaccurate accommodation (Gardner & Weitzman, 1967).

Some subjects at some times start nystagmus voluntarily, but the velocity and frequency of that nystagmus does not resemble the optokinetic nystagmus induced by a visual stimulus (Alpern, 1962b; Lipman, 1972; Spector, 1971).

B. Summary of the Data from Infants

Optokinetic nystagmus is easily found in infants—even new-borns—with only a slight change of technique: The stripes should be presented not merely in front of the infant, but instead totally surrounding him (Gorman, Cogan, & Gellis, 1959). OKN is much more easily found than ordinary fixation or ordinary following (Brazelton, Scholl, & Robey, 1966; McGinnis, 1930). McGinnis (1930) observed the response in all the babies he tested (newborns to 42 days) as long as the field was rotating not faster than 10° or 20° per second. Gorman, Cogan, and Gellis (1957) found it in 93% of 100 babies younger than 5 days, although some showed it only after retesting. And in a second study (Gorman *et al.*, 1959) they found it in 93% of 60 babies aged 8 days to 4 months, with one of those who did not show it known to be blind and another suspected to be blind.

In fact, OKN is so common, its absence may be related to neurological pathology. One study seems to indicate this: Seventy-six percent of 29 normal 1-year-olds had shown OKN at birth, while none of the eight abnormal or questionable babies had shown it (Brazelton *et al.*, 1966).

Few more details are known about OKN in infants because most studies have used no more precise a method than an unaided observer trying to detect its presence or absence.[15] An exception is McGinnis (1930), who photographed the eyes and measured their

---

[15] Dayton *et al.* (1963; Dayton, Jones, Aiu, Rawson, Steele, & Rose, 1964) did use electrooculography, but since they did not calibrate the response or restrict head movement, their data are little better.

movements on stripes 20° apart. At speeds of 10° and 20° per second, the infants tended to saccade toward each bar when it first appeared in the visual field. At 40° per second they refixated only every second or third bar. The frequency of refixation increased with age up to 6 weeks, but then decreased as the infants turned their heads to prolong fixation.

Optokinetic nystagmus has also been used to study whether babies can detect apparent motion. Tauber and Koffler (1966) showed newborns a field of stationary stripes lighted by a moving stroboscopic light so that the stripes appeared to an adult to be moving. Sixty-five percent of the 19 babies showed OKN.

Doris and Cooper (1966) varied the intensity of the stripes to determine the minimum brightness that would elicit OKN. All babies (4 to 69 days) responded to the brightest stripes (.4 foot-candles), but as babies got older they were more likely to respond to dimmer stripes. In a subsequent study (Doris, Casper, & Poresky, 1967) they varied the contrast between black and white stripes. The minimal contrast necessary for OKN decreased rapidly over the first 4 months.

One last use of OKN has been to measure the visual acuity of infants. The strategy is to find the most narrow stripes that will elicit a response (see Table 1.4 for a summary of the data). The best modal values for newborns are 20/400 (Fantz, Ordy, & Udelf, 1962) and 20/450 (Dayton, Jones, Aiu, Rawson, Steele, & Rose, 1964), although Fantz *et al.* used subjects up to a month old.

There is also some question about the suitability of OKN for measuring acuity: Kiff and Lepard (1966) varied their infant subjects' accommodation with both cycloplegic drugs and corrective lenses and found no effects whatsoever. Yet Fantz *et al.* (1962), found OKN predicted almost perfectly the most narrow stripes the same infants would look at in preference to a gray panel of equal brightness.

C.   Interpretation of Results

The slow phase of OKN does not require the ability to track normal moving stimuli, at least in babies (Brazelton *et al.*, 1966; McGinnis, 1930). Nor does the slow phase require macular vision: It persists in patients with partial lesions of the macula or with no central vision whatsoever (Walsh & Hoyt, 1969). But macular vision does seem to be necessary for one aspect of the fast phase: With

TABLE 1.4 VISUAL ACUITY IN NEWBORNS AS DETERMINED BY OKN

Study	N	Age	Velocity (degrees per second)	Distance of stripes (inches)	Best acuity		Modal acuity		Percentage of subjects showing modal acuity
					Minutes of arc	Snellen value	Minutes of arc	Snellen value	
Dayton, Jones, Aiu, Rawson, Steele, & Rose, 1964	32	birth–8 days	16.0	14.5	7.5	20/150	22.3	20/440	50
Fantz, Ordy, & Udelf, 1962	7	4 days–1 month	Variable	10.0	20.0	20/400	20.0	20/400	100
Gorman, Cogan, & Gellis, 1957	100	birth–5 days	8.5	6.0	33.5	20/670	33.5	20/670	93
Gorman, Cogan, & Gellis, 1959	100	birth–5 days	7.0	6.0	30.0	20/600	30.0	20/600	93
Gorman, Cogan, & Gellis, 1959	100	birth–3 days	7.0	6.0	17.5	20/350	22.5	20/450	100
Kiff & Lepard, 1966	44	premature 5–82 days	—	7.0	41.4	20/820	41.4	20/820	54

macular vision intact, when the movement of the stimuli is reversed, the reversal of OKN begins with the fast phase; yet if macular vision is reduced (by disease or by exposure to only ultraviolet light), the reversal starts with the slow phase (Cawthorne *et al.*, 1968).

The fast phase is not related in any other direct way to perception. The saccades do not redirect fixation to the exact center of the field; instead they take the eyes past the midline (Cawthorne *et al.*, 1968; Dix & Hood, 1971). They do not necessarily move the eyes to a line seen in the periphery, since they will move the eyes into the blind side in patients with homonymous hemianopsia (Davson, 1972). And the distance of the saccade is not correlated with the distance of the preceding slow movement; instead it is correlated (.86) with the distance of the succeeding slow movement (Stark, 1971).

The fast phase is, however, caused by at least some of the same physiological mechanisms as voluntary saccades: Unilateral lesions of the frontomesencephalic areas which eliminate voluntary leftward saccades also eliminate leftward fast phases (Hoyt & Daroff, 1971); and with paralysis of voluntary gaze, no fast phase occurs (Ling & Gay, 1968).

Just what parts of the brain mediate the response is not known; almost every part has been implicated by some theorist or other. Table 1.5 is a summary of the findings. There is general agreement

TABLE 1.5   PARTS OF THE BRAIN INVOLVED IN OPTOKINETIC NYSTAGMUS

Part of brain	Author	Effect of lesions (unilateral)		Effect of lesions (bilateral)	
		Human	Animal	Human	Animal
Optic tract	Smith, 1963	00[a]			
	Cogan, 1966	00			
	Duke-Elder & Scott, 1971	00			
Lateral geniculate	Smith, 1963	00			
	Duke-Elder & Scott, 1971	00			
Geniculo-calcarine tract	Duke-Elder & Scott, 1971	Maybe −0[b]			

(continued on next page)

fixating. The ratio of *(1)* the distance between two lamps in the visual field, to *(2)* the distance between their reflections on the eye, is a scale by which all distances on the eye can be related to distances in the visual field. Take the distance between the center of the pupil and the reflection of a lamp, multiply it by the scale, and the result is the distance of the subject's fixation point from that lamp. Calculate the distance from a second lamp, and the fixation point is located exactly.

Alternately, Cartesian coordinates can be superimposed on the visual field and on the eye. Once the scale of these coordinates is known, only one reflection is needed to locate a fixation point. If more than one reflection is visible, the best one to use is the one closest to the center of the subject's pupil: An extensive calibration with adults has shown that using this reflection gives the most accurate results (Haith, personal communication).

Exact determinations of fixation point require exact measurements of distances on the eye. The easiest way to do this is to use a movie camera instead of an observer[20]: The film can be projected frame by frame and distances measured on the screen. Alternatively, a videotape of the eye can be stopped as it is played back and measurements made electronically from the video signal (Haith, 1969).

In adults, the reflections should be measured about four times per second to pick up the shortest fixations—200 to 300 msec—that occur under normal circumstances (Khomskaya & Denisovskiy, 1970; Westheimer, 1968). Since there is no reason to suppose infants can fixate more frequently than adults, four frames per second should be right for them too.

The exposure time of each frame must be sufficiently long that an eye photographed in transit will appear blurred; otherwise it would be scored as a fixation. The exposure time should be about 50 msec: Adults' saccades last 20 msec to 50 msec (Westheimer, 1968), and preliminary data on infants suggest their eyes move almost as quickly (Aslin & Salapatek, 1973).

In most cases the experimenter wishes to make the lamps invisible so the subject will see only the stimulus. He can do this by *(1)* shining them either through window screening to which the

---

[20] In most studies of infants' visual preferences, an observer simply notes whether the reflection of the stimulus falls over the center of the pupil. The same principles apply as when the reflections are measured, but this chapter does not deal with them.

stimuli are attached, or through a half-silvered mirror in which the stimuli are reflected, and *(2)* filtering out all the visible wavelengths, recording only the infrared with an infrared video tube or infrared film. Filters often used are the Corning 769, which transmits most light between 700 mμ and 1000 mμ, and about 1% of light above 2100 mμ; the Kodak Wratten 87C, which transmits some light below 400 mμ, some light between 790 mμ and 940 mμ, and all light above 940 mμ; and a filter made from three sheets of Polaroid filter type HN7, rotated with respect to one another until they transmit no light visible to an adult. A filter such as the Corning, that eliminates hot wavelengths, should always be used and, if combined with other filters, placed nearest the bulb. The Wratten eliminates some of the visible light transmitted by the Corning, and the Polaroid eliminates all of it. However, the Polaroid cannot be used with infrared films, for they are too insensitive; so, when a movie camera is used, the subject may see slight red glows unless the stimulus is bright enough to flood them out.

The greatest source of error with corneal reflection is the false assumption that the line of sight passes through the center of the pupil, or that the visual and optic axes are the same. The visual axis is the line connecting the fixation point, the nodal point of the eye, and the fovea; the optic axis is the line connecting the centers of all the refracting planes of the eye and passing close to the center of the pupil. The angle between the visual and optic axes at the nodal point of the eye is called the angle alpha. In human adults this angle is about 5°: The fovea is temporal to where the optic axis strikes the back of the eye (the posterior pole) by about 5°, and is also about 1½° below it (Alpern, 1962a; Bennett & Francis, 1962; Kestenbaum, 1963; Scheie & Albert, 1969) (see Figure 1.9). In human newborns the fovea might be even more temporal (Keibel & Mall, 1912; Kestenbaum, 1963; Knighton, 1939; Mann, 1964).

Adults differ greatly from one to another in how far the fovea is from the posterior pole: Distances range from 1° nasal to 10° temporal (Slater & Findlay, 1972a). Note that the discrepancy in most cases will make the subject appear to be fixating more temporally than he actually is. There are no comparable data from infants, nor are there data on how the deviation changes postnatally.

Another source of error is parallax: The virtual image of the reference lamp rarely falls right on the pupil, yet the observer always sees it as if it did. If the camera and the lamp were

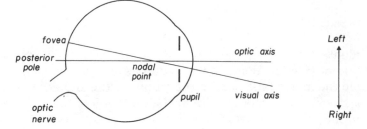

Figure 1.9 The discrepancy between the optic and visual axes in the left eye.

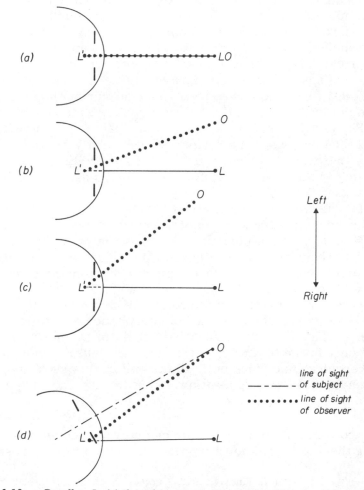

Figure 1.10 Parallax. In (a) the subject is staring at LO where there is both a lamp and the observer. The virtual image L′ is formed behind the pupil. Nevertheless the observer sees it in the center of the pupil. In (b) the observer has moved to the left of the lamp. The virtual image now appears farther to the left than it would if it were formed on the pupil. If the observer moves even farther over, as in (c), then the virtual image appears even farther to the left. Where the subject looks is not important: Even if he looks directly at the observer, as in (d), the virtual image still appears too far left.

coincident, this displacement would not matter; but in most cases they cannot be coincident, so there will usually be parallax. Most of the time the image falls behind the pupil, so the subject is scored as fixating too far from the camera in the direction of the lamp, and the farther the camera is from the lamp the greater is the error (see Figure 1.10).[21]

Just how much error is hard to estimate because as the subject fixates more peripherally from the camera, the pupil observed by the camera (the entrance pupil) changes shape and position. Also, as the subject fixates more peripherally from a lamp, the position of the virtual image changes—for two interacting reasons. First, because of spherical aberration, rays reflected off the periphery of the cornea (or any other convex spherical mirror) form a virtual image farther forward in the eye than rays reflected off the center (see Figure 1.11). Yet the cornea is not perfectly spherical; it is slightly flatter toward the periphery, particularly in adults. To an unknown extent this counteracts spherical aberration, causing rays reflected off the periphery to form a virtual image farther back in the eye (see Figure 1.12).

Slater (1973) estimated the error caused by parallax by using average figures for the location of the entrance pupil and assuming no effects from the asphericity of the cornea or, in infants, from spherical aberration. Given these assumptions, when the fixation point and a coincident reference lamp are 20° from the camera, the average error should be 4.4° in the adult and 6.5° in the newborn, in each case in the direction of the reference lamp. When the fixation point is away from the reference lamp, spherical aberration should cause parallax to be reduced considerably in the newborn, especially since his more nearly spherical cornea causes greater spherical aberration. And since both adults and infants show individual differences in the pupil's location and in the cornea's shape, there should be individual differences in parallax.

The corneal reflection technique can be validated with adults by asking them to fixate known points in the visual field, then scoring

---

[21] Slater (1973; Slater & Findlay, 1972a) argues that parallax (which he calls "projective distortion") is caused by the subject's looking away from the camera, so he predicts that the error will be greater the farther from the camera the subject looks. But he is wrong. In his analysis he has the fixation point and reference lamp coincident, so when the camera is away from the fixation point (the variable he claims is important), it is equally far away from the reference lamp. And it is this distance—from camera to reference lamp—that is the important one.

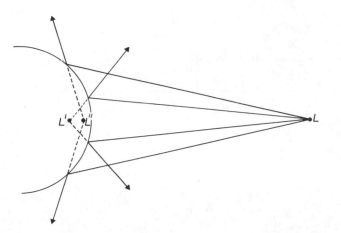

Figure 1.11   Spherical aberration. Rays of light reflected by the periphery of the cornea form a virtual image (L″) closer to the cornea than rays reflected by the center of the cornea.

Figure 1.12   The asphericity of the cornea. The cornea is not perfectly spherical, but instead is slightly flatter toward the periphery. This causes rays from a lamp reflected off the periphery (*l*) to form a virtual image (*l′*) farther back in the eye than rays from a lamp (L) reflected off the center.

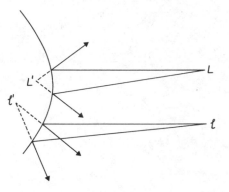

the film and noting any differences between the calculated fixation point and the real one. Parallax varies with the arrangement of the reference lamps, but several different calibrations consistently show the average error to be ±3° to 6° (Salapatek, 1967; 1968; Salapatek & Kessen, 1969; Slater & Findlay, 1972a), with variations among individuals (Salapatek, Haith, Maurer, & Kessen, 1972) (see Figure 1.13). In most cases it is in the expected direction: The calculated fixation point is too temporal.[22]

[22] Note, though, that in all these studies the reference lamps were fairly far from the camera (31° in Slater & Findlay [1972a] and Salapatek [1967, 1968; Salapatek & Kessen, 1969]; 26° in Salapatek *et al.* [1972]), so there should be a lot of parallax. With closer lamps less error would be expected.

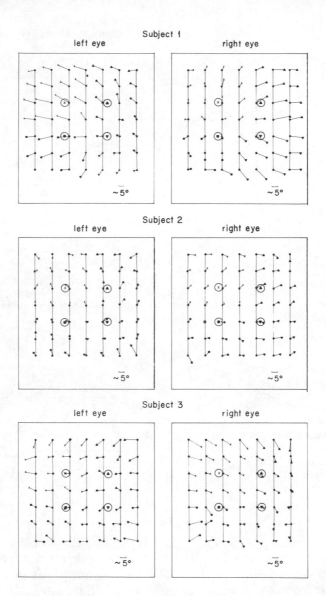

Figure 1.13　Calibration plots for the left and right eyes of three adults. Each adult fixated 49 points spaced at 3-inch intervals on a field 10 inches from the eye. These points are marked by dots and joined by vertical lines. The circled symbols indicate the locations of the reference lamps.) Each dot is also connected to a symbol representing the derived fixation point. These short lines represent the error of measurement. In all three subjects error is mostly in the temporal direction, but each subject shows different amounts: Subject 3 shows a relatively constant error; Subject 1 shows a large error which is larger toward the periphery; and Subject 2 shows much less error, but with greater variability. [From Salapatek, Haith, Maurer, & Kessen, 1972, p. 494.]

Slater and Findlay (1972a) noticed another error in their data: a tendency when the stimulus is away from the midline to derive the fixation even farther from the midline. When the stimulus was on midline the error for each eye was about as expected, $4\frac{1}{2}°$. But when the stimulus was toward one side, the error was larger for the ipsilateral eye (the eye on the same side as the stimulus) and smaller for the contralateral eye (the eye on the side opposite the stimulus). Thus, a tendency to derive the fixation too far from midline combined with the error caused by the discrepancy between the optic and visual axes to produce the measured results (see Figure 1.14).

This tendency to calculate fixation points farther from midline than they actually were can probably be explained by the variations in parallax caused by scoring from different reference lamps when the subject is looking at different parts of the field: When the subject looks to the right of the camera, a reference lamp on the right is used because its reflection is closest to the center of the pupil, so because of parallax the subject is scored as looking too far to the right. Conversely, when the subject looks to the left of the camera, a reference lamp on the left is used, and parallax causes the fixation to be derived too far to the left.

Slater and Findlay (1972a) attempted to do a similar validation with newborn infants. The newborns wore a gauze patch over one or the other eye, and were shown strings of colored lights located in

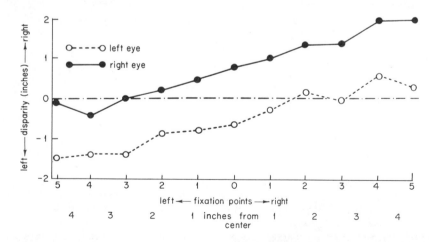

Figure 1.14   The average horizontal error of the corneal reflection technique when used to determine the fixation points of adults with the stimuli in the center and both sides of the field. [Reprinted from Slater & Findlay, 1972a, p. 352.]

the center of the field, or $1\frac{5}{16}$ or $3\frac{1}{2}$ inches toward the side of the uncovered eye. In a later experiment, newborns were held upright and *directly* facing "contralateral" stimuli which were 2 and $3\frac{1}{2}$ inches on the other side of center. Slater and Findlay found twice as much error as in adults ($8\frac{1}{3}°$ for central stimuli) and they inferred the same two types: the systematic temporal deviation (probably caused by the discrepancy between the optic and visual axes) and the tendency to derive any point too far from midline (probably caused by parallax). They also imply that the error differed up to 10° among different newborns.

But there is a major problem with this study which confounds these errors with several others. Slater and Findlay did not know when the infant was looking at each target, so they assumed a subject was looking at it if his fixations clustered somewhere in the visual field while the target was present. The fact that the fixations clustered could mean the subject actually was looking at the stimulus—but it could also mean that he looked part way toward the stimulus but not directly at it, or that he looked at one region of the field while totally ignoring the stimulus. Aslin and Salapatek (1973) found that 1- and 2-month-old babies do sometimes look part way toward a peripheral stimulus without looking directly at it. In addition, the tendency to look toward a stimulus varies systematically with its location in the visual field: The probability of a movement from the center of the field to the side of the field where a stimulus was presented was greater than 80% when the stimulus was 10° to the side but no different from chance when it was 40° to the side. And newborns do spend a lot of time staring at nothing, totally ignoring any stimulus (Doris *et al.*, 1967). So all in all, it seems reasonable to assume that part of what Slater and Findlay measured was the probability of fixations in various parts of the field (Salapatek *et al.*, 1972).[23]

[23] Slater and Findlay (1972b) "answer" this criticism: ". . . We have no reason to suppose that our subject loss was related in any systematic way to the position of the array of lights in the babies' visual field." But the issue is not subject loss; it is knowing whether the subjects who were included were actually looking at the stimulus—a question which is definitely not answered. Moreover, because they eliminated subjects who were so unattracted by the stimulus that they did not even look in the field does not mean all the remaining subjects who did look somewhere in the field looked right at the stimulus. Rather, some of those subjects could have been attracted by the stimulus—but others could have looked only near the stimulus (as in Aslin and Salapatek's study) or simply ignored the stimulus and stared somewhere else in the field.

This problem is exacerbated by monocular fixations. As Slater and Findlay note, infants when wearing a patch over one eye fixate farther to the temporal side than when they can see with both eyes. The same phenomenon can be seen by comparing two studies of fixations on a blank, homogeneous field: Fixations were much more temporal in the monocular study (Salapatek, 1968) than in the binocular study (Salapatek & Kessen, 1966). Thus Slater and Findlay may have documented the nature of looking under monocular conditions and not the optical error of the corneal reflection technique (Salapatek *et al.*, 1972).[24]

Finally, there is one considerable advantage of the corneal reflection technique besides its accuracy without calibration: It tolerates a great deal of head movement. Cowey (1963) filmed an adult who repeatedly fixated a point while moving his head sideways up to five-eighths of an inch. The distances of four reflections from the center of the pupil did not change observably— while the distances did change when the subject fixated a different point only 5° away. And Cowey had his reference lamps considerably behind the stimulus. If he had placed them in the same plane as the stimulus, the effects of head movement would have been even smaller (see Figure 1.15).

B. Summary of the Data from Infants

1. EYE MOVEMENTS OVER A BLANK FIELD

When a newborn is shown a blank and homogeneous field he scans broadly in all directions, but his horizontal eye movements are more widely dispersed than his vertical eye movements (Salapatek, 1968; Salapatek & Kessen, 1966). This broad scanning occurs even if the field is dark (Haith, 1968). So far it has been impossible to collect comparable data in older infants: When shown a blank field they fuss, fall asleep, or look off to the side (Salapatek, 1969).

---

[12] Slater and Findlay's (1972b) answer (?) is that they were well aware of the phenomenon and, therefore *(1)* presented their stimuli in the initial experiment only in central and ipsilateral positions (to the right for the right eye; to the left for the left eye); and *(2)* in another experiment presented "contralateral" stimuli by turning each baby's head so it was contralateral to the camera—but pointing right at the stimulus. All this, of course, merely facilitates viewing the stimuli; it does not correct for the tendency of infants to look at the temporal side.

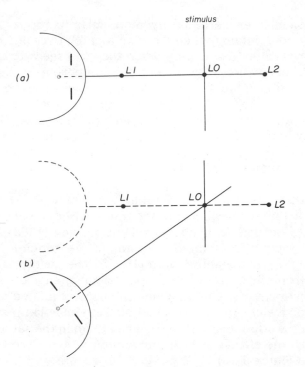

Figure 1.15   The effect of head movement on corneal reflections. In (a) the subject is looking at point LO on the stimulus where there is both a lamp and the observer. The lamp at LO appears to the observer to be in the center of the pupil, as would lamps L1 and L2, located in front of and behind the stimulus. In (b) the subject has moved his head but is still looking at point LO on the stimulus. Lamp L still appears in the center of the pupil—but lamps L1 and L2 would not. As long as the stimulus and reference lamps are approximately the same distance from the eye, head movements will not matter.

2.   Eye Movements over a Patterned Stimulus

When a stimulus is introduced, the broad scanning stops and the newborn looks at it. He frequently concentrates his scanning on a small part of the contour—particularly an angle if one is present—even if the exposure is prolonged and repeated. This is true for both circles of various sizes (Salapatek, 1967, 1968) and triangles (Nelson & Kessen, 1969; Salapatek, 1967, 1968; Salapatek & Kessen, 1966, 1969, 1973). Angles alone are not so effective in capturing his attention as closed figures like triangles, even though he rarely looks at sides (Nelson & Kessen, 1969). And an open figure made up of sides only (⌂) does not elicit any fixations.

Nor do straight edges (◗ ◢) always attract fixations (Kessen, Salapatek, & Haith, 1972). When the edge is oriented horizontally and introduced 3 inches above or below the center of the field, the subject does not fixate it; instead he continues to scan as broadly as he did on the blank field. When the edge is oriented vertically and appears 3 inches to the right or left of center, the subject does fixate it and he repeatedly crosses the contour with small horizontal eye movements.

Like the newborn, the 1-month-old baby also looks at only a limited part of a stimulus, particularly an angle. He does this even if the stimulus is complicated and/or irregular in design (Salapatek, 1969).

Between 1 and 2 months there is an increase in the scanning of some geometric shapes: The 2-month-old scans all parts of them repeatedly with few long fixations (Salapatek, 1969). But when the stimulus is a shape enclosing a smaller shape (▣), infants at *both* 1 and 2 months fixate only some part of it (Salapatek, 1969, 1973). There is a development from fixating mostly the external contour at 1 month to fixating mostly the internal contour at 2 months; but this has nothing to do with where the infant is capable of looking: If either contour is presented without the other, a child at both ages will fixate it (Salapatek, 1969).

This development is found in all three studies of how infants scan faces (Bergman, Haith, & Mann, 1971; Donnee, 1973; Maurer, 1969). A 1-month-old does not often look at a face, but when he does he looks at some part of its perimeter, usually the hairline or the chin. In contrast, a 2-month-old looks longer at the internal features (at both the eyes and the mouth with perhaps a preference for the eyes). The tendency to fixate internal features may decrease again after 2 months: Donnee (1973) reports a return by 10 weeks to fixating the perimeter.

3. BINOCULAR CONJUGATION AND CONVERGENCE

A newborn's horizontal eye movements are frequently conjugate —45% to 50% of the time when one eye moves to the right or left, so does the other eye (Wickelgren, 1969). Nevertheless, a newborn's eyes are rarely convergent: The right eye tends to look toward the right side of the visual field, while the left eye tends to look toward the left (Wickelgren, 1967, 1969). The amount of divergence depends on the stimulus: 17° for a small blinking light; 25° to 27° for a small blinking light either stationary or moving among three positions; 20° for two squares, one gray and one red; and 11° for a dim gray square paired with a panel of black and white stripes.

C. Interpretation of Results

When interpreting any study using corneal reflection, one question must come first: Did the many errors of measurement alter the results? For most studies of eye movements the consensus is no. Salapatek *et al.* (1972) note that corrections for parallax, spherical aberration, and the discrepancy between the visual and optic axes would not change their conclusions about the scanning of patterns, although the effects would be stronger for some subjects if such corrections were applied. Slater and Findlay (1972b) agree that the conclusions stand, but they do suggest an average correction should be applied to the data from each subject. If one knew the average correction for every age of infant, then applying them would make averaged, group data more correct. But scanning plots are normally analyzed subject by subject, and an average correction would not make an individual's plots accurate. Moreover, no one knows the average correction for any age of infant; the one Slater and Findlay (1972a) suggest for newborns is not well founded. And parallax varies with the arrangement of the reference lamps, so a correction derived from one setup would not be correct for any other setup. For the moment it seems best to leave the data as they are and note the probable direction of the error.

On the other hand, Slater and Findlay (1972a) suggest that the divergence reported by Wickelgren (1967, 1969) may be artifactual: The error caused by the discrepancy between the visual and optic axes causes the fixations to be derived too far to the temporal side of each eye, and parallax can cause the same effect. But some of the divergences Wickelgren reports are larger than the predicted errors. And more importantly, she obtained different amounts of divergence on different figures, while the error caused by the discrepancy between the visual and optic axes is constant.[25]

Studies which compare different age groups would be affected more. This is because the greatest source of error decreases

---

[25] This is not necessarily so for the error caused by parallax. It stays constant only *(1)* if the fixations are always scored using the same reference lamp, and *(2)* the subject always looks in roughly the same part of the field, keeping the amount of spherical aberration about the same. Unfortunately, Wickelgren doesn't say whether these conditions were met.

substantially with age: the discrepancy between the visual and optic axes.[26]

Almost all the data gathered with corneal reflection refute the long-standing opinion that babies are blind, or that they are just barely sensitive to light, or that they can fixate only under unusual circumstances (Gesell, Ilg, & Bullis, 1949; Guernsey, 1929; Nelson, 1959; Peiper, 1963; Rand & Vincent, 1946; Rasmussen, 1920; Stone, 1938). Instead, newborns will frequently look at figures and even at selected parts of figures.

Most physiologists would conclude from the corneal reflection data that newborns have a functioning occipital cortex. Their saccadic eye movements and long fixations on visual stimuli as small as 12° indicate this, since in many organisms, ablations of the occipital cortex prevent saccadic eye movements and the discrimination of forms (Held, 1970; Schneider, 1969). But there is evidence that some ability to discriminate forms and make eye movements is possible even without an occipital cortex. Schneider's hamsters, for example, could discriminate a bright form from a black one, and a speckled form from a gray one. Trevarthan (1968) reports that monkeys with lesions of the striate cortex can make a number of discriminations involving the amount of black and white contour, can reach for objects on the basis of visual cues, and will respond to small moving targets or fluctuating patterns of light. And Humphrey (1970, 1972) reports that after a long recovery period (6 years), a monkey with an ablated cortex can detect stationary targets and can even discriminate spots differing by only a few millimeters in diameter or by only 10% in brightness. (See Bronson, 1969, for an argument that all the visual abilities demonstrated at birth are subcortical.)

For unknown reasons, horizontal eye movements are easier for newborns than vertical eye movements. On a blank field they scan more broadly sideways than up and down, and they can pursue targets horizontally before they can pursue them vertically (Jones, 1926). This may explain why the newborns in the study by Kessen *et al.* (1972) looked at the vertical contour rather than the horizontal: Only horizontal eye movements were necessary first to reach the target and then to scan it.

The implication of the corneal reflection data for peripheral vision is disputed. Salapatek (1969) believes the rapid localization of a

---

[26] Although this should be mitigated slightly by increased spherical aberration as the cornea assumes its mature shape.

stimulus newly introduced into the field means the newborn discriminates the stimulus with his peripheral retina. Additional support for this position is the observation that newborns often cross one part of the figure to get to another. On the other hand, Haith (1968) maintains that newborns scan randomly until they happen upon a stimulus. This argument can be resolved only by a detailed analysis of the initial approach to a stimulus.

VIII. CONCLUSION

Although each of the methods discussed in this chapter has serious limitations, that does not mean there is no good way to study infants' visual perception, nor that the methods are useless. It means only that for any given question the method of study must be chosen with care.

Each of the methods can be used to gain information about some questions. Many questions about eye movements and fixations require that one know only approximately how far an eye moved, or approximately where it is looking, or whether both eyes moved at the same time; and either electrooculography or corneal reflection can provide this information. Anatomical studies give background information and may suggest when to expect improvements in visual acuity, accommodation, tracking, etc. The electroretinogram can be used to ascertain what parts of the infant's retina are functioning. Optokinetic nystagmus can show if the infant responds to apparent motion. And even the visually evoked potential can be useful. So far it has provided little interpretable data because of the many parameters affecting it, but these parameters may be interesting phenomena in their own right, and may shed light on questions of perception. For example, the influence of the intensity of light on the newborn's VEP may show its intensity affects his visual system in the same way it affects that of the older infant or adult.

The criteria for judging a method should be not only the method's precision but also its appropriateness for the particular question asked. Each of the methods discussed is appropriate for some questions about infants' visual perception.

ACKNOWLEDGMENTS

I wish to thank John Armington, Ed Ballik, Glenn Dayton, Bernard Karmel, and Linda Siegel who read and commented on sections of the manuscript; and my husband, Charles Maurer, who edited it.

REFERENCES

Aantaa, E. Light-induced and spontaneous variations in the amplitude of the electro-oculogram. *Acta Oto-laryngologica (Stockholm)*, 1970, Supplement 267.

Aantaa, E., & Elenius, V. Diurnal variation in the amplitude of the corneo-fundal potential. *Practica Oto-rhino-laryngologica (Basel)*, 1968, *30*, 245.

Adrian, E. Rod and cone components in the electric response of the eye. *Journal of Physiology*, 1946, *105*, 24–37.

Algvere, P., & Zetterstrom, B. Size and shape of the electroretinogram in newborn infants. *Acta Ophthalmologica*, 1967, *45*, 399–410.

Alpern, M. Specification of the direction of regard. In H. Davson (Ed.), *The eye*. Vol 3. *Muscular mechanisms*. New York: Academic Press, 1962. Pp. 7–13. (a)

Alpern, M. Types of movements. In H. Davson (Ed.), *The eye*. Vol. 3. *Muscular mechanisms*. New York: Academic Press, 1962. Pp. 63–151. (b)

Alpern, M. Effector mechanisms in vision. In J. Kling, & L. Riggs (Eds.), *Woodworth and Schlosberg's experimental psychology*. New York: Holt, 1971. Pp. 369–394.

Arden, G., & Barrada, A. Analysis of the electro-oculograms of a series of normal subjects. *British Journal of Ophthalmology*, 1962, *46*, 468–482.

Arden, G., & Kelsey, J. Changes produced by light in the standing potential of the human eye. *Journal of Physiology*, 1962, *161*, 189–204.

Armington, J. Spectral sensitivity of simultaneous electroretinograms and occipital responses. In H. Burian, & J. Jacobsen (Eds.), *Clinical electroretinography: Proceedings of the Third International Symposium (1964)*. Oxford: Pergamon Press, 1966. Pp. 225–233.

Armington, J. The electroretinogram, the visually evoked potential, and the area-luminance relation. *Vision Research*, 1968, *8*, 263–276.

Aserinsky, E. Effects of illumination and sleep upon amplitude of the electrooculogram. *Archives of Ophthalmology*, 1955, *53*, 542–546.

Aslin, R., & Salapatek, P. Saccadic localizations of peripheral visual targets by the very young human infant. Paper presented at the meeting of the Psychonomic Society, St. Louis, November, 1973.

Barber, A. *Embryology of the human eye*. St. Louis: C. V. Mosby, 1955.

Barnet, A., Lodge, A., & Armington, J. Electroretinogram in newborn human infants. *Science*, 1965, *148*, 651–654.

Barnet, A., Lodge, A., Armington, J., Shanks, B., & Newcomb, C. Newborn infants' electroretinograms and evoked electroencephalographic responses to short and long wave length light. *Neurology (Minnesota)*, 1968, *18*, 304.

Bembridge, B. The problem of myelination of the central nervous system with specific reference to the optic nerve. *Transactions of the Opthalmological Society of the United Kingdom*, 1956, *76*, 311–322.

Bennett, A., & Francis, J. The eye as an optical system. In H. Davson (Ed.), *The eye*. Vol. 4. *Visual optics and optical space sense*. New York: Academic Press, 1962. Pp. 101–131.

Bergman, T., Haith, M., & Mann, L. Development of eye contact and facial scanning in infants. Paper presented at the meeting of the Society for Research in Child Development, Minneapolis, April, 1971.

Brazelton, T., Scholl, M., & Robey, J. Visual responses in the newborn. *Pediatrics*, 1966, *37*, 284–290.

Bronson, G. Vision in infancy: Structure-function relationships. In R. Robinson (Ed.), *Brain and early behavior*. New York: Academic Press, 1969. Pp. 207–210.

Brown, K. The electroretinogram: Its components and their origins. *Vision Research,* 1968, *8,* 633–677.

Bruner, J. Pacifier-produced visual buffering in human infants. *Developmental Psychobiology,* 1973, *6,* 45–51.

Brunette, J. A standardizable method for separating rod and cone responses in clinical roretinography. *American Journal of Ophthalmology,* 1973, *75,* 833–845.

Byford, G. Non-linear relations between the corneal-retinal potential and horizontal eye movements. *Journal of Physiology,* 1963, *168,* 14.

Cawthorne, T., Dix, M., & Hood, J. Recent advances in electronystagmographic technique with specific reference to its value in clinical diagnosis. In J. Smith (Ed.), *Neuro-opthalmology.* Vol. 4. St. Louis: C. V. Mosby, 1968. Pp. 81–109.

Cogan, D. *Neurology of the visual system.* Springfield, Illinois: Thomas, 1966.

Collins, W. Some characteristics of optokinetic eye-movement patterns: A comparative study. *Aerospace Medicine,* 1972, *41,* 1251–1262.

Conel, J. *The postnatal development of the human cerebral cortex.* Vol. 1. *The cortex of the newborn.* Cambridge, Massachusetts: Harvard Univ. Press, 1939.

Conel, J. *The postnatal development of the human cerebral cortex.* Vol. 2. *The cortex of the one-month infant.* Cambridge, Massachusetts: Harvard Univ. Press, 1941.

Conel, J. *The postnatal development of the human cerebral cortex.* Vol. 3. *The cortex of the three-month infant.* Cambridge, Massachusetts: Harvard Univ. Press, 1947.

Conel, J. *The postnatal development of the human cerebral cortex.* Vol. 4. *The cortex of the six-month infant.* Cambridge, Massachusetts: Harvard Univ. Press, 1951.

Conel, J. *The postnatal development of the human cerebral cortex.* Vol. 5. *The cortex of the fifteen-month infant.* Cambridge, Massachusetts: Harvard Univ. Press, 1955.

Conel, J. *The postnatal development of the human cerebral cortex.* Vol. 6. *The cortex of the twenty-four-month infant.* Cambridge, Massachusetts: Harvard Univ. Press, 1959.

Cowey, A. The basis of a method of perimetry with monkeys. *Quarterly Journal of Experimental Psychology,* 1963, *15,* 81–90.

Davson, H. *The physiology of the eye.* New York: Academic Press, 1972.

Dayton, G., & Jones, M. Analysis of characteristics of fixation reflex in infants by use of direct current electrooculography. *Neurology,* 1964, *14,* 1152–1156.

Dayton, G., Jones, M., Aiu, P., Rawson, R., Steele, B., & Rose, M. Developmental study of coordinated eye movements in the human infant: I. Visual acuity in the newborn human: a study based on induced optokinetic nystagmus recorded by electro-oculography. *Archives of Opthalmology,* 1964, *71,* 865–870.

Dayton, G., Jones, M., & Dizon, L. Electrooculography, technique and clinical application. *Transactions of the Pacific Coast Oto-ophthalmology Society,* 1963, *44,* 65–80.

Dayton, G., Jones, M., Steele, B., & Rose, M. Developmental study of coordinated eye movements in the human infant: II. An electro-oculographic study of the fixation reflex in the newborn. *Archives of Ophthalmology,* 1964, *71,* 871–875.

Dix, M., & Hood, J. Further observations upon the neurological mechanism of optokinetic nystagmus. *Acta Oto-laryngologica (Stockholm),* 1971, *71,* 217–226.

Donnee, L. Infants' developmental scanning patterns to face and nonface stimuli under various auditory conditions. Paper presented at the meeting of the Society for Research in Child Development, Philadelphia, March, 1973.

Doris, J., Casper, M., & Poresky, R. Differential brightness thresholds in infancy. *Journal of Experimental Child Psychology*, 1967, *5*, 522–535.

Doris, J., & Cooper, L. Brightness discrimination in infancy. *Journal of Experimental Child Psychology*, 1966, *3*, 31–39.

Duffy, F., & Rengstorff, R. Ametropia measurements from the visual evoked response. *American Journal of Optometry*, 1971, *48*, 717–728.

Duke-Elder, S., & Cook, G. *System of opthalmology.* Vol. 3. *Normal and abnormal development.* Part 1. *Embryology.* London: Henry Kimpton, 1963.

Duke-Elder, S., & Scott, G. *System of ophthalmology.* Vol. 12. *Neuro-ophthalmology.* London: Henry Kimpton, 1971.

Eason, R., Harter, M., & White, C. Effects of attention and arousal on visually evoked cortical potentials and reaction time in man. *Physiology and Behavior*, 1969, *4*, 283–290.

Eason, R., Oden, D., & White, C. Visually evoked cortical potentials and reaction time in relation to site of retinal stimulation. *Electroencephalography and Clinical Neurophysiology*, 1967, *22*, 313–324.

Eason, R., White, C., & Bartlett, N. Effects of checkerboard pattern stimulation on evoked cortical responses in relation to check size and visual field. *Psychonomic Science*, 1970, *21*, 113–115.

Eason, R., White, C., & Oden, D. Averaged occipital responses to stimulation of sites in the upper and lower halves of the retina. *Perception and Psychophysics*, 1967, *2*, 423–425.

Edwards, D. Comparison of first-eye movement detection methods. *Perceptual and Motor Skills*, 1971, *32*, 435–441.

Ehlers, N., Matthiessen, M., & Anderson, H. The prenatal growth of the human eye, *Acta Ophthalmologica (Kobenhavn)*, 1968, *46*, 329–349.

Ellingson, R. Electroencephalograms of normal, full-term newborns immediately after birth with observations on arousal and visual evoked responses. *Electroencephalography and Clinical Neurophysiology*, 1958, *10*, 31–50. (a)

Ellingson, R. Occipital evoked potentials in human newborns. *Electroencephalography and Clinical Neurophysiology*, 1958, *10*, 189. (b)

Ellingson, R. Cortical electrical responses to visual stimulation in the human infant. *Electroencephalography and Clinical Neurophysiology*, 1960, *12*, 663–677.

Ellingson, R. Cerebral electrical responses to auditory and visual stimuli in the infant (human and subhuman studies). In P. Kellaway, & I. Peterson (Eds.), *Neurological and electroencephalographic correlative studies in infancy.* New York: Grune and Stratton, 1964. Pp. 78–116. (a)

Ellingson, R. Studies of the electrical activity of the developing human brain. In W. Himwish, & H. Himwish (Eds.), *Progress in brain research.* Vol. 9. *Developing brain.* Amsterdam: Elsevier, 1964. Pp. 26–53. (b)

Ellingson, R. Development of visual evoked responses in human infants recorded by a response averager. *Electroencephalography and Clinical Neurophysiology*, 1966, *21*, 403–404.

Ellingson, R. Methods of recording cortical evoked responses in the human infant. In A. Minkowski (Ed.), *Regional development of the brain in early life.* Oxford: Blackwell Scientific Publications, 1967. Pp. 413–435. (a)

Ellingson, R. The study of brain electrical activity in infants. In L. Lipsitt, & C. Spiker (Eds.), *Advances in child development and behavior.* Vol. 3. New York: Academic Press, 1967. Pp. 53–97. (b)

Ellingson, R. Clinical applications of evoked potential techniques in infants and children. *Electroencephalography and Clinical Neurophysiology*, 1968, *24*, 293.

Ellingson, R. Variability of visual evoked responses in the human newborn. *Electroencephalography and Clinical Neurophysiology*, 1970, *29*, 10–19.

Ellingson, R., Lathrop, G., Danahy, T., & Nelson, B. Variability of visual evoked potentials in human infants and adults. *Electroencephalography and Clinical Neurophysiology*, 1973, *34*, 113–124.

Ellingson, R., Lathrop, G., Nelson, G., & Danahy, T. Visual evoked potentials of infants. *Revue E.E.G., Paris,* 1972, *2*, 395–400.

Engel, R. Electroencephalographic responses to photic stimulation and their correlation with maturation. *Annals of the New York Academy of Science*, 1964, *117*, 407–412.

Engel, R. Maturational changes and abnormalities in newborn electroencephalogram. *Developmental Medicine and Child Neurology*, 1965, *7*, 498–506.

Engel, R. Electroencephalographic responses to sound and light in premature and full term neonates. *The Journal-Lancet*, 1967, *87*, 181–186.

Engel, R. Acoustic and photic response latencies in Oriental neonates. *Electroencephalography and Clinical Neurophysiology*, 1968, *24*, 394–395.

Engel, R., & Benson, R. Estimate of conceptional age by evoked response activity. *Biologia Neonatorum*, 1968, *12*, 201–213.

Engel, R., & Butler, B. Appraisal of conceptual age of newborn infants by electroencephalographic methods. *Journal of Pediatrics*, 1963, *63*, 386–393.

Engle, R., Crowell, D., & Nishijima, S. Visual and auditory response latencies in neonates. *Felicitation volume in honour of C. C. DeSilva*, 1968.

Engel, R., & Fay, W. Visual evoked responses at birth, verbal scores at three years, and IQ at four years. *Developmental Medicine and Child Neurology*, 1972, *14*, 283–289.

Fantz, R., Ordy, J., & Udelf, M. Maturation of pattern vision in infants during the first six months. *Journal of Comparative and Physiological Psychology*, 1962, *55*, 907–917.

Ferriss, G., Davis, G., Dorsen, M., & Hackett, E. Changes in latency and form of the photically induced average evoked response in human infants. *Electroencephalography and Clinical Neurophysiology*, 1967, *22*, 305–312.

Fichsel, H. Visual evoked potentials in prematures, newborns, infants and children by stimulation with colored light. *Electroencephalography and Clinical Neurophysiology*, 1969, *27*, 660.

Fleming, D., Wilson, C., & Merrill, H. Photic intermittency, pupillary diameter, and the visually evoked potential. *Vision Research*, 1972, *12*, 487–493.

Francois, J. Maculopathies. In H. Henkes (Ed.), *Perspectives in ophthalmology.* Amsterdam: Excerpta Medica Foundation, 1968. Pp. 65–78.

Francois, J., & de Rouck, A. The electroretinogram in young children (single stimulus, twin flashes and intermittent stimulation). *Documenta Ophthalmologica*, 1964, *18*, 330–343.

Gaboresek, V. Choice of binocular or monocular deviations in electronystagmography. I. General remarks. *Electroencephalography and Clinical Neurophysiology*, 1968, *25*, 511.

Gaboresek, V. Choice of binocular or monocular deviations in electronystagmography. II. The influence of vertical eye movements. *Electroencephalography and Clinical Neurophysiology*, 1969, *26*, 637.

Gardner, R., & Weitzman, E. Examination for optokinetic nystagmus in sleep and waking. *Archives of Neurology (Chicago)*, 1967, *16*, 415–420.

Gesell, A., Ilg, F., & Bullis, G. *Vision. Its development in infant and child.* New York: Hafner, 1949.

Gonshor, A., & Malcolm, R. Effect of changes in illumination level on electro-oculography. *Aerospace Medicine*, 1971, *42*, 138–140.

Gorman, J., Cogan, D., & Gellis, S. An apparatus for grading the visual acuity of infants on the basis of opticokinetic nystagmus. *Pediatrics*, 1957, *19*, 1088–1092.

Gorman, J., Cogan, D., & Gellis, S. A device for testing visual acuity in infants. *Sight-Saving Review*, 1959, *29*, 80–84.

Gottlieb, G. Ontogenesis of sensory function in birds and mammals. In E. Tobach, L. Aronson, & E. Shaw (Eds.), *The biopsychology of development.* New York: Academic Press, 1971. Pp. 67–128.

Gouras, P. Electroretinography: Some basic principles. *Investigative Ophthalmology*, 1970, *9*, 557–569.

Granit, R. The components of the retinal action potential in mammals and their relation to the discharge in the optic nerve. *Journal of Physiology*, 1933, *77*, 207–239.

Groth, H., Weled, B., & Batkin, S. A comparison of monocular visually evoked potentials in human neonates and adults. *Electroencephalography and Clinical Neurophysiology*, 1970, *28*, 478–487.

Guernsey, M. A quantitative study of the eye reflexes in infants. *Psychological Bulletin*, 1929, *26*, 160–161.

Haith, M. Visual scanning in infants. Paper presented at the regional meeting of the Society for Research in Child Development, Worcester, Massachusetts, 1968.

Haith, M. Infrared television recording and measurement of ocular behavior in the human infant. *American Psychologist*, 1969, *24*, 279–283.

Harter, M. Evoked cortical responses to checkerboard patterns: Effect of check-size as a function of retinal eccentricity. *Vision Research*, 1970, *10*, 1365–1376.

Harter, M. Visually evoked cortical responses to the on- and off-set of patterned light in humans. *Vision Research*, 1971, *11*, 685–695.

Harter, M., & Suitt, C. Visually-evoked cortical responses and pattern vision in the infant: a longitudinal study. *Psychonomic Science*, 1970, *18*, 235–237.

Harter, M., & White, C. Effects of contour sharpness and check-size in visually evoked cortical potentials. *Vision Research*, 1968, *8*, 701–711.

Harter, M., & White, C. Evoked cortical responses to checkerboard patterns: Effect of check-size as a function of visual acuity. *Electroencephalography and Clinical Neurophysiology*, 1970, *28*, 48–54.

Heck, J., & Zetterstrom, B. Analyse des photopischen Flimmerelektroretinogramms bei Neugeborenen. *Ophthalmologica*, 1958, *135*, 205–210. (a)

Heck, J., & Zetterstrom, B. Electroencephalographic recording of the on- and off-response from the human visual cortex. *Ophthalmologica*, 1958, *136*, 258–265. (b)

Held, R. Two modes of processing spatially distributed visual stimulation. In F. Schmitt (Ed.), *The neurosciences: Second study program.* New York: Rockefeller Univ. Press, 1970. Pp. 317–324.

Henderson, J., & Crosby, E. An experimental study of optokinetic nystagmus. *Archives of Ophthalmology (Chicago)*, 1952, *47*, 43–54.

Henderson, N., & Engel, R. Neonatal visual evoked potentials as predictors of psychoeducational tests at age seven. *Developmental Psychology*, 1974, *10*, 269–276.

Horsten, G., & Winkelman, J. Development of the ERG in relation to histological differentiation of the retina in man and animals. *Archives of Ophthalmology*, 1960, *63*, 232–242.

Horsten, G., & Winkelman, J. Electrical activity of the retina in relation to histological differentiation in infants born prematurely and at full-term. *Vision Research*, 1962, *2*, 269–276.

Horsten, G., & Winkelman, J. Electro-retinographic critical fusion frequency of the retina in relation to the histological development in man and animals. *Documenta Ophthalmologica*, 1964, *18*, 515–521.

Hoyt, W., & Daroff, R. Supranuclear disorders of ocular control systems in man. In P. Bach-y-rita, & C. Collins (Eds.), *The control of eye movements*. New York: Academic Press, 1971. Pp. 175–236.

Hrbek, A. Evoked responses of different sensory modalities in newborn infants. *Electroencephalography and Clinical Neurophysiology*, 1969, *27*, 669.

Hrbek, A., Hrbkova, M., & Lenard, H. Somato-sensory, auditory, and visual evoked responses in newborn infants during sleep and wakefulness. *Electroencephalography and Clinical Neurophysiology*, 1969, *26*, 597–603.

Hrbek, A., Karlberg, P., & Olsson, T. Development of visual and somato-sensory evoked responses in pre-term newborn infants. *Electroencephalography and Clinical Neurophysiology*, 1973, *34*, 225–232.

Hrbek, A., & Mares, P. Cortical evoked responses to visual stimulation in full-term and premature newborns. *Electroencephalography and Clinical Neurophysiology*, 1964, *16*, 575–581.

Humphrey, N. What the frog's eye tells the monkey's brain. *Brain, Behavior, and Evolution*, 1970, *3*, 324–337.

Humphrey, N. Seeing and nothingness. *New Scientist*, 1972, *53*, 682–684.

Hymes, C. The postnatal growth of the cornea and palpebral fissure and the projection of the eyeball in early life. *Journal of Comparative Neurology*, 1929, *48*, 415–440.

Jansson, F. Measurements of intraocular distances by ultrasound. *Acta Ophthalmologica (Kobenhavn)*, 1963, Supplement 74.

Jensen, D., & Engel, R. Statistical procedures for relating dichotomous responses to maturation and EEG measurements. *Electroencephalography and Clinical Neurophysiology*, 1971, *30*, 437–443.

John, E., Herrington, R., & Sutton, S. Effects of visual form on the evoked response. *Science*, 1967, *155*, 1439–1442.

Jones, M. The development of early behavior patterns in young children. *Pedagogical Seminary and Journal of Genetic Psychology*, 1926, *33*, 537–585.

Karmel, B. Brain mechanisms involved in early visual perception. Paper presented at the meeting of the Society for Research in Child Development, Philadelphia, March, 1973.

Karmel, B., Hoffman, R., & Fegy, M. Processing of contour information by human infants evidenced by pattern-dependent evoked potentials. *Child Development*, 1974, *45*, 39–48.

Karmel, B., White, C., Cleaves, W., & Steinsiek, K. A technique to investigate evoked potential correlates of pattern perception in infants. Paper presented at the meeting of the Eastern Psychological Association, Atlantic City, April, 1970.

Karpe, G. The basis of clinical electroretinography. *Acta Ophthalmologica*, 1945, Supplement 24.

Kawasaki, K., Tsuchida, Y., & Jacobson, J. The direct current component of the electroretinogram in man. *American Journal of Ophthalmology*, 1972, *73*, 243–249.

Keibel, F. Development of the sense organs. In F. Keibel, & F. Mall (Eds.), *Human embryology*. Philadelphia: J. B. Lippincott, 1912. Pp. 180–290.

Kelsey, J. Electrodiagnostic methods in ophthalmology. *Transactions of the Ophthalmological Society of the United Kingdom*, 1967, *87*, 239–246. (a)

Kelsey, J. Variations in the normal electrooculogram. *British Journal of Ophthalmology*, 1967, *51*, 44–49. (b)

Kessen, W., Salapatek, P., & Haith, M. The visual response of the human newborn to linear contour. *Journal of Experimental Child Psychology*, 1972, *13*, 9–20.

Kestenbaum, A. *Applied anatomy of the eye*. New York: Grune and Stratton, 1963.

Khomskaya, E., & Denisovskiy, G. Individual features of eye macromovements in a prolonged series of fixation points. *Soviet Psychology*, 1970, *8*, 179–197.

Kiff, R., & Lepard, C. Visual response of premature infants. *Archives of Ophthalmology*, 1966, *75*, 631–633.

Knighton, W. Development of the normal eye in infancy and childhood. *Sight-Saving Review*, 1939, *9*, 3–10.

Kooi, K., & Bagchi, B. Visually evoked responses in man: normative data. *Annals of the New York Academy of Science*, 1964, *112*, 254–269.

Kris, C. Corneo-fundal potential variations during light and dark adaptation. *Nature (London)*, 1958, *182*, 1027.

Kris, C. Vision: Electrooculography. In O. Glasser (Ed.), *Medical physics*. Vol. 3. Chicago: Yearbook Publishers, 1960. Pp. 692–700.

Kris, E. Bi-dimensional, binocular eye-position and motion electrooculogram measurement in infants and children with nystagmus and strabismus. *Digest of the Seventh International Conference of Medical and Biological Engineering*, 1967. P. 248.

Langworthy, V. Development of behavior patterns and myelinization of the nervous system in the human fetus and infant. *Contribution to embryology*, 1933, *24*, No. 139.

Larroche, J. Part II. The development of the central nervous system during intrauterine life. *Human Development*, 1966, *9*, 257–276.

Larsen, J. The sagittal growth of the eye. I. Ultrasonic measurement of the depth of the anterior chamber from birth to puberty. *Acta Ophthalmologica*, 1971, *49*, 239–262. (a)

Larsen, J. The sagittal growth of the eye. II. Ultrasonic measurement of the axial diameter of the lens and the anterior segment from birth to puberty. *Acta Ophthalmologica*, 1971, *49*, 427–440. (b)

Larsen, J. The sagittal growth of the eye. III. Ultrasonic measurement of the posterior segment (axial length of the vitreous) from birth to puberty. *Acta Ophthalmologica*, 1971, *49*, 441–453. (c)

Larsen, J. The sagittal growth of the eye. IV. Ultrasonic measurement of the axial length of the eye from birth to puberty. *Acta Opthalmologica*, 1971, *49*, 873–886. (d)

Larson, W. Clinical electrooculography with suitable apparatus. *American Journal of Optometry*, 1970, *47*, 295–303.

Last, P. *Eugene Wolff's anatomy of the eye and orbit*. London: H. K. Lewis, 1968.

Ling, W., & Gay, A. Optokinetic nystagmus: a proposed pathway and its clinical application. In J. Smith (Ed.), *Neuro-opthalmology.* Vol. 4. St. Louis: C. V. Mosby, 1968. Pp. 117–123.

Lipman, I. "Voluntary nystagmus"—ocular shuddering. *Diseases of the Nervous System*, 1972, *33*, 200–201.

Lodge, A., Armington, J., Barnet, A., Shanks, B., & Newcomb, C. Newborn infants' electroretinograms and evoked electroencephalographic responses to orange and white light. *Child Development*, 1969, *40*, 267–293.

Ludlam, W., & Meyers, R. The use of visually evoked responses in objective refraction. *Transactions of the New York Academy of Science* 1972, *34*, 154–170.

Mann, I. *The development of the human eye.* London: British Medical Association, 1964.

Marg, E. Development of electrooculography. *Archives of Opthalmology (New York)*, 1951, *45*, 169–185.

Maurer, D. The scanning of faces by infants. Unpublished manuscript, 1969.

McGinnis, J. Eye-movements and optic nystagmus in early infancy. *Genetic Psychology Monographs*, 1930, *8*, 321–430.

Miles, W. The steady polarity potential of the human eye. *Proceedings of the National Academy of Science*, 1939, *25*, 25–36.

Miller, R., & Dowling, J. Intracellular responses of the Müller (glial) cells of mudpuppy retina: Their relation to b-wave of the electroretinogram. *Journal of Neurophysiology*, 1970, *33*, 323–341.

Mirzoyants, N. Changes in the electrical activity of the brain in early childhood in response to a flicker stimulus. *Pavlov Journal of Higher Nervous Activity*, 1961, *11*, 31–36.

Nakayama, K. Studies on the myelination of the human optic nerve. *Japanese Journal of Opthalmology*, 1968, *11*, 132–140.

Nelson, K., & Kessen, W. Visual scanning by human newborns: Responses to complete triangle, to sides only, and to corners only. Paper presented at the meeting of the American Psychological Association, 1969.

Nelson, W. *Textbook of pediatrics.* Philadelphia: Saunders, 1959.

Noell, W. The origin of the electroretinogram. *American Journal of Ophthalmology*, 1954, *38*, 78–93.

Parks, M. Growth of the eye and development of vision. In S. Liebman, & S. Gellis (Eds.), *The pediatrician's ophthalmology.* St. Louis: C. V. Mosby, 1966. Pp. 15–25.

Peiper, A. *Cerebral function in infancy and childhood.* New York: Consultants Bureau, 1963.

Prechtl, H., & Lenard, H. A study of eye movements in sleeping newborn infants. *Brain Research*, 1967, *5*, 477–493.

Rabinowicz, T. The cerebral cortex of the premature infant of the eighth month. *Progress in Brain Research*, 1964, *4*, 39–92.

Rabinowicz, T. Quantitative appraisal of the cerebral cortex of the premature infant of eight months. In A. Minkowski (Ed.), *Regional development of the brain in early life.* Oxford: Blackwell Scientific Publications, 1967. Pp. 91–124. (a)

Rabinowicz, T. Techniques for the establishment of an atlas of the cerebral cortex of the premature. In A. Minkowski (Ed.), *Regional development of the brain in early life.* Oxford: Blackwell Scientific Publications, 1967. Pp. 71–90. (b)

Rand, W., & Vincent, E. *Growth and development of the young child.* Philadelphia: Saunders, 1946.

Rasmussen, V. *Child psychology.* Vol. I. *Development in the first four years.* London: Glydendal, 1920.

Reinecke, R., & Cogan, D. Standardization of objective visual acuity measurements. *Archives of Ophthalmology,* 1958, *60,* 418–421.

Riesen, A. Problems in correlating behavioral and physiological development. In M. Sterman, D. McGinty, & A. Adinolfi (Eds.), *Brain development and behavior.* New York: Academic Press, 1971. Pp. 59–70.

Rietveld, W., Tordoir, W., Hagenouw, J., Lubbers, J., & Spoor, T. Visual evoked responses to blank and to checkerboard patterned flashes. *Acta Physiologica et Pharmacologica Neerlandica,* 1967, *14,* 259–285.

Riggs, L. Electroretinography in cases of night blindness. *American Journal of Ophthalmology,* 1954, *38,* 70–78.

Riggs, L. Electrophysiology of vision. In C. Graham (Ed.), *Vision and visual perception.* New York: Wiley, 1965. Pp. 81–131.

Riggs, L., & Wooten, B. Electrical measures and psychophysical data on human vision. In D. Jameson & L. Hurvich (Eds.), *Visual psychophysics.* Berlin: Springer-Verlag, 1972. Pp. 690–731.

Robinson, R. Cerebral hemisphere function in the newborn. In R. Robinson (Ed.), *Brain and early behavior.* New York: Academic Press, 1969. Pp. 343–349.

Rodieck, R. Components of the electroretinogram—a reappraisal. *Vision Research,* 1972, *12,* 773–780.

Rose, C. Relationship of electrophysiological and behavioral indices of visual development in mammals. In M. Sterman, D. McGinty, & A. Adinolfi (Eds.), *Brain development and behavior.* New York: Academic Press, 1971. Pp. 145–183.

Salapatek, P. Visual scanning of geometric figures by the human newborn. Unpublished Ph.D. thesis, Yale Univ., New Haven, Connecticut, 1967.

Salapatek, P. Visual scanning of geometric figures by the human newborn. *Journal of Comparative and Physiological Psychology,* 1968, *66,* 247–258.

Salapatek, P. The visual investigation of geometric pattern by the one and two month old infants. Paper presented at the meeting of the American Association for the Advancement of Science, Boston, December, 1969.

Salapatek, P. Visual investigation of geometric form by the human infant. Paper presented at the meeting of the Society for Research in Child Development, Philadelphia, March, 1973.

Salapatek, P., Haith, M., Maurer, D., & Kessen, W. Error in the corneal-reflection technique: A note on Slater and Findlay. *Journal of Experimental Child Psychology,* 1972, *14,* 493–497.

Salapatek, P., & Kessen, W. Visual scanning of triangles by the human newborn. *Journal of Experimental Child Psychology,* 1966, *3,* 155–167.

Salapatek, P., & Kessen, W. Prolonged investigation of a plane geometric triangle by the human newborn. Paper presented at the meeting of the Society for Research in Child Development, Santa Monica, California, April, 1969.

Salapatek, P., & Kessen, W. Prolonged investigation of a plane geometric triangle by the human newborn. *Journal of Experimental Child Psychology,* 1973, *15,* 22–29.

Scammon, R., & Armstrong, E. On the growth of the human eyeball and optic nerve. *Journal of Comparative Neurology,* 1925, *38,* 165–219.

Scammon, R., & Hesdorffer, M. Growth in mass and volume of the human lens in postnatal life. *Archives of Ophthalmology*, 1937, *17*, 104–112.

Scheibel, M., & Scheibel, A. Selected structural-functional correlations in postnatal brain. In M. Sterman, D. McGinty, & A. Adinolfi (Eds.), *Brain development and behavior*. New York: Academic Press, 1971. Pp. 1–21.

Scheie, H., & Albert, D. *Adler's textbook of ophthalmology*. Philadelphia: Saunders, 1969.

Schneider, G. Two visual systems. *Science*, 1969, *163*, 895–902.

Schulman, C. Eye movements in infants using dc recording. *Neuropädiatrie*, 1973, *4*, 76–87.

Shackel, B. Review of the past and present in oculography. Medical electronics. *Proceedings of the Second International Conference on Medical Electronics (Paris, June 1959)*. London: Ilifte, 1960. Pp. 57–62.

Shackel, B. Electro-oculography: The electrical recording of eye position. *Proceedings of the Third International Conference on Medical Electronics*. London: International Federation for Medical Electronics, 1961.

Shipley, T., & Anton, M. The human electroretinogram in the first day of life. *Journal of Pediatrics*, 1964, *65*, 733–739.

Slater, A. Causes of the disparity of the pupil centre from the target position. Unpublished manuscript, 1973.

Slater, A., & Findlay, J. The measurement of fixation position in the newborn baby. *Journal of Experimental Child Psychology*, 1972, *14*, 349–364. (a)

Slater, A., & Findlay, J. The corneal-reflection technique: a reply to Salapatek, Haith, Maurer, and Kessen. *Journal of Experimental Child Psychology*, 1972, *14*, 497–499. (b)

Smith, J. L. *Optokinetic nystagmus*. Springfield, Illinois: Thomas, 1963.

Smith, J. M. The relative brightness value of three hues for newborn infants. *University of Iowa Studies in Child Welfare*, 1936, *12*, 91–140.

Sorsby, A., & Sheridan, M. The eye at birth: Measurement of the principal diameters in forty-eight cadavers. *Journal of Anatomy*, 1960, *94*, 192–197.

Sorsby, A., & Sheridan, M. Refraction and its components during the growth of the eye. *Special Report Series Medical Research Council*, 1961, No. 301.

Spector, M. Horizontal nystagmus in routine subjects on electronystagmography. *Journal of Laryngology and Otology*, 1971, *85*, 1039–1045.

Spehlmann, R. The averaged electrical responses to diffused and to patterned light in the human. *Electroencephalography and Clinical Neurophysiology*, 1965, *19*, 560–569.

Stark, L. The control system for versional eye movements. In P. Bach-y-rita, and C. Collins (Eds.), *The control of eye movements*. New York: Academic Press, 1971. Pp. 363–428.

Stone, E. *The newborn infant. A manual of obstretrical pediatrics*. Philadelphia: Lea and Febiger, 1938.

Tauber, E., & Koffler, S. Optomotor response in human infants to apparent motion: evidence of innateness. *Science*, 1966, *152*, 382–383.

Todd, T., Beecher, H., Williams, G., & Todd, A. The weight and growth of the human eyeball. *Human Biology*, 1940, *12*, 1–20.

Trevarthen, C. Two mechanisms of vision in primates. *Psychologische Forschung*, 1968, *31*, 299–337.

Trevarthen, C., & Tursky, B. Recording horizontal rotations of head and eyes in spontaneous shifts of gaze. *Behavior Research Methods and Instrumentation,* 1969, *1,* 291–293.

Trincker, D., & Trincker, I. Development of brightness vision in infants. In Y. Brackbill, & G. Thompson (Eds.), *Behavior in infancy and early childhood.* New York: Free Press, 1967. Pp. 179–188.

Tronick, E., & Clanton, C. Infant looking patterns. *Vision Research,* 1971, *11,* 1479–1486.

Umezaki, H., & Morrell, F. Developmental study of photic evoked responses in premature infants. *Electroencephalography and Clinical Neurophysiology,* 1970, *28,* 55–63.

Vanzulli, A., Bogacz, J., Handler, P., & García-Ausst, E. Evoked responses in man. I. Photic responses. *Acta Neurologica Latinoamericana,* 1960, *6,* 219–231.

Vanzulli, A., Wilson, E., & García-Ausst, E. Visual evoked responses in the newborn infant. *Acta Neurologica Latinoamericana,* 1964, *10,* 129–136.

Vitova, Z., & Hrbek, A. Cerebral responses to repetitive photic stimulation during waking and sleep in children. *Activitas Nervosa Superior,* 1970, *12,* 295–303. (a)

Vitova, Z., & Hrbek, A. Ontogeny of cerebral responses to flickering light in human infants during wakefulness and sleep. *Electroencephalography and Clinical Neurophysiology,* 1970, *28,* 391–398. (b)

Vitova, Z., & Hrbek, A. Developmental study on the responsiveness of the human brain to flicker stimulation. *Developmental Medicine and Child Neurology,* 1972, *14,* 476–486.

Walls, G. *The vertebrate eye.* Bloomfield Hills, Michigan: The Cranbrook Press, 1942.

Walsh, F., & Hoyt, W. *Clinical neuro-ophthalmology.* Vol. 1. (3rd ed.) Baltimore: Williams and Wilkins, 1969.

Walton, D. The visual system. In U. Stave (Ed.), *Physiology of the perinatal period.* Vol. 2. New York: Appleton, 1970. Pp. 875–888.

Watanabe, K., Iwase, K., & Hara, K. Maturation of visual evoked responses in low-birthweight infants. *Developmental Medicine and Child Neurology,* 1972, *14,* 425–435.

Watanabe, K., Iwase, K., & Hara, K. Visual evoked responses during sleep and wakefulness in pre-term infants. *Electroencephalography and Clinical Neurophysiology,* 1973, *34,* 571–577.

Westheimer, G. The eye. In V. Mountcastle (Ed.), *Medical physiology.* Vol. 2. St. Louis: C. V. Mosby, 1968. Pp. 1532–1553.

Wickelgren, L. Convergence in the human newborn. *Journal of Experimental Child Psychology,* 1967, *5,* 74–85.

Wickelgren, L. The ocular response of human newborns to intermittent visual movements. *Journal of Experimental Child Psychology,* 1969, *8,* 469–482.

Wilmer, H., & Scammon, R. Growth of the components of the human eyeball. I. Diagrams, calculations, computation and reference tables. *Archives of Ophthalmology,* 1950, *43,* 599–619.

Winkelman, J., & Horsten, G. The ERG of premature and full-term born infants during their first days of life. *Ophthalmologica,* 1962, *143,* 92–101.

Yakovlev, P., & Lecours, A. The myelogenetic cycles of regional maturation of the brain. In A. Minkowski (Ed.), *Regional development of the brain in early life.* Oxford: Blackwell Scientific Publications, 1967. Pp. 3–70.

Yamada, E., & Ishikawa, T. Some observations on the submicroscopic morphogenesis of the human retina. In J. Rohen (Ed.), *The structure of the eye. II. Symposium.* Stuttgart: F. K. Schattauer, 1965. Pp. 5–16.

Yarbus, A. *Eye movements and vision.* New York: Plenum Press, 1967.

Young, L. Measuring eye movements. *American Journal of Medical Electronics,* 1963, *2,* 300–307.

Young, L. Pursuit eye tracking movements. In P. Bach-y-rita, & C. Collins (Eds.), *The control of eye movements.* New York: Academic Press, 1971. Pp. 429–443.

Zetterstrom, B. The clinical electroretinogram. IV. The electroretinogram in children during the first year of life. *Acta Ophthalmologica,* 1951, *29,* 295–304.

Zetterstrom, B. The electroretinogram in prematurely children. *Acta Ophthalmologica,* 1952, *30,* 405–408.

Zetterstrom, B. Flicker electroretinography in newborn infants. *Acta Ophthalmologica,* 1955, *33,* 157–166.

Zetterstrom, B. *Studies on the postnatal development of the electroretinogram in newborn infants.* Stockholm: Tryckeri AB Thule, 1956.

Zimmerman, A., Armstrong, E., & Scammon, R. The change in position of the eyeballs during fetal life. *Anatomical Record,* 1934, *59,* 109–134.

chapter 2: A Neuronal Activity Model for Infant Visual Attention[1]

BERNARD Z. KARMEL
The University of Connecticut, Storrs

EILEEN B. MAISEL
The University of Connecticut, Storrs

The nervous system has phylogenetically developed structural and functional organizations that predetermine stimulus saliency. Such organization is evidenced at birth or shortly thereafter by selective attention and orienting reactions. This chapter will examine the question of how the infant's developing nervous system differentially processes stimuli by concentrating on one aspect of the attention process, visual fixation to patterns. An attempt will be made to show what stimulus properties control visual reactions to patterns, what systematic changes in these reactions occur over development, and finally, what relationships exist between visual attention and the developing nervous system.

[1] This research was supported by grants from the University of Connecticut Research Foundation and by a research grant, #HD-05282, to the first author, from the National Institute of Child Health and Human Development.

I. BEHAVIORAL PREFERENCES

A. Properties of Patterned Stimuli Important for Orienting or Attention

Fantz (1958) and Berlyne (1958) established significant avenues of investigation into early visual attention when they found that infants fixated longer (i.e., preferred) certain visual stimuli over others. The major feature of preferred stimuli was that they were patterned. Response measures such as greater total looking on a fixed trial (cf. Fantz, Ordy, & Udelf, 1962; Karmel, 1969a,b), longer length of first look on a trial (cf. Berlyne, 1958; McCall & Kagan, 1967), and longer average duration of a look (cf. Cohen, 1969) have been used to indicate greater attention. Not only have these measures shown that patterns are preferred to nonpatterned stimuli, but they also indicate that some patterns are looked at more than others.

The mechanisms controlling selective visual attention have been the subject of much speculation and recent experimentation. Many studies have attempted to relate total looking time or duration of fixation to the "complexity" of the stimulus as defined by the number of checks or angles in patterns. However, in defining complexity, retinal angle often has been totally or partially confounded with number of checks or number of angles (cf. Brennan, Ames, & Moore, 1966; Greenberg & O'Donnell, 1972; Hershenson, 1964; Jones-Molfese, 1972; Miranda, 1970; Hershenson, Munsinger, & Kessen, 1965).

Generally, preferences are found to increase as size of check elements decreases down to some specific element size (cf. Brennan *et al.*, 1966). Additional decreases in element size result in decreased preference (Brennan *et al.*, 1966; Greenberg & O'Donnell, 1972; Fantz *et al.*, 1962; Karmel, 1969a,b). If the area of a pattern is held constant, preference for particular element sizes can also be interpreted as related to the number of elements in the array rather than element size. When the total area of stimulation is manipulated, element size and element number may be independently varied. However, a problem arises when a choice must be made between equating for size of element or equating for total stimulus area. The total amount of light impinging on the retina will vary. Consequently, pattern preferences can be interpreted to relate to luminance differences, a nonpattern aspect of the stimulus field, rather than "complexity."

An alternative explanation for preferences is that contour is the major factor in pattern sensitivity in the first half year of life (cf. Bond, 1972). McCall, Kagan, and Melson (McCall, 1971; McCall & Kagan, 1967; McCall & Melson, 1970) have suggested that preferences vary not on the basis of stimulus "complexity" but as a function of the number of contrast borders. While studies by Karmel, Maisel, and McCarvill (Karmel, 1969a,b; Maisel & Karmel, 1973; and McCarvill, 1973) have suggested that when patterns are equated for area, the "amount of contour" (the sum of the lengths of all black–white transitions contained in a pattern) controls looking preferences. The importance of contour in determining visual reactions is also suggested by the work of Salapatek, Haith, and Kessen (Salapatek & Kessen, 1966; Kessen, Salapatek, & Haith, 1972; and Salapatek, Chapter 3, in this volume) who have indicated that saccadic eye movements are primarily directed onto a contrast border (i.e., a contour) in the stimulus field.

B. The Case for Contour Density

In order to contrast infants' relative preferences for patterned stimulus fields, we have generated a set of stimuli (Figure 2.1) by manipulating pattern features involving element orderliness and element size (Karmel, 1969a,b). Manipulation of patterns along these two stimulus attributes produces a range of patterned surfaces of equal luminance that can be scaled along two independent dimensions, "complexity" and "amount of contour." Using stimuli taken from the basic set shown in Figure 2.1, contrasts of looking preferences between these stimulus dimensions were assessed.

For the first dimension, the "complexity" of stimuli was determined by a paired comparison technique where adult judges were presented all possible pairs of stimuli and were asked to choose which stimulus was "more complex" (Karmel, 1969a). "Complexity" ratings were generally found to be based on a two-rule system: (1) Random check patterns are judged more "complex" than redundant checkerboards, regardless of check size. (2) Within configuration type, patterns with smaller checks are judged more "complex."

The second independently scaled dimension, "amount of contour"

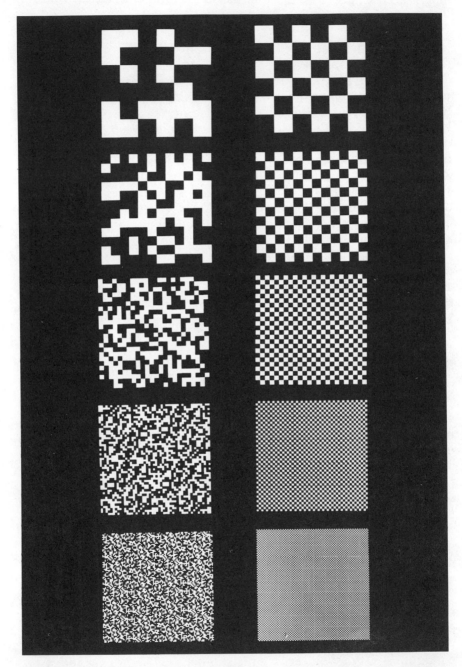

Figure 2.1 General set of checkerboard (Column 1) and random check patterns (Column 2) used in various studies. The eight stimuli used in Karmel (1969a) were a subset of these stimuli which excluded Row 2 patterns.

is obtained without subjective judgments by measuring the length of black–white transitions contained in projected patterns.[2] "Amount of contour" differs from "complexity" in that "amount of contour" is a true equal interval scale with a real zero value. Further, the two dimensions produce two rankings of patterns that appear to be orthogonal to one another.

In order to assess the relative effectiveness of "complexity" as opposed to "amount of contour" on infant visual attention, Karmel (1969a) measured the total looking time of 13- and 20-week-old subjects for all possible pairs of the eight stimuli listed in Table 2.1. Patterns subtended 27° of retinal arc at the 20-inch viewing distance. Stimulus "complexity" based on adult "complexity" ratings did not predict infant visual looking preferences nearly as well as "amount of contour." Specifically, it was found that: (1) Infant preference responses constitute an inverted U-shaped quadratic function of the "amount of contour" in the stimulus; (2) predictions of infant preferences based on adult judgments of "complexity" require a less parsimonious polynomial expression of the fourth order (quartic equation) to account for any significant variance; (3) older subjects prefer patterns having greater "amount of contour" (*not* greater "complexity") than younger subjects; and (4) element arrangement has no differential effect on attention independent of the "amount of contour" at either age.

In order to find the highest correlation between measures of contour contained in the stimulus and looking responses, various transformations on the "amount of contour" dimension were performed and the lowest order polynomial expression accounting for the highest significant proportion of variation in looking was determined. A square root transformation on the total amount of contour in a pattern was found to describe best the stimulus dimension with respect to total looking time. Since the amount of contour increases exponentially as the retinal angle of elements in the stimulus decreases linearly, a square root transformation on the amount of contour reduces intervals in the stimulus dimension to linearly varying estimates of the retinal angles subtended by the elements of the pattern. Thus, preferences are best described as

---

[2] A 12 × 12 checkerboard matrix containing 1-inch black and white squares on a black background contains 288 inches of black–white transition (see Karmel, 1974, for a further discussion of this measure as standardized for retinal angles and subject–stimulus distances).

TABLE 2.1 "COMPLEXITY" AND "AMOUNT OF CONTOUR" ORDERINGS[a]

| | Complexity: Randomness Supersedes size of element | | | Amount of contour | | | |
	Check size	Order	"Complexity" rankings by adults[b]	Check size	Order	Inches of contour in pattern	Square root contour (in CDUs)[c]
least	1. 2 inch	redundant	1.38	1. 2 inch	random	100	10.0
	2. 1 inch	redundant	2.14	2. 2 inch	redundant	144	12.0
	3. $\frac{1}{2}$ inch	redundant	3.38	3. 1 inch	random	166	12.9
	4. $\frac{1}{8}$ inch	redundant	4.82	4. 1 inch	redundant	288	17.0
	5. 2 inch	random	3.96	5. $\frac{1}{2}$ inch	random	299	17.3
	6. 1 inch	random	5.68	6. $\frac{1}{2}$ inch	redundant	576	24.0
	7. $\frac{1}{2}$ inch	random	6.80	7. $\frac{1}{8}$ inch	random	1163	34.1
most	8. $\frac{1}{8}$ inch	random	7.84	8. $\frac{1}{8}$ inch	redundant	2304	48.0

[a] Adapted from Karmel, 1969a.

[b] Rank of 8 represented highest possible "complexity."

[c] Contour density units (CDUs) equal the square root of the amount of contour: (1 where the amount of contour is expressed in terms of the total inches of black–white transition contained in the pattern; (2) where internal elements are equated for retinal angle of the viewed pattern; (3) where the viewed pattern is assumed to fill a 1-foot square area at a 20-inch distance from the subject.

varying curvilinearly along an interval scale reflecting subtended retinal angles of elements.

Theoretical inverted U-shaped curvilinear functions were then generated for different age groups by taking ordinal relationships of checkerboard preferences reported by Brennan *et al.* (1966) and Hershenson (1964) in which the retinal angle of check elements varies. The curves derived from this study served as a basis against which empirically derived preference functions could be contrasted either in predicting future data or in generating the most preferred contour density level at a given age. The solid lines of Figure 2.2 show these curves (from Karmel, 1969a) while the dotted lines reflect curves subsequently generated (Karmel, 1974) for stimuli used by Greenberg and O'Donnell (1972). These hypothetical curves represent preferences for the square root of the total amount of

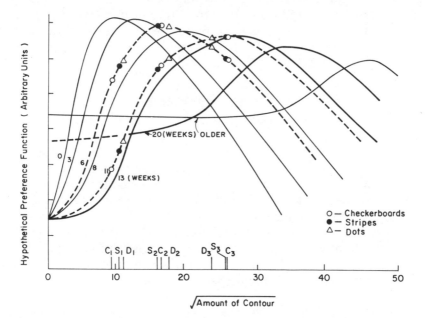

Figure 2.2 Hypothetical preference functions over development as a function of contour density expressed as the square root of contour standardized for visual angle and area of stimulus (CDUs). Solid curves are reproduced from Karmel (1969a) and were extrapolated from data reported by Brennan *et al.* (1966), Hershenson (1964), and Karmel (1969a). The dashed-line curves are hypothetical curves assumed to depict 6- and 11-week-old subjects' functions. Points along these curves for checkerboards, stripes, and dots were plotted to demonstrate how theoretical predictions for Greenberg and O'Donnell's (1972) stimuli might be obtained. [From Karmel, 1974.]

contour when contour lengths are standardized for retinal angle of elements contained in a 1-square-foot area viewed from a standard 20-inch distance (cf., the square root of contour values in terms of contour density units [CDUs] listed in the last column of Table 2.1). Preferences are inverted curvilinear functions of the square root of contour. The maxima of these functions shift toward greater contour density values with development. In general, for a given age, ordinal relationships of responses to individual stimulus patterns reported in Brennan *et al.* (1966), Hershenson (1964), and Karmel (1969a) can be accounted for by the hypothetical curves. Two ends of a contour continuum hold for each age, the ends being a Ganzfeld on one hand and a pattern exceeding acuity threshold on the other—both effectively patternless stimulus fields.

Since the hypothetical curves fit the data only if we assume that stimuli contain the same retinal angle of elements across studies and since the square root of contour as opposed to the total amount of contour best reflects looking behavior, it was concluded that contour density at the retina is a major determinant of infant preferences over development (Karmel, 1969a).[3]

C. Mathematical Functions Relating Contour Density to Looking Behavior

The usefulness of contour density in describing looking behavior can be tested by applying theoretical predictions from the hypothetical contour density response curves to data collected from other infant preference studies. Many infant preference studies do not contain a sufficient number of points along the stimulus dimension or report too few parametric dependent scores along the response dimension to analyze for true interval response differences between stimulus values. This design problem has been noted earlier (Bond, 1972; Greenberg & O'Donnell, 1972; Hershenson, 1967). However,

---

[3] Although spatial frequency, the number of cycles per degree of area measured at the retinal surface of a projected spatial grating, has been used to describe such a stimulus dimension (Blakemore, Garner, & Sweet, 1972; Campbell & Robson, 1968), we prefer to utilize Gibson's (1966) idea of contour (texture) density since accurate physical operations describing spatial frequency for patterns with mixed retinal angle elements have not been performed upon stimuli used in preference studies. The use of Fourier spectral density analysis may prove useful in this regard, but it remains to be demonstrated whether such a Fourier spectral density analysis can predict preference behavior more accurately than contour density, as described here.

polynomial regression analyses[4] could be performed on the data from the following studies: Greenberg and O'Donnell (1972) for total time spent looking at stimuli by 6- and 11-week-old subjects; Cohen (1972) for duration of unrestricted looking in 18-week-old subjects (but only for stimuli 10° or greater in total size); Karmel (1969a) for average total looking time shown by 13- and 20-week-old subjects; and McCarvill (1973) for average total looking time of 9- and 13-week-old subjects. A polynomial regression analysis for parametric studies describes the best fitting equation for the relationship between stimuli and responses for a given subject group. The most preferred value for the square root of contour is obtained by differentiating each regression equation for the curve maximum. Table 2.2 summarizes these parametric analyses describing preference functions in terms of contour density.

In studies where four or fewer stimuli are used, only monotonic or bitonic nonparametric trends could be estimated (Gaito, 1965). The curve maximum is obtained by visual inspection. The following data were viewed using nonparametric, ordinal preference relationships: Brennan *et al.* (1966) for 3-, 8-, and 14-week-old subjects; Hershenson (1964), Jones-Molfese (1972), and Miranda (1970) for premature and newborn subjects; and Maisel and Karmel (1973) for 6- and 10-week-old subjects. Obviously, this selection of studies is not exhaustive; however, it represents a collection of comparable reports using two-dimensional patterned stimuli in which contour density is somewhat systematically varied. Table 2.3 summarizes these nonparametric analyses.

1. Results of Polynomial Regression Analyses

The polynomial equation describing total looking time as a function of checkerboard and random check patterns taken from Karmel (1969a) can account for 90% of the variance in looking in 13-week-old subjects and 79% of the variance in 20-week-old subjects. Table 2.2 contains the appropriate equations. Differentiation of these equations predicts the preferred contour density level in these two age groups (see Table 2.2, last column).

---

[4] This regression analysis can be obtained as part of the Biomedical Statistical Programs (BMD-05R) supplied by the UCLA computer facility (Dixon, 1971). A more detailed description of the use of this analysis in preference studies can be found in Karmel (1974) and McCarvill (1973).

TABLE 2.2   CONTOUR DENSITY PREFERENCES EXTRAPOLATED FROM POLYNOMIAL REGRESSION ANALYSIS

Age in weeks	Study	Number of stimuli	Measure	Stimulus range in contour density units (CDUs)
6	Greenberg & O'Donnell, 1972	9	TL[b]	9.4 to 26.6
9	McCarvill, 1973	8	ATL[c]	10.0 to 48.0
11	Greenberg & O'Donnell, 1972	9	TL	9.4 to 26.6
13	Karmel, 1969a	8	ATL	10.0 to 48.0
13	McCarvill, 1973	8	ATL	10.0 to 48.0
18	Cohen, 1972	6	DL[d]	8.0 to 39.2
20	Karmel, 1969a	8	ATL	10.0 to 48.0

[a] Percentage of the variation accounted for by the polynomial expression.
[b] TL   = Total looking across trials.
[c] ATL = Average total looking time per trial.
[d] DL   = Duration of a look (unlimited time)

Using stimuli similar to those used by Karmel (1969a), McCarvill (1973) found that a cubic polynomial expression best describes average total looking (ATL) for 9-week-olds. The cubic polynomial equation indicates a preference maximum (20.0 CDUs) close to the predicted CDU value for 9-week-olds inferred from the set of hypothetical functions shown in Figure 2.2. Similarly, a quadratic equation with a maximum at 29.9 CDUs replicates the effect and maximum (30.0 CDUs) previously reported by Karmel (1969a) for 13-week-olds.

Greenberg and O'Donnell (1972) showed 6- and 11-week-old subjects three different configurations of patterns: checkerboards, dots, or stripes. Each configuration type was shown at three roughly equivalent levels of contour density. A re-analysis of these data in terms of contour density yields an inverted U-shaped quadratic equation predicting the obtained looking behavior in both age groups (Karmel, 1974). The proportion of variation, the regression expression, and the predicted value for the most preferred contour density level are listed in Table 2.2.

Cohen (1972) presented nine stimuli varying in a 3 × 3 design to 18-week-old subjects. Stimuli consisted of three checkerboard patterns comprised of matrices of 2 × 2, 12 × 12, or 24 × 24 checks. Three sizes of patterns subtending 5°, 10°, and 20° of retinal angle were used. Thus, the number of checks varied at each level of

TABLE 2.2 (continued)

Best fitting polynomial expression	Correlation coefficient (r) for polynomial expression	Percent variation[a]	Maximum predicted (Y) value for square root contour value (X) in CDUs
$Y = -.032X^2 + 1.07X - 3.21$	+.69	(48%)	17.1
$Y = .0008X^3 - .0834X^2 + 2.38X - 11.40$	+.97	(94%)	20.0
$Y = -.04^2 + 1.71X - 11.41$	+.90	(82%)	21.4
$Y = -.009X^2 + .54X - 1.16$	+.95	(90%)	30.0
$Y = .012X^2 + .73X - 1.94$	+.81	(65%)	29.9
$Y = .066X + 2.89$	+.95	(90%)	39.2
$Y = .003X^3 + .02X^2 - .37X + 5.72$	+.89	(79%)	37.0

TABLE 2.3　CONTOUR DENSITY PREFERENCES EXTRAPOLATED FROM NONPARAMETRIC TRENDS FOR INFANTS OVER SIX WEEKS CA

Age in weeks	Study	Number of stimuli	Measure	Nonparametric trend function	Stimulus range in terms of contour density units (CDUs)	Most preferred CDU level
8	Brennan et al., 1966	3	ATL[a]	bitonic (inverted curvilinear)	10.0 to 32.0	20.0
10	Maisel & Karmel, 1973	3	DL[b]	monotonic (increasing as amount of contour increases)	10.2 to 25.3	25.3
14	Brennan et al., 1966	3	ATL	monotonic (increasing as amount of contour increases)	10.0 to 32.0	32.0

[a] ATL = Average total looking time per trial.
[b] DL　= Duration of a look (unlimited time).

pattern size. He found that the total amount of contour independent of area could not be used to predict duration of an unrestricted look (DL) since patterns with equal total contour but differing sizes of checks resulted in significantly different durations of fixation. However, total stimulus area interacts with check size and contour density in Cohen's study. If the means for "medium"- and "large"-sized stimuli having 10° and 20° total retinal angles are plotted in terms of the square root of contour standardized in CDUs, a highly significant linear relationship can be shown to exist between DL and the square root of contour ($r = +.95$). The proportion of variation, polynomial expression, and most preferred stimulus reported by Cohen are also listed in Table 2.2.

Although contour density within a pattern can be shown to have systematic relationships to looking in the above studies, these relationships may not hold if the area of stimulation (total pattern size) varies within a study. Cohen (1972) reported lower average DL in 18-week-old subjects to stimuli whose total retinal size subtended 5° of arc. Incorporation of 5° stimuli into the regression analysis eliminates any consistent relationship between DL and contour density. Further, the latency of looking (LL) depends on stimulus area. The effect of area on LL was replicated by Maisel and Karmel (1973) for 5-week-old subjects, using 37° and 18° stimuli, but not for 10-week-old subjects whose LL scores did not significantly differ for 18° versus 37° stimuli. Thus, LL is apparently sensitive to the retinal angle of the entire stimulus as well as to age but not necessarily to contour density within a pattern.

The relationship between total stimulus size and age requires further study. Although the data are not extensive, overall area of stimulation appears to affect the latency of a look such that a larger stimulus is looked at more quickly than a smaller one. This may contribute to average total looking time since, in a fixed trial interval, a longer latency of look reduces the total possible looking time whereas a shorter latency of look would tend to increase the total looking time. Nonetheless, contour density predicts Cohen's DL data as well as total looking time measures for subjects 5 weeks and older when total stimulus area is 10° or larger.

2. RESULTS OF NONPARAMETRIC TREND ANALYSES

Although nonparametric trend analysis is statistically less powerful than polynomial regression analysis, nonparametric trends may also indicate response functions when few stimulus points exist.

Estimates of curve maxima can be obtained from studies utilizing few stimulus points by noting the type of nonparametric trend and contour preference maxima present. This was done for 8-week-old subjects (20.0 CDUs) and 14-week-old subjects (32.0 CDUs) reported by Brennan *et al.* (1966) and for checkerboard stimuli used by Maisel and Karmel (1973) for 10-week-old subjects (25.3 CDUs). Nonparametric trends and preference maxima are reported in Table 2.3. As with parametric analyses the most preferred stimulus appears to shift toward greater contour density levels with age.

Response functions reported for subjects below 6 weeks of age are not as clearly defined with respect to contour density as functions for older subjects. Hershenson's (1964) data for newborns, the data of Brennan *et al.* (1966) for 3-week-old subjects, and Maisel and Karmel's (1973) data for 5-week-old subjects all indicate that preferences are greater as the size of elements in pattern stimuli increases up to a point where stimuli contain checks subtending 7° or more of retinal arc (see Table 2.4). There is some evidence which suggests that preference maxima may not be linearly related to contour density in very young subjects. Miranda (1970), for example, has reported that both newborn and premature subjects prefer a stimulus containing element sizes between 5° and 10° as opposed to a homogeneous gray square stimulus subtending approximately 25° of retinal arc. Similarly, Jones-Molfese (1972) reports no differences between premature subjects and full-term subjects in the stimulus most preferred. Since large retinal areas are involved in the size of any one check element in these studies, pattern preferences may reflect a response based primarily upon brightness or intensity rather than contour density in infants less than 6 weeks old. This possibility is reinforced by Hershenson's (1964) report of an inverted curvilinear effect of intensity on total looking in neonates. Thus light intensity may play some role in pattern preferences when there are large element sizes. However, no parametric study has been reported that examines the interaction of intensity, area, and contour density.

In summary, below 6 weeks, preferences appear to decrease as contour density increases, but this effect may reflect a response to the brightness of large check elements and requires further study for verification. Preference functions for subjects 6 weeks and older for patterns subtending 10° or more of visual arc appear to be curvilinearly related to contour density represented by the square root of contour. The maximum of the preference function for a

TABLE 2.4   CONTOUR DENSITY PREFERENCES EXTRAPOLATED FROM NONPARAMETRIC TRENDS FOR INFANTS UNDER SIX WEEKS CA

Age in weeks	Study	Number of stimuli	Measure	Nonparametric trend function	Stimulus range in terms of contour density units (CDUs)	Most preferred CDU level
.5 (Newborns)	Miranda, 1970	4	TL[a]	bitonic (inverted curvilinear)	8.1 to 11.2	9.5
−4.0 (Prematures)[b]	Miranda, 1970	4	TL	bitonic (inverted curvilinear)	8.1 to 11.2	8.6[c]
Newborns (.5) and prematures	Jones-Molfese, 1972	4	TL	"related to the amount of contour"	6.8 to 11.0	9.1 or less
Newborn (.5)	Hershenson, 1964	3	ATL[d]	monotonic (decreasing as amount of contour increases)	10.0 to 24.0	10.0
3	Brennan et al., 1966	3	ATL	monotonic (decreasing as amount of contour increases)	10.0 to 32.0	10.0
5.5	Maisel & Karmel, 1973	3	DL[e]	monotonic (decreasing as amount of contour increases)	10.2 to 25.3	10.2

[a] TL = Total looking across trials.
[b] Four weeks prior to full-term birth.
[c] No significant differences were reported between premature and full-term infants by Miranda (1970). However, inspection of the means for total looking at each stimulus tentatively suggests this value for premature infants.
[d] ATL = Average total looking time per trial.
[e] DL = Duration of a look (unlimited time).

given age shifts to patterns with increasing contour density values as a function of age, especially after 6 weeks.

D. Equation Relating Maximally Preferred Contour Density Level to Age

The mathematical function relating shifts in contour preference maxima to development can be obtained by using a scatter plot of the preference maximum at a given chronological age (CA) for the set of studies summarized in Section I-C. Figure 2.3 plots this relationship for all age samples listed in Tables 2.2, 2.3, and 2.4. A strong linear relationship ($r = +.97$) exists between the predicted preference maximum value for contour density and CA. The linear expression reflecting the relationship between CA and the contour density level most preferred after 6 weeks is (as computed by regressing the first column onto the last column of both Tables 2.2 and 2.3 taken together): $Y = .6X - 4.0$, where $Y = $ CA in weeks and $X = $ square root of contour in CDUs. The regression equation for the most preferred stimulus for subjects less than 6 weeks CA as abstracted from Table 2.4 is: $Y = 4.4X - 42.0$. The apparent difference in slope of the regression lines for young and old subjects evidences a sharp break occurring after 5 weeks. This strongly suggests two distinct processes or mechanisms controlling looking

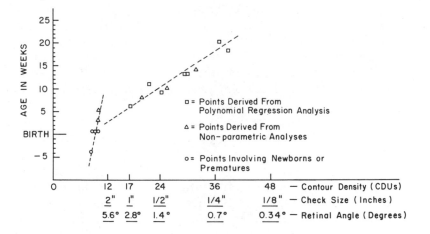

Figure 2.3   Regression functions indicating the relationship of the maximally preferred level of contour density (expressed in CDUs) to chronological age (CA). The check size and retinal angle of a check element within redundant checkerboard stimuli at a 20-inch distance are also given to facilitate contrasts among studies.

preference functions in infants; one operating up until 5–6 weeks, the other taking over after this point in development. However, application of the function below 6 weeks to newborn and premature subjects may require the use of stimuli containing element sizes whose retinal angles vary extensively between 5° and 15°. Other evidence suggests that a significant developmental discontinuity occurs at about 2 months. For instance, bull's-eye preferences emerge (Fantz, 1967), changes in the ability to habituate to visual stimuli occur (Cohen & Gelber, Chapter 5 in this volume), and saccadic eye movements appear to differ from those found in younger infants (Salapatek, Chapter 3 in this volume).

It should be pointed out that contour density is not the sole determinant of preferences but rather a major source of stimulation around which various looking responses are clearly ordered. Other stimulus variables such as light intensity, motion, three-dimensionality, total stimulus size, and stimulus depth may all affect looking behavior. However, responsiveness to these factors is assumed to intereact predictably with contour density preferences.

E.   Contour Density Effects on Visually Dependent Choices in Developing Animals

There are common developing mechanisms among diverse species that may well be involved in determining early visual attention and suggest a strong genetic component underlying preference responses. Animal preference functions obtained from subjects having little experience with patterned surfaces are similar to contour density preference functions reported for human infants. Rats and chicks, given a choice to descend to either of two equally shallow patterns on a visual cliff, will choose a pattern containing an intermediate amount of contour independent of element orderliness. However, the most preferred level of contour density appears to be species-specific (Karmel, 1966, 1969b). Preference shifts also have been reported in various species. Simner (1967), using checkerboard stimuli, demonstrated that chicks' visual preference functions shift toward patterns containing smaller checks during the first few days of life when, as Simner indicates, the rate of neural maturation in the visual system is the greatest.

Contour density appears to be basic to depth avoidance in that the ability to detect contour must exist so that motion parallax can be utilized to indicate a depth (Walk, 1965; Walk & Gibson, 1961). In this regard, Karmel, Miller, Dettweiler, and Anderson (1970) have shown that the density of elements of textured surfaces on the visual cliff interacts with development of shallow choice preferences. In cats and two species of rabbits, deep surfaces with greater texture density (smaller retinal angles) are avoided later in development than deep surfaces containing coarser texture density. Also, Walk and Walters (1971), using chicks, and DeHardt (1969), using rats, have shown that contour density preferences interact with depth avoidance such that the contour density level most preferred is chosen over a less preferred, but closer surface.

Finally, a genetically dependent characteristic of preferences has been indicated by both Fantz, Fagan, and Miranda (see Chapter 4 in this volume) and Sigman and Parmelee (1974) who have shown that preferences for contour density are the same for a given developmental group when conceptional age (age based on mother's report of last menstruation) rather than CA is used to group a sample of full-term and premature subjects.

Thus the conclusion that contour density as a major stimulus feature generally affecting spontaneous orienting to visual stimuli is reinforced by animal preference or choice response functions. Further, shifts of preferences over development as a function of contour density are generally suggested by the similarity in response functions in animal and infant data. However, the exact time and manner in which these developmental shifts occur and the contour density level preferred at a given age appear to be species-specific.

II. VISUAL SYSTEM MATURATION RELATED TO PATTERN PROCESSING AT THE NEUROLOGICAL LEVEL

There are several factors other than systematic developmental transitions in preference responses which suggest that orienting reactions are related to neurological maturation within the visual system. These factors include myelination, development of dendritic branching in various levels of the visual system, as well as increased maturation of receptors in the macular region of the eye.

Visual behaviors in diverse species have been shown to relate to maturation of regions of the visual system. For instance, the most rapid changes in chicks' visual preference during the first 3 days of life coincide with major tectum development (Simner, 1967). Sacket (1963) has hypothesized that tectum development also is correlated with imprinting to visual stimuli. Similarly, development of electro-physiological response to visual stimulation in cats (Rose & Lindsley, 1968; Rose, 1971) corresponds to development of depth avoidance in cats (Karmel, Miller *et al.*, 1970; Karmel & Walk, 1965) as well as visual acuity development (Warkentin, 1937). Finally, correlations among developing behavioral, neurological, and brain electrical responses have been shown to exist in dogs (Fox, 1971), rats (Schapiro, 1969), and rabbits (Stewart & Riesen, 1972).

In humans, there is evidence for myelination of the primary visual system during the first 6 months of life (Conel, 1939, 1941, 1947). In addition, foveal receptors undergo rapid development between 1 and 2 months (Mann, 1964). Ellingson (1967) has suggested that maturation of scotopic and photopic vision is strongly correlated with the development of the electrophysiological response to light. McGraw (1945) and Bronson (1965) have suggested that much of early infant behavior can be accounted for by the differential development of cortical as opposed to subcortical systems. However, little is known of the maturation of subcortical and cortical structures as they relate to behavior in humans.

Neurological maturation is likely to place specific constraints on developing visual and visual-motor behaviors. Consequently, contour processing capacity is expected to be bounded by neurological development within the visual system, regardless of which specific neuroanatomical or neurophysiological effects are used to measure this capacity. We have assumed this to be the case (Karmel, 1969b,c) and have argued that developing properties of the neurological substrate as related to contour processing abilities determine behavioral attention.

A. Single Neuron Response to Contour in Mature Visual Systems

In order to determine how contour stimulation can result in differential visual orienting responses over development, an analysis of the manner in which contour stimulation affects certain neurophysiological reactions is necessary. Response to contours at the single neuron level has been extensively documented by Hubel and Wiesel (1962, 1965a) following the work of Kuffler (1953). Inhibitory and facilitory effects of a spot of light projected onto a circumscribed retinal region, called a receptive field, converge onto a single neuron beyond the receptor level. These effects alter the spontaneous spiking activity recorded at the higher level neuron when retinal stimulation is present (Kuffler, 1953). Hubel and Wiesel (1962, 1965a) have mapped retinal receptive fields which, when stimulated, produce spiking rate activity changes in neurons in progressively ascending loci of the visual system from the ganglion layers through the lateral geniculate nucleus (LGN) and then into striate cortex. More recently stimulus contour effects in regions equivalent to Brodmann's areas 18 and 19 have been mapped (Hubel & Wiesel, 1965b, 1968). Investigation of properties of neurons in other regions affected by visual stimulation have been reported for inferotemporal cortex (cf. Gross, Rocha-Miranda, & Bender, 1972) and for the superior colliculus (cf. Schiller & Koerner, 1971; Sprague, 1966; McIlwain & Buser, 1968; McIlwain & Fields, 1971).

Regardless of the area involved most visual neurons possess retinal receptive field organization such that light of a specific intensity falling on one area facilitates spiking, but the same light intensity falling on another area inhibits spiking activity. If the same intensity of light falls on both areas simultaneously there would be no net spiking rate change since facilitory and inhibitory effects would summate across the total receptive field to cancel each other. Retinal receptive fields of neurons in lower visual regions such as the LGN are usually circular fields with a center functionally oppossed to the surround (Kuffler, 1953). Changes in the shapes and sizes of circular receptive fields have been shown to occur as one ascends the primary visual projection system (Hubel & Wiesel, 1962). For example, elongated receptive fields for cortical neurons have been reported. Such neurons would functionally respond to slits or edges of light projected onto the retina in a given orientation and have been termed "contour cells."

In additon to functional differences shown for receptive field organization in the various anatomical loci, receptive fields are known to undergo developmental change. For example, it has been shown that receptive fields are more diffusely organized in "young, inexperienced" cats (Hubel & Wiesel, 1963) and in subcortical as opposed to cortical structures (Hubel & Wiesel, 1962; Schiller & Koerner, 1971). In addition, receptive fields extend over smaller regions of the retina as one ascends the visual system from optic tectum and LGN to the visual cortex (Maffei & Fiorentini, 1973). Environmental events can also influence receptive field development. As is the case for immature subjects, neuron spiking is "sluggish" and hard to obtain after dark-rearing or diffuse light restricted experience (Ganz & Fitch, 1968; Wiesel & Hubel, 1965). Receptive field orientation characteristics (i.e., vertical or horizontal) can also be directly determined by exposure to vertical or horizontal lines (Blakemore & Cooper, 1970; Hirsch & Spinelli, 1970).

The development of receptors at the retinal level is also suggestive of developmental changes in receptive field organization. The macula is relatively undeveloped in the young infant (Mann, 1964). Thus, before 2 months of age vision may be dependent upon peripheral rather than foveal receptors. Indeed, in the mature visual system most of the retinal receptors are concentrated in the fovea rather than in the periphery. In further emphasis of this distinction, Hubel and Wiesel (1962) found that most cortical cells have connections to receptive fields located in the fovea. Receptive fields for cells in the superior colliculus are smaller the closer the fields are to the fovea and are organized to contain foveal representation (Schiller & Koerner, 1971).

If these data can be generalized to humans, a sluggish response to large-sized retinal stimuli may be the dominant condition in the contour neurons of visually immature subjects, while a more rapid response to smaller-sized retinal stimuli would be assumed to be the case in contour neurons of more mature subjects. Influence of subcortical cells may dominate during early life if development of subcortical regions precedes that of cortical regions (cf. Jacobson, 1970). Further, if cortical regions connected to the fovea are immature, peripheral retinal stimulation may have a greater relative influence on behavior.

B. Hypothetical Output of Size-Dependent Receptive Fields Related to Contour Density

Assuming that the receptive field of a contour neuron contains an antagonistic center-surround organization of restricted size, spiking activity in the form of changes from some spontaneous firing level would show an inverted U-shaped function if the change were plotted against a contour density stimulus dimension. The degree of spike rate change (activity) would necessarily contain at least two minima (i.e., no rate change) and at least one maximum (i.e., maximum rate change). One minimum would occur when a pattern containing very small elements is projected onto the retina. In this case small dark and light elements would project dark and light spots onto both the center and the surround simultaneously.

Summation across the inhibitory and facilitatory effects would produce little change in firing rate. A second minimum would occur when very large texture elements are present since an eye fixation would simultaneously project the same light intensity onto both the center and the surround of a receptive field. This condition would also result in a cancellation of facilitatory and inhibitory effects and, thus, no net change in the firing rate. At least one maximum activity rate change would occur somewhere between these extremes. The maximum activity would depend on anatomical locus and retinal connections of the neuron being stimulated.

Figure 2.4a depicts the proposed inverted U-shaped relationship between contour density of checkerboard stimuli and spike rate change in a single neuron where the limits of contour density range from element sizes approaching a Ganzfeld condition at one end and an acuity threshold at the other.

If contour density varies from low to high, the change in the rate

Figure 2.4 (a) Hypothetical function relating change in spiking of a single contour-dependent neuron to variations in contour density. (b) Hypothetical functions relating developmental changes in spiking of a pool of contour-dependent neurons to variations in contour density.

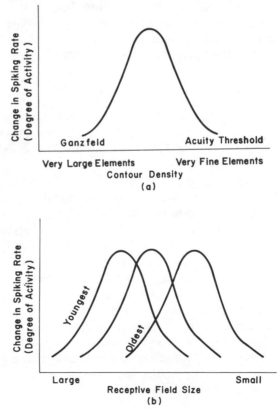

of firing of a single contour neuron would increase up to some point of contour density well above threshold and then decrease again as greater density in the stimulus approaches the subjects' ability to detect contour. For random patterned stimuli (i.e., random checkerboards) it is assumed that the visual system responds to the average contour density value by integrating contour over area. This has been demonstrated to be the case in the ommatidia system of insects (Reichardt, 1961) and in the visual system of cats (Pollen, Lee, & Taylor, 1971). The peak of the inverted U-shaped function corresponding to the maximum spike rate change for any single neuron would depend on the neuron's receptive field size. The average maximum point across many neurons would depend on how activity across receptive fields is pooled by the nervous system. A series of shifting inverted U-shaped curves (Figure 2.4b) would describe activity across neurons as CA increases if: *(1)* the average receptive field size in the system controlling behavior becomes smaller as CA increases, and *(2)* the effects of spike rate changes of individual neurons are cumulative when the whole system of neurons controlling behavior is stimulated. Such conditions would exist in any visual area where the receptive fields of neurons are restricted to specific retinal sizes.

III. MEASUREMENT OF GROSS ELECTRICAL PHENOMENA ASSUMED TO CORRELATE WITH ACTIVITY IN POOLS OF NEURONS

Our research is ultimately directed at the question of how neurological responses are transformed into attentional behaviors in developing humans. Although the importance of the neurological substrate for infant behavioral development has long been recognized by early investigators such as McGraw (1945), Conel (1939, 1941, 1947), and Peiper (1963), details of the relationship between neurological functions and complex behaviors have been demonstrated only at the level of the reflex. However, in order to demonstrate how specific neurological responses correlate with perception and attention, both *qualitative* and *quantitative* relationships to active, ongoing behaviors must be presented. Therefore, an attempt will be made to show that there are plausible and measurable correspondences between pattern stimulation and neural functioning as hypothesized in Section II. Single neuron responses cannot be recorded in infants. However, correspondence between activity at the single unit level and activity at a more gross neurophysiological level correlated with activity at the single unit level, can be inferred from slow-wave evoked potentials (John, 1967; Elul, 1968). These latter potentials are small changes in electrical potential embedded within the electroencephalogram (EEG).

The measurement of single neuron spiking recorded with micro-electrodes is typically accomplished by presenting a stimulus and noting the changes in distribution of action potentials over time after stimulus presentation. If the distribution of response is expressed in the form of the probability of a spike at a given instance after stimulation, a post-stimulus-probability-histogram (PSPH) of average probabilities of spiking response over time can be generated for that stimulus. Since neurons always have some spontaneous level of spiking, a zero probability of response would generally indicate inhibitory effects while a 1.0 probability would generally indicate that facilitatory effects were acting on the neuron at that point in time. A temporal "envelope" (Fox & O'Brien, 1965) of changing spiking probabilities can be constructed for any single neuron when a stimulus is presented. These temporal "envelopes" represent complex "waves" containing frequencies of change similar to those found in the EEG frequency domain, i.e., they are very slow. Thus, the PSPH appears to represent a summary response of the pattern of spiking in a neuron over time, given a specific stimulus.

Several investigators have indicated that slow frequency potentials recorded in regions in the vicinity from which single neuron responses are recorded show some direct correlation with the complex PSPH "envelope." Slow potentials, either spontaneous or evoked by stimulation, probably arise from some form of integration of dendritic excitatory and inhibitory postsynaptic potentials (EPSPs and IPSPs; Creutzfeldt, Watanabe, & Lux, 1966). This conclusion has been reached by a number of other investigators. Fox, O'Brien, and Norman (Fox & O'Brien, 1965; Fox & Norman, 1968) have shown that a single neuron's spiking rate can be directly predicted by observing the much slower evoked potentials recorded near the single unit from which PSPHs are generated. Verzeano, Dill, Vallecalle, Groves, and Thomas (1968), Wozniak, Ham, Vanzini, and Garcia-Austt (1970), and John (1967) have suggested that a high correlation exists between the first derivative of amplitude changes in evoked slow potentials and the changes in the "envelope" of the PSPH. Finally, Thompson (1970), recording from insect pin electrodes that measure multiple units discharging simultaneously, reported a close relationship between the probability of multi-unit discharges and slow potentials recorded from the same site. Thus, a direct relationship is assumed to exist between single neuron activity and the amplitudes of slow evoked potentials. Presumably, then, the greater the amplitude of the components of the evoked potential, the greater would be the synchronous activity of neurons reflected in that component (John, 1967).

IV. CORTICALLY EVOKED POTENTIALS

A. General Discussion

Evidence for spontaneously occurring synchronized spiking activity across neurons presumably as some form of spontaneously occurring slow potentials, can be recorded from scalps of humans as the EEG (Creutzfeldt et al., 1966; John & Thatcher, in press). Specific stimulus-related potentials are generally recorded from the scalps of humans as cortically evoked potentials (CEPs). These cortically evoked responses are defined as reliably occurring potentials found within the more variable EEG that are contingent on the occurrence of a stimulus.

If evoked potentials are strong relative to the background EEG, a single presentation of the stimulus will elicit a reliable response. If the evoked signal is weak relative to the background EEG, some form of averaging of the evoked event is necessary in order to produce a statistically stable response. Time-dependent averaging of the EEG makes possible the detection of changes in potentials which are correlated with the stimulus as opposed to those changes merely reflecting random EEG fluctuation.

Ellingson (1967) has summarized CEP measurements as they apply to infants. Other good summaries describe methods and basic findings regarding visual CEPs in adults (cf. Donchin & Lindsley, 1969; MacKay, 1970; Perry & Childers, 1969; Regan, 1972). Briefly, a CEP is established by separately averaging the momentary EEG potential every few milliseconds after each stimulus occurrence for a fixed period, usually for $\frac{1}{2}$ sec or more. Random positive and negative fluctuations in potential at each time point approach zero, while any potential that is routinely greater (or less) than zero is reflected in a positive (or negative) voltage value for that specific time point after the stimulus.

Important features of the visually evoked potential (VEP) are commonly identified as a series of oscillating positive and negative peaks (or components) varying in amplitude (in microvolts) and latency (in milliseconds) from stimulus onset. Measurement of the response to stimulus variation is reflected in differences in the dependent values for the amplitude and latency of various components (also see Maurer, Chapter 1 in this volume, for a detailed methodological summary of VEP techniques).

B. Effects of Contour Stimulation on VEPs in Human Adults

The effect of contour stimulation on VEP component amplitude and latency has been extensively reviewed by Perry and Childers (1969), MacKay (1970), and Regan (1972). The response to contour stimulation is clearly defined in an individual subject's VEP record. Clynes and Kohn (1967) and Harter and White (1968, 1970), among others, have demonstrated that changes in VEP components systematically reflect the degree to which a stimulus is focused on the retina. The size of a check within checkerboard stimuli also affects components systematically. In pattern VEP studies, a pattern is generally tachistoscopically exposed for the brief duration of a stroboscopic light flash. Other techniques such as sine-wave modulation of the exposing light can be employed and yield essentially similar results (cf. Spekreijse, 1966). In adults, when VEPs are recorded from the occipital pole, the amplitudes of a negative component at about 100 msec and a positive component between 160 and 200 msec after the onset of light vary such that sharply focused checks between 5 min and 20 min of arc result in maximization of the negative component amplitude at 100 msec and the positive component at 160–200 msec (Harter & White, 1968, 1970). Figure 2.5 shows this effect and also is a typical presentation of VEP records. The response function to stimuli varying in check size is an inverted U-shaped curve of component amplitudes having two minima: one at large check sizes and one at the acuity threshold or when patterns are blurred beyond detection (Spehlmann, 1965; Harter & White, 1968, 1970). The maximum occurs at what has been referred to as the "optimal check size" (Harter & White, 1970).

Because of the inverted U-shape of the component amplitude response function to variations in check size, both Harter and

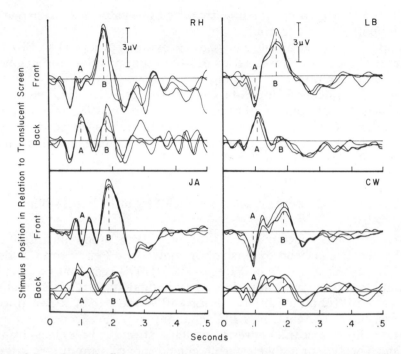

Figure 2.5   Typical effects of sharply defined contours on adult VEPs. Individual checks of the stimulus pattern subtended visual angles of about 20′; overall pattern subtended about 20° x 15°. The subjects binocularly fixated the center of a translucent screen. Flash rate was 1 per sec. VEPs were obtained by means of a single scalp electrode placed 2.5 cm above the inion and 2.5 cm to the right of midline, referenced to the right earlobe. One hundred responses were summed for each average. Contour sharpness was varied between sharp focus and degraded focus simply by placing the stimulus pattern in *front* or in *back* of a translucent screen, respectively. Points A and B indicate latency where amplitude measures (indicated by dotted lines) reflect contour in the stimulus. *Negative downward.* [Adapted with permission of Pergamon Publishing Company from M. R. Harter & C. T. White, Effects of contour sharpness and check-size on visually evoked cortical potentials. *Vision Research*, 1968, *8*, 701–711, Fig. 1.]

White (1968, 1970) and Armington, Corwin, and Marsetta (1971) have hypothesized a form of neural tuning similar to our arguments in Sections II-A and II-B such that a particular "optimal size" of checks, which corresponds to receptive field size results in the greatest amplitude of certain VEP components. Furthermore, using psychophysical procedures, Jung and Spillman (1970) have estimated that receptive field sizes in adult humans probably lie somewhere between 10 min and 20 min of visual arc at the fovea, values where maximum VEP effects have been recorded by Harter and White (1968, 1970). Thus, if arguments regarding single unit activity and evoked responses are tenable, it is not unreasonable to assume that component amplitude variation as a function of contour density correlates with underlying synchronous single unit activity in one or more brain regions in humans, at least in those units for which contour density is an important determinant of receptive field characteristics. Since VEPs contain contour-sensitive components, recording pattern-dependent components in infant VEPs can be used to determine how response at the neurophysiological level is translated into orienting behaviors.

C. Infant VEPs: Response to Unpatterned Stimuli[5]

Ellingson (1967) has provided a summary of the infant VEP literature. A major criticism of this literature is that the data are poorly anchored to specific behaviors other than state (cf. Hrbek, Hrbkova, & Lenard, 1969). In addition, interpretation of behavior based on these studies is limited since unpatterned flashes have been used as stimuli. However, although the effects of patterned stimuli may be different from those produced by an unpatterned flash of light (the typical method used to generate VEPs), it may be useful to examine VEP studies which use unpatterned flashes in order to identify important components in infant VEPs.

Ellingson (1960, 1964) first successfully recorded VEPs in infants. He defined the newborn VEP as containing a visual component identified as a positive peak at the occipital pole. The latency of this component was found to decrease rapidly with development. Fogarty and Reuben (1969) and Ferris, David, Dorsen, and Hackett (1967) have summarized this as well as other data showing major identifiable VEP component peaks over a longer period of development in infants. The positive-going peak labeled P_2 in Figure 2.6, is the only consistent wave reported at all ages and is the visual peak referred to by Ellingson (1964, 1967). Development of an earlier positive peak (P_1), in addition to two negative peaks labeled N_1 and N_2, respectively (Ellingson, 1970; Ferris *et al.*, 1967) occurs as CA increases. Other components also have been shown to develop after P_2 and N_2 but are not reported in all studies.

---

[5] The preparation of this section was aided by an unpublished paper written by Christine McKay.

Both Ellingson (1960) and Ferris *et al.* (1967) report that P_2 latency changes are more closely related to conceptional age than to CA. Thus P_2 latency changes are probably a function of neurological maturation, since latency reflects transmission speeds, and are likely genetically linked. Figure 2.7 reproduces this relationship and indicates a sharp transition in the changes in latency of P_2 beginning about 4 weeks of age, an age perhaps reflecting some dichotomy of functioning previously indicated by the slopes of preferred contour density levels over CA (refer to Figure 2.3).

Other experimenters, including Weinmann, Creutzfeldt, and Heyde (1965), Dustman and Beck (1966, 1969), and Ellingson (1967) have followed development of the diffuse flash VEP through infancy and into early childhood. Weinmann *et al.* (1965) report a steady decrease in the latency of all components during the first 3 months as does Ellingson (1964). By the fourth month, however, the VEP waveform to diffuse flashes of light is essentially mature.

V. INFANT PATTERN-DEPENDENT VEPs

Although diffuse light VEPs help define the neural response to visual stimuli in infants, such measures offer little quantitative correspondence to ongoing behavior. Further, the implicit assumption that complex perceptual responses are based on a system of light detection is suspect in view of findings that response to luminance values independent of contour is weak. It is much more likely that the basic system is organized around contour detection. Thus, a concentration on pattern stimuli may prove useful in understanding early brain and behavior relationships.

Two initial reports have related pattern-dependent VEP component variation to pattern stimuli. Karmel, White, Cleaves, and Steinsiek (1970) using subjects varying between 8 and 21 weeks of age have indicated that pattern stimuli strongly affect VEP component amplitudes, primarily as a function of contour density. In addition, Harter and Suitt (1970) indicate that P_2 amplitude maxima shift as a function of check size as CA increases. Although suggestive of a correlation to preference behavior, these reports do not provide sufficient data to allow direct evaluation of whether component variation in the VEP reflects quantitative aspects of visual behavioral development. The following studies investigated this problem more systematically.

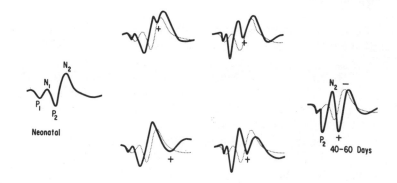

Figure 2.6 Idealized series of changes in the VEP from birth to 60 days showing the decrease in latency of all components and the emergence of P_2. Two types of changes are shown from the neonatal representation to the 40- to 60-day representation. *Negative upward.* (Top two as opposed to the bottom two central VEPs.) Changes indicate the differentiation of the P_2–N_2 complex subsequently followed by a second positive–negative complex. Broken line indicates the neonatal form. Line length equals 500 msec in each VEP waveform. [Adapted from G. S. Ferris, G. D. Davis, M. M. Dorsen, & E. R. Hackett, changes in latency and form of the phonetically induced average evoked response in human infants. *Electroencephalography and Clinical Neurophysiology*, 1967, *22*, 305–312, Fig. 4.]

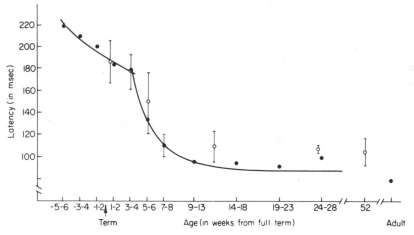

Figure 2.7 Mean latency of P_2 as function of conceptional age. The solid dots and continuous line are a plot of data derived from ink-writer tracings. The open dots are derived by means of an averaging computer ($N = 21$). The open dots for 3–4 and 7–8 weeks are obscured because they fall directly on top of closed dots. The vertical lines passing through the open dots signify ± 1 S.D. for the group of 21 subjects. Latency to a (presumable) comparable component of the adult evoked response is shown at the far right for comparison. [Adapted from Ellingson, 1967.]

A. Study I: Tachistoscopic Presentation of Redundant Checkerboard Patterns

Karmel, Hoffmann, and Fegy (1974) presented checkerboard patterns tachistoscopically to infants between 55 and 107 days of age. The stimulus set contained four pattern stimuli and one nonpattern (or blank) stimulus. There were four 12- × 12-inch square checkerboards (retinal angle = 27°) with $\frac{1}{8}$-, $\frac{1}{4}$-, $\frac{1}{2}$-, and 2-inch checks and a 27° square blank equated to the other stimuli in total luminance. Retinal sizes of checks in the pattern stimuli were approximately: 20′, 40′, 1°10′, and 5°, respectively. The EEG was simultaneously recorded from the midline occipital pole (1–2 cm above the inion) referenced to the back of one ear (O_z—A). VEPs were computed for a 1-sec duration after stimulus onset for 32 movement-free trials during which the subject was judged to be looking at the stimulus. Eye fixations at different parts of the patterns were assumed to produce essentially equivalent stimulation regardless of fixation point since the average contour density for any portion of the fixated pattern is the same.

At least four reliable components of the VEP could be established by visual inspection of each subject's records. Figure 2.8 illustrates

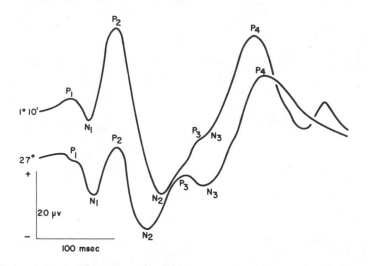

Figure 2.8   Sample occipital VEP following tachistoscopic presentation of pattern (1°10′ checks) and nonpattern (27°) stimuli from selected subjects depicting major identifiable component peaks. Downward deflection represents negative going voltage. Patterns were 12 inches square viewed from approximately 20 inches. [Adapted from Karmel, Hoffmann, & Fegy, 1974.]

these components for a selected subject as well as other components that were not evident in all records. The four reliable components were: N_1 (the most negative peak after 60 msec but prior to P_2); P_2 (the most positive peak between 100 and 200 msec); N–after–P_2 (the most negative *point* after P_2 but prior to the first most positive peak occurring after 300 msec); and P_4 (the first most positive peak after 300 msec). When two positive peaks occur at P_2, amplitude and latency measurements are taken from the larger of the two. A P_1 (a positive peak after 50 msec but prior to N_1) occurs in some but not all records. A negative–positive–negative complex ($N_2P_3N_3$) is also evident in some but not all records. N_2 is defined as the first negative peak after P_2. P_3 is defined as a positive peak between 200 and 300 msec with N_3 defined as a negative peak between P_3 and P_4. The components appear to correspond to those suggested by Ferris *et al.* (1967) shown in Figure 2.7 with the addition of a fourth positive peak. The N–after–P_2 *point* was established since not all records contained discernible $N_2P_3N_3$ complexes.

For quantitative amplitude analyses, the average of the mean voltage values at 20, 25, 30, and 35 msec after stimulus onset was used as an arbitrary zero for each VEP. Amplitudes from zero for the five stimuli for each separate reliable component (N_1, P_2, N–after–P_2, P_4) were converted to z-scores to standardize responses across subjects. Each component was analyzed separately using multivariance analysis of covariance for repeated measures (Finn, 1969) with age as the independent factor and response to stimuli as a 5-variable covariate. This analysis treats the response measures to the five stimuli as correlated dependent variables correcting the error term for the exact correlation among the five response measures.[6] Unequal interval polynomial trend analyses across the stimulus dimension were also performed by transforming the response to the five stimuli by appropriate contrast weights that reflect the contour density in CDUs of each pattern.

The amplitude of P_2 was strongly affected by contour density. A significant quadratic trend (inverted U-shaped function) best described relative changes in P_2 amplitude as a function of square root of contour. A similar relationship also exists for the magnitude of the P_2–(N–after–P_2) peak-to-peak amplitude difference. However,

[6] This analysis exists as a Fortran IV program with extensive documentation for users from J. D. Finn, State University of New York at Buffalo, titled, *Multivariance, Covariance, and Regression: A Fortran IV Program, Version 4, June, 1968.* See also McCall and Appelbaum (1973) for a discussion of the use of multivariate analysis of variance as opposed to a univariate analysis of variance with repeated measures.

there were no significant polynomial trends for N_1, N–after–P_2, or P_4 amplitudes. Thus, the major correlation between response strength and stimuli appears to be in response measures affected by P_2, the visual component peak identified earlier by Ellingson (1967), the latency of which appears to reflect visual system maturation.

Component peaks occurring after N_1 have significantly longer latencies from stimulus onset in younger CA subjects. However, changes in contour density have no apparent systematic effects on component latencies after N_1. Thus, although component latencies are found to decrease with CA, no systematic decrease in latency was detected as a function of stimulus differences in contour density.

A CA-by-stimulus (CA × S) interaction effect was analyzed using young and old CA groups. The means and standard deviations in milliseconds for component latencies for the younger CA subjects for N_1, P_2, N–after–P_2, and P_4, respectively, were: 79 ± 13, 146 ± 22, 226 ± 46, and 483 ± 73. Similar measures for older subjects were: 79 ± 14, 133 ± 30, 227 ± 48, and 392 ± 40. Z-score transformation across all five stimulus values for each component eliminates the main effect of age on component amplitude as a factor in statistical analysis but not the CA × S interaction effects. Since shifts in the maximum point of the behavioral fixation preference function occur as a result of changes in CA, the CA × S interaction for differences in polynomial trends was analyzed to determine if a similar shift in P_2 amplitudes could be found for this VEP component. A significant age difference between cubic trends across stimuli was found in P_2 amplitude. In younger CA subjects P_2 amplitude is greatest for large check sizes. No significant differences in quadratic or cubic trends were found for other components. These results were interpreted by Karmel *et al.* (1974) to indicate that the maximum point of the function relating P_2 amplitude to contour density shifts toward higher CDU values as CA increases.

Ellingson (1967) has argued that P_2 latency reflects neurological development and thus is a good measure of conceptional age. Therefore, subjects were divided into three neurological age (NA) groups on the basis of P_2 latency in order to obtain a maturation-dependent grouping other than CA. This subject grouping produces a significant difference in cubic trends to contour density among groups. This significant effect is mainly due to the differences in cubic trends of the "youngest" NA subjects versus the remaining subjects. Differentiation of the equation for the best fitting polynomial functions for these three groups indicates progressively higher predicted maxima for square root of contour as NA increases (18.8, 21.2, and 29.4 CDUs, respectively).

In summary of Study I, the data indicate that contour density effects are primarily associated with dependent measures involving the amplitude of the P_2 component. Inverted U-shaped functions relate contour density to P_2 amplitude. And, the maxima of these inverted U-shaped functions shift to patterns that contain greater contour density when CA increases as well as when the latency of P_2 becomes shorter.

B. Study II: Intensity Modulation of Random and Redundant Patterns

Only a limited number of checkerboard stimuli were used in Study I and the results could be criticized in that they may reflect responses to a single stimulus configuration, redundant checkerboards. However, preference studies as previously discussed have shown that total looking time to pattern stimuli does not depend on pattern configuration unless it affects contour density. Inspection of incomplete pilot VEP records ($N = 5$) has indicated that an inverted U-shaped function relating $P_2 - (N\text{–after–}P_2)$ amplitude differences to contour density is found whether checkerboards or random patterns are used (Karmel et al., 1970).

Study II uses both random and redundant patterns. When VEPs are obtained using a minimum 1-sec interflash interval, the number of VEPs that can be collected is limited because the total testing time is too long for a majority of infants. However, modulation of light intensity instead of a tachistoscopic source to illuminate patterns allows for more speedy data collection. When a sine-wave modulated source of light is substituted for the flash source of Study I the stimulus pattern appears to change continuously in brightness. Both Regan (1966, 1972) and Van der Tweel and Verduyn Lunel (1965) have described this technique, while Spekreijse (1966) demonstrated that these techniques produce VEP response information comparable to that obtained using tachistoscopic presentation of patterned stimuli.[7]

In Study II, recording procedures for EEG and VEP for seven

---

[7] Cornsweet (1970) has discussed this technique in detail, and Spekreijse (1966) has utilized these procedures to develop a theoretical model pertaining to a systems analysis of evoked potential effects.

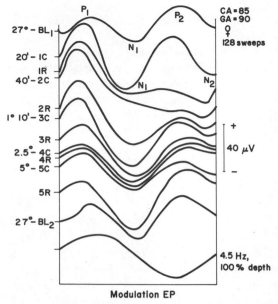

Modulation EP

Figure 2.9 Sample sine-wave intensity modulation VEPs across the range of pattern stimuli from a selected subject. Light onset occurs at lowest portion of sine wave. Approximately one cycle of information is provided. Numerals 1–5 correspond to $\frac{1}{16}$-, $\frac{1}{8}$-, $\frac{1}{4}$-, $\frac{1}{2}$-, and 1-inch checks, respectively, viewed from 9 to 12 inches. (C) and (R) refer to redundant checkerboard and random patterns respectively. The retinal angles of elements with the (C) patterns are provided. No scale was used for y-axis in order to fit all VEPs onto the figure. *Negative downward.* [Adapted from Karmel, Hoffmann, & Fegy, 1974.]

subjects (average CA = 93 days) were the same as those used previously. Response averaging was synchronized to the trough of the sine-wave light source, a point representing the beginning of light onset. Subjects viewed 6-inch square patterns from a 9- to 12-inch distance. Each subject viewed first a set of five checkerboard (C) patterns, four of which were similar to those used in Study I, then a set of five random (R) patterns shown in Figure 2.1. A blank stimulus was interspersed in each set of "C" and "R" patterns. A single frequency of light modulation (4.5 Hz) was used. The average luminance was 1 foot-Lambert changing from off to on between 0 and 2 foot-Lamberts.

Four components appeared reliably across stimuli. One positive peak (P_1) occurred approximately 100 msec after light onset in all records. P_1 was followed successively by a negative–positive–negative complex with peaks labeled N_1, P_2, and N_2, respectively.[8] A typical set of VEPs for one subject condensed to approximately one cycle of light change (approximately 225 msec) is reproduced in Figure 2.9. Stimulus effects are reflected in the peak-to-peak amplitude difference between P_1 and P_2 (P_1–P_2) and between P_1 and

[8] P_1 and P_2 refer here to the first and second positive peak found and do not correspond to the P_1 or P_2 found in flash VEP recordings. P_1 and P_2 are used here merely to distinguish these peaks in the records.

N_1 (P_1–N_1). The P_1–N_1 difference appears to be more variable than the P_1–P_2 difference across subjects at the age and modulation frequency used. A multivariate analysis of z-transformed P_1–P_2 scores similar to that described in Study I was used to test contour density effects. This analysis treats the 12-variable stimulus dimension (instead of the 5 as in Study I) as a correlated set of repeated measures for each subject. When the square root of contour is used to depict points along the stimulus dimension, inverted U-shaped functions for both P_1–P_2 and P_1–N_1 amplitude differences account for roughly 80% ($r \geq .90$) or more of the variation due to the stimulus factor. Standardized P_1–P_2 amplitude differences for each stimulus across subjects are plotted in Figure 2.10. Separate effects of "C" and "R" configurations are minimal when compared to contour density.

In summary, use of modulation procedures indicates that contour density predicts modulation VEP component variation by a function similar to that found for the P_2 component when tachistoscopic presentation is used. At the same time, this technique indicates that VEP component variations are similar to fixation preferences in that pattern configuration, random or redundant, does not play a role independent of contour density.

C. Contrasts between Behavioral Preferences and VEP Components

If VEP component variation is linked to preference behavior, then a positive quantitative relationship should exist between preference magnitude and VEP component amplitudes sensitive to contour

Figure 2.10 Mean peak-to-peak (P_1–P_2) amplitude difference to range of pattern stimuli across infants. Stimulus check size listed in inches and according to pattern types redundant (C) or random (R). Numeral represents element size in inches if viewed from 18 to 24 inches. Retinal angles were 5°, 2.5°, 1°10′, 40′, and 20′; CDU values were 12, 17, 24, 34, and 48, for the 2C, 1C, ½C, ¼C, and ⅛C respectively. [Adapted from Karmel, Hoffmann, & Fegy, 1974.]

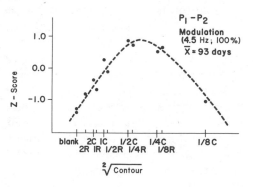

density. In order to test this proposition, the regression equation used to predict the behaviorally preferred stimulus after 6 weeks CA (Section I-D, Figure 2.3) was used to predict the expected VEP component amplitude maxima for the three ages tested in the two-pattern VEP studies reviewed previously. For 8- to 10-week-old subjects in Study I, predicted contour density preference maxima range from 20.0 CDUs to 23.3 CDUs. The maximum P_2 amplitude derived from a polynomial regression analysis of P_2 variation to stimuli for the younger CA groups of Study I was 24 CDUs, a value close to the preference prediction. For 11- to 14-week-old subjects in Study I, the predicted most preferred CDU values range from 25.0 CDUs to 30.0 CDUs. The maximum P_2 amplitude occurs between 24.0 CDUs and 32.0 CDUs, a reasonable prediction from the preference functions. In Study II, CAs ranged from 13 to 14 weeks. The predicted preference CDU maximum varies between 28.3 CDUs and 30.0 CDUs. The observed maximum P_1–P_2 amplitude difference falls within this range at 28.4 CDUs.

Given these outcomes, the maximum for the P_2 amplitude or P_1–P_2 amplitude difference functions falls at similar points along the contour density continuum as do preferences for a given CA in subjects more than 8 weeks of age. Thus, the relationship between curves for both preferences and VEP component variation are both *qualitatively* and *quantitatively* similar over CA. Common underlying mechanisms are probably involved.

D. Further Replication and Extensions

Thus far, only VEPs recorded from the O_Z site have been discussed. However, the distribution of the response to visual stimulation is not restricted to the occipital pole. For example, Rose (1971) and Rose and Lindsley (1968) recording from young kittens identify two major sources for VEP components that change over development: a short latency, positive–negative complex attributed to sources within the primary, or specific, geniculostriate projection system, and a long latency, negative component attributed to nonprimary subcortical sources and having a more indirect route to cortical tissue. The latter component is thought to involve neurons in the superior colliculus or midbrain reticular formation and other nonprimary subcortical visual nuclei. According to Rose and Lindsley, the geniculostriate component only can be observed directly over the primary visual cortex which corresponds to the O_Z lead used in infant studies reported above. The nonprimary subcortical component can be observed over a wide scalp area including the O_Z site.

In order to determine whether pattern-sensitive VEP component variation can be obtained from sites other than O_Z in human infants, Hoffmann (1973) evaluated pattern sensitivity at four cortical loci: an occipital lead, O_Z (1–2 cm above the inion); a midline central lead, C_Z (at the vertex); a parietal lead, P_Z (a site midway between O_Z and C_Z along the midline); and a left temporal lead, T_3 (a lateral lead 20% of the distance between C_Z and the left preauricular point, approximately at the middle of the left ear). Procedures and stimuli similar to those in Study I were used with the exception that three rather than four checkerboard stimuli along with the blank were presented. Check element sizes were 2 inches, $\frac{1}{2}$ inch, and $\frac{1}{4}$ inch, and subtended 5°, 1°10′, and 40′ of visual angle respectively. Twenty-six subjects from two age groups (5- and 12-week-old subjects) were tested. However, NA as defined by P_2 latency derived from the O_Z lead rather than CA was used to divide subjects into two equal groups ($N = 13$) for data analysis. This was done because NA is more sensitive to conceptional age than to CA (Ellingson, 1967) and conceptional age is more closely tied to contour preferences (Fantz, Fagan, & Miranda, Chapter 4, in this volume; Sigman & Parmelee, 1974). Two composite VEPs for each brain site were generated for each NA group by standardizing and combining VEPs across subjects and stimuli.[9]

Composite waveforms obtained at O_Z for the two NA groups are shown in Figure 2.11. The waveform (solid line) of younger NA subjects (P_2 latency > 155 msec; $\overline{X} = 180$ msec; $\overline{CA} = 6.2$ weeks) is primarily composed of an early positive–negative complex (P_2–N) followed by a late–negative wave (L–N). A similar composite waveform (dashed line) was found for older NA subjects (P_2 latency < 155 msec; $\overline{X} = 130$ msec; $\overline{CA} = 10.4$ weeks). The latency of the first positive peak (P_2 in Figure 2.11) corresponds to the latency of the positive peak labeled P_2 in Figure 2.8

The P_2–N component was observed only over the visual cortex (O_Z) while the L–N component was observed over widely differing

[9] To calculate a composite VEP, Hoffmann first calculated the average root mean square (rms) value across the VEPs from a given scalp location for a given subject. Then this value was used as the estimate of variance to obtain a standardized magnitude for each time point along the VEP. Finally, all such standardized VEPs for a given NA group for a given site were averaged across subjects as if each subject's VEP were a single sample of an evoked brain event.

scalp areas (O_Z, P_Z, C_Z, and T_3). Thus, Hoffmann concluded that P_2–N may correspond to the biphasic positive–negative VEP complex observed by Rose and Lindsley and might be attributed to sources involving the geniculostriate system, while the L–N component may correspond to the late–negative component observed by Rose and Lindsley and might be attributed to sources involving the superior colliculus or midbrain reticular formation projected onto wide cortical areas.

A polynomial regression analysis utilizing the P_2 component amplitudes of the P_2–N complex found for the different patterns indicates no significant trend for P_2 amplitude in younger NA subjects. However, an inverted U-shaped function with a maximum of 25.3 CDUs was found for P_2 amplitude in older NA subjects. A similar analysis of the late–negative component (L–N) yields a maximum CDU value of 16.2 for younger NA subjects and an 18.5 CDU value for older NA subjects. On the basis of the behavior

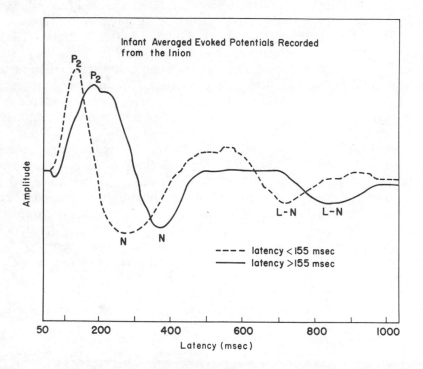

Figure 2.11   Composite RMS occipital pole VEPs across infants and stimuli where infants are grouped on the basis of P_2 latency (NA). Average CA was 6 and 10 weeks for the longer and shorter NA groups, respectively. *Negative Downward.* [Adapted from Hoffmann, 1973.]

contour density preference function [Y = +.6X − 4.0], the 6.2-week-old subjects are expected to prefer stimuli with contour density value of 17.0 CDUs while 10.4-week-old subjects are expected to prefer a stimulus having a 24.0 CDU value. Therefore, it appears that, although both cortical and subcortical components can be identified, the P_2 amplitude maximum corresponds to preferences only in older NA subjects while the L–N maximum corresponds to preferences only in younger NA subjects.

The fact that P_2 amplitude shows significant sensitivity to contour density differences in older subjects but not younger subjects suggests that there may be a major change in the functioning of the visual cortex between 6 and 10 weeks of age. However, even though the visual cortex may not be sensitive to contour density in less developed subjects, nonprimary influences as evidenced by variations in L–N amplitude are sensitive to contour density. Further, there appears to be little indication of change in the nonprimary component sensitivity to contour density after 6 to 10 weeks although the latency of all VEP components still decreases and is assumed to indicate some form of development.

Whether other neuroanatomical structures influence early visual behavior is unclear. However, Lieb and Karmel (1974) using bipolar electrode implants in adult rhesus monkeys have shown that multiple cortical regions, including visual association regions such as the inferotemporal cortex, generate VEP components which systematically reflect contour density. The functional significance of these effects remains to be determined. Also, Hoffmann (1973) has identified visually dependent components in sites other than O_Z in infants. But, response reliability, anatomical distribution, and behavioral significance also remain to be specified. Standardization of infant VEP amplitudes linked to NA groupings should prove useful in this respect. Indeed, L–N was not clearly identified by visual inspection until standardization procedures were applied. Reliance on visual inspection for component identification in Karmel *et al.* (1974) may account for their failure to identify L–N in that study while the use of nonpattern flashes may have prevented Ellingson (1967) from reporting nonoccipital visual effects prior to 12 weeks.

E. Summary of VEP Effects Related to Contour Density

In summary, pattern-dependent components in infant VEPs measured from over the occipital cortex contain at least two components associated with visual attention, P_2 and L–N, the amplitudes of which are sensitive to differences in contour density. After 6 weeks, changes in P_2 amplitude occur such that the maximum P_2 amplitude corresponds to stimuli which have greater contour density as CA or NA increases. At any point in development after 6 weeks CA, maximum P_2 amplitude is also associated with the greatest behavioral attention. Prior to 6 weeks CA the amplitude of L–N but not P_2 reflects contour density with the maximum L–N amplitude corresponding to the preferred contour density values for a given CA. In recent studies we have found that the P_2 component is restricted to the O_Z area of the occipital pole along the midline, and is believed to stem from the primary geniculostriate projection system while the L–N component has a wider distribution over the scalp and is believed to stem from the nonprimary system. Other VEP components have been found, but their amplitudes do not relate systematically to contour density and their relationship to behavior has not been determined. Development is associated with decreasing latency of all components, the behavioral significance of which also has not yet been determined.

These data lend support to a neuronal activity hypothesis for visual attention in infants. That is, they provide empirical evidence which suggests that VEP component amplitudes correlate with variation in attention to contour density. Assuming that component amplitudes reflect synchronous activity based on contour-dependent neurons, then it is reasonable to conclude that contour-dependent neuronal activity underlies the magnitude of visual attention. Furthermore, since changes in both VEP component amplitudes and visual attention to contour density covary over development, changes in attention probably reflect changes in the activity of developing contour-dependent neurons.

F. Temporally Varying Stimulation

Since at any point in the development of a given infant a particular contour density level is preferred, a form of neuronal "tuning" with respect to the contour density continuum appears to exist and to change in a progressive fashion over development. The degree of "tuning" in the neuron pool at any time is thought to control visual attention to stationary pattern stimuli in a relatively mechanistic fashion. This mechanistic process may be similar to that reported for very simple forms of life such as invertebrates. For instance, in the beetle *Chlorophanus,* a specific distribution of stimulation of the ommatidia system can be used to predict the magnitude and direction of the optomotor response (Reichardt, 1961). Interestingly, this optomotor response is directly proportional not only to the spatial density of contours distributed across the insect's visual field but also to the temporal rates of stimulus movement across the visual receptors.

The effect of temporally changing stimulation can also be handled within the framework of a neuronal activity model of infants' responses to pattern stimulation. A stationary pattern, the stimulus thus far used in pattern preference studies, does not change over time, yet attention is continuous over several seconds to a given stimulus. The correspondence between attention and neuronal activity has been inferred from a brief pattern flash transient that excites neurons as reflected in VEP components whose momentary amplitudes covary with visual attention and contour density. Although for technical reasons a VEP cannot be obtained under the continuous, nonchanging stimulus presentation conditions used in preference studies, if one were to infer the type of neuronal activity sustaining continuous attention from the flash evoked potential data, one would predict continuous driving of P_2 in older infants and possibly L–N in younger infants because these components have been found to correspond to looking behavior and contour density. Therefore, in order for the neuronal activity model to account for continuous attention, an operational mechanism is needed to link the behavioral effect, continuous attention, with the transient neuronal activity, VEP components, elicited by a brief occurrence of a stimulus.

Continuous neuronal activity resulting from pattern stimulation can be inferred to occur as infants scan stimuli. For instance, Armington (1973) has shown that in adults, saccadic eye movements produce VEPs that are time-dependent on the saccades. Amplitudes of certain components of these saccade-linked VEPs systematically reflect the contour density of the stimulus over which the eye moves. Thus, a mechanism producing continuous eye saccades would result in the maintenance of continuous attention to stationary patterns as is observed during preference studies. Assuming this mechanism holds for infants, then a temporally varying visual pattern would be predicted to elicit attention as does a stationary pattern because it would simulate the temporal change in stimulation that ordinarily results from eye movements. And, based on a neuronal activity hypothesis, those temporal rates of change that continuously maximized contour-dependent amplitudes in the VEP would be predicted to maximize attention.

Anecdotal evidence indicates that temporally varying stimuli elicit some form of fixation response related to attention. Repetitious flashing lights have been used in several studies of infant visual attention in order to control fixation during an intertrial interval (cf. Cohen, 1972; Maisel & Karmel, 1973), as a form of "attention-getting" operation to direct attention to a desired stimulus (Cohen, 1972; Aslin & Salapatek, 1973), or to elicit visual fixation (Sigman & Parmelee, 1974).

In order to investigate the rate effect on total looking time, 12- to 13-week-old infants were presented two stimulus fields, each containing a checkerboard with $\frac{1}{2}$-inch checks viewed from 20 inches (McCarvill, Brown, & Karmel, 1975). A square-wave of light intensity changing from on to off was used to turn the pattern stimulus on and off. Eight rates of change from 1 Hz to 20 Hz were presented in a paired comparisons design using presentation controls and fixation observations similar to that used to obtain preferences to stationary patterns reported by Karmel (1969a). Each pair remained on for 16 sec. A significant rate effect was obtained ($F = 4.71$, $df = 7/105$, $p < .001$). A quadratic equation, $Y = -0.3X^2 + 1.5X + 3.0$ accounts for 79% of the variation due to rate ($r = +.89$) and predicts a maximum preferred stimulus rate of 5.7 Hz where $Y =$ mean looking time in seconds and $X = \log_2 X'$ where X' is the rate in hertz. Figure 2.12 shows this function along with the looking time means for various rates of change. Although this study indicates an inverted U-shaped preference curve for temporal rates of change, further data are required to specify rate preference functions more exactly as well as to specify changes in these functions over development.

VEP studies also suggest a relationship between temporal rates of change, attention, and underlying neuronal activity. Using sine-wave modulation techniques, occipitally recorded VEPs in 12- to 14-week-old infants contain components which vary as a function of contour density when 4.5 Hz is used as the stimulation frequency (Study II, Section V-B). Two positive peaks usually occur for each cycle of stimulation (see Figure 2.9). The first positive peak appears to correspond to P_2 produced by the short pattern flash used in Study I (Section V-A) since its latency is approximately 100 msec after pattern onset (see Figure 2.8). As contour density shifts away from preferred levels, an increased likelihood of obtaining the second positive peak is found. In subsequent unpublished studies, it

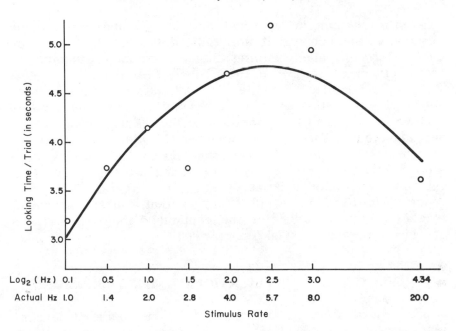

Figure 2.12   Looking preference for rate of stimulus change expressed as a function of mean total looking time per trial versus rate of stimulus change for 12- to 13-week-old infants.

was found that an increase to approximately 7 Hz produces a single positive component. A similar frequency effect on presence or absence of components and component amplitudes is evidence in 8- to 10-week-old subjects, but slower frequencies must be used (2.25 Hz and 4.5 Hz, instead of 4.5 Hz and 7.0 Hz). These data are consistent with the decrease in latency of all VEP components as the nervous system matures, reported by Ellingson (1967) and Hrbek *et al.* (1969). Extrapolation from the preference function for rate (Figure 2.12) suggests that a 5.7 Hz rate of change would tend to maximize attention at 12–13 weeks. Although VEP studies involving rate require extension and replication, we can tentatively point to the correspondence among these data and the rate preference data that suggest that visual attention varies with the rhythmic driving of VEP component amplitudes reflecting contour density with preferences maximized at rhythmic driving rates that maximize the fundamental frequency of the stimulus rhythm in the recruited brain response.

The finding that temporal effects play systematic and testable roles in maintaining infant visual attention is consistent with the observation that component amplitudes are essentially temporally coded effects of spatially varying stimuli, a position consistent with that of others (cf. Spekreijse, 1966; Pollen *et al.*, 1971; Campbell & Robson, 1968; Maffei & Fiorentini, 1973). Contours possessing finite spatial characteristics, as reflected here by contour density measurements, are in constant motion over the retinal surface due to saccadic eye movements, head movements, and eye tremor. Hence, changing stimulation of the receptive field contour cells by some finite frequency occurs even when patterns are stationary. With regard to this factor, it is interesting to note that in their initial reports, Hubel and Wiesel (1962) suggest that constant movement is a necessary condition for the continuous maintenance of a specific firing rate of a single contour cell.

VI. GENERAL IMPLICATIONS AND CONCLUSIONS

Infant visual attention follows a predictable course of development related to contour density and temporal rates of change of stimulation. At least two neuronal systems, one nonprimary and the other primary, are postulated to be involved in early attention reactions.

Until 6 weeks of age, the L–N component of the VEP derived from the nonprimary system correlates with attention. The nonprimary system has been shown to include visual sensory projections to the midbrain reticular formation (with subsequent projections to wide cortical areas) and/or to the secondary optic system that includes projections from the retina into the superior colliculus via the brachium of the superior colliculus that bypass the LGN. Stimulation of the midbrain reticular formation results in a general cortical arousal effect, while stimulation of the superior colliculus produces eye saccades which function to bring the source of peripheral contour stimulation onto the fovea at the end of the saccade. In addition, cells in the superior colliculus respond to contours of specific retinal sizes and loci as do cortical contour cells, but they possess larger receptive field sizes than do cortical cells and respond only to the general size characteristics of the contour elements rather than to the form or organization of stimulus elements (Schiller & Koerner, 1971). Thus, the nonprimary system forms an integrated feedback network where the effective stimulus element size tends to be larger than that for the primary system.

Further, visual stimulation results in a general arousal effect as well as in activity of superior colliculus neurons that, in turn, produce saccadic eye movements. These eye movements serve to place the fovea of the eye over the source of contour stimulation in the visual field.

These nonprimary system effects can be related to magnitudes of neuronal activity. VEP components sensitive to contour density are elicited by eye movements across pattern stimuli. The magnitude of their amplitudes are correlated with the length of the eye movement and the density of contours traversed (Armington, 1973). Thus, an eye movement of any length over a pattern produces activity in at least the nonprimary system in young infants proportional to the eye movement length and the contour density of the pattern over which the eye moves. This activity in turn would result in locating the source of stimulation over the fovea. Simultaneously, a general cortical arousal would occur that would be proportional to the magnitude of the L–N component and distributed over a wide cortical region. This cortical arousal then would interact with arousal effects produced by other sources of stimulation including stimulation derived directly from the geniculostriate system.

An eye movement would also provide a source of stimulation for the primary, geniculostriate system if contours were brought onto the fovea by an eye saccade and if receptors in the fovea were sufficiently developed. Foveal stimulation, in turn, would selectively result in activity in the geniculostriate system since a large proportion (about 95%) of all cortical striate cells are innervated from the foveal region. Evidence for an intact geniculostriate system is present from birth in that a P_2 component can be detected in neonatal as well as older infants (see Figures 2.6 and 2.11). However, P_2 amplitudes do not selectively reflect differences in contour density prior to 6 weeks providing evidence that the geniculostriate system, although intact, is not sufficiently developed to control behavior. Correlated with this finding is the fact that receptor cells in the fovea are not well developed until at least 2 months (Lodge, Armington, Barnet, Shanks, & Newcomb, 1969; Mann, 1964). Thus, constant foveation of contoured stimulation produced by eye movements linked to contours in the stimulus would occur even prior to the development of a mature P_2 response generated by the geniculostriate system. The infant's behavior prior to 6 weeks in turn would appear to be a continuous general arousal response given the existence of contour stimulation of sufficient density to stimulate the large majority of contour cells outside the geniculostriate system. This conclusion is directly supported by the observation that the level of contour density preferred by 6 weeks CA is represented by a check size larger than the 2° to 3° size of the fovea. Thus, the nonprimary system would provide a mechanism of eye movement control as well as a means by which extrafoveal stimulation would be brought onto the foveal region of the retina where 95% or more of the mature receptors in the eye will eventually be located. Ordinarily, pattern stimuli that infants encounter subtend a large retinal angle or contain elements of a sufficient retinal angle to continually arouse the nonprimary system and thereby capture the young infant's gaze.

In addition to controlling eye movements producing foveation, a functional nonprimary system response to pattern stimulation at birth would act to bring about pattern stimulation to an immature, diffusely organized geniculostriate visual system. Stimulation of the primary sensory system brought about by foveation of contours as a result of the nonprimary eye movement control system might then act to further organize receptive field characteristics in cortical cells since early experience has been shown to dictate to some degree subsequent receptive field characteristics (Hirsch & Spinelli, 1970; Blakemore & Cooper, 1970). A report by Greenberg (1971) to the effect that preference responses to checkerboard stimuli are shifted toward patterns containing smaller checks as a result of prior exposure to checkerboards would suggest that receptive field characteristics in humans might also be affected by exposure history, especially if our arguments on preferences and receptive fields holds true.

After 6 weeks of age, the P_2 component of the VEP derived from the primary system correlates with visual attention. As this geniculostriate system develops, contour stimulation resulting from stimulation of the fovea would bring about activity in the sensory-specific occipital regions of the cortex. The magnitude of this activity would correlate positively with the amplitude of the P_2 component and would relate at least to the degree of maturation of cortical neurons connected to the fovea. The occurrence of P_2 amplitudes correlated with attention suggests that once contours are foveated after 6 weeks of age, control of the duration of looking at a stimulus is shifted from the nonprimary system to the primary system. A possible mechanism by which this could be accomplished can be inferred from single neuron activity in the superior colliculus. Superior colliculus activity associated with eye saccades is directly inhibited by activity and stimulation within area 18 (McIlwain &

Fields, 1971). In primates, area 18, directly connected to area 17, is associated with the superior colliculus through interconnections with the pulvinar, a subcortical visual association region in the posterior thalamus. The absence of cortical inhibition on eye movements of visually naive organisms is also evidenced by increasing nystagmus responses after dark-rearing (Riesen, 1961) which is presumed to inhibit the development of visual cortical neurons (Wiesel & Hubel, 1965). Increased nystagmus responses are also recorded when visual cortex is damaged in infants (Cogan, 1966). The effect of cortical stimulation on looking behavior then might be to delay the initiation of a subsequent eye movement and bring about an increase in the duration of fixation as well as to delay initiation of a subsequent eye movement. This, in turn, would result in an increase in measures related to the duration of looking. In addition, the degree of inhibition would be directly proportional to the magnitude of activity reflected by the amplitude of P_2 and, thus, would correspond to looking behavior reflected in developmentally changing response to contour density after 6 weeks. Constantly changing externally imposed stimulation in the form of temporally varying patterns would act continuously to inhibit eye movements. The results of this stimulation condition would be to generate a continuous state of neuronal activity in the cortical regions of the primary system with subsequent continuous inhibition of eye movements which would result in a corresponding behavioral condition of continuous attention.

In summary, the nonprimary system present at birth controlling general arousal and saccadic eye movements is suggested to control visual attention prior to 6 weeks CA. Subsequent development of the primary projection system could act directly to control the magnitude and direction of ongoing eye excursions after 6 weeks CA by means of an inhibitory loop between area 18 to the superior colliculus. These developmentally changing effects would act to control the magnitude of the neural activity produced to stationary patterns.

Eventually older children can shift attention away from visual stimuli altogether. Obviously some other form of control must supersede or momentarily interact with stimulus-produced neuronal activity due to visual pattern inputs. This control could correlate with development of acts of intention. Thus, an interaction of the primary and nonprimary visual projection systems with those systems related to intention is likely to occur.

In an analogous manner, the mechanisms controlling changes in attention to visual stimulation over development might be used as a model to understand similar developing responses occurring to other stimulus invariances in the visual system as well as other modalities either in infancy or during other periods in development. Such adaptive changes are presumed to underlie adult cognition to the point where the adult is much less under the influence of the external stimulus than is the infant and is more under internal control as to which stimulus captures his attention.

The special case of how neuronal activity interacts in two or more modalities simultaneously might prove to be a fruitful problem to pursue in future analyses where neurological processes related to early function may be involved. If development of a child's knowledge about the world is encoded by the developing nervous system, then fundamental to the development of adult knowledge is a clear understanding of the specific structural and functional details of the transitions that occur in the nervous system as cognitive structures undergo change. The amount of neuropsychological knowledge to be gained is thus immense since neuropsychological structures, as Piaget suggests to be the case for cognitive structures, must be undergoing continuous alteration as perceptual and cognitive development proceed.

VII. SUMMARY

1. Contour density at the retina is a major determinant of infant visual preferences over development. Preferences are best described as inverted U-shaped functions relating visual attention to contour density at any specific age. The maxima of the inverted U-shaped preference functions systematically shift toward greater contour density levels with development.

2. Neurological maturation is thought to constrain and determine early visual attention. Visual attention is postulated to be related to neuronal activity resulting from the interaction over development of contour stimulation and receptive field characteristics of visually dependent neurons that are assumed to be reflected in component amplitudes of the VEP.

3. The amplitudes of both an early positive component and a late negative component of the VEP in infants are sensitive to differences in contour density and can be related to behavioral attention. The amplitude of the late negative component (assumed to arise from activity of nonprimary, extra-geniculostriate sources) is corre-

lated with behavioral attention only prior to 6 weeks of age. The amplitude of the early positive component (assumed to arise from activity of geniculostriate sources) is correlated with behavioral attention after 6 weeks of age.

4. A mechanism related to control of eye movements by the primary and nonprimary system was postulated to relate the hypothetical neuronal activity underlying VEP components to the phenomenon of continuous visual attention and inspection of pattern stimulation by infants.

ACKNOWLEDGMENTS

The authors wish to express their sincere appreciation to numerous colleagues who over the years have helped generate this chapter, especially Donna Apter, Pamela Brown, Wallace Cleaves, Michael Dorman, Martin Fegy, Robert Hoffmann, Sharon McCarvill, and Christine McKay. Their suggestions and insightful comments have helped in formulating the ideas contained in these pages. We also wish to express our gratitude to Carol Service who typed and retyped the manuscript.

REFERENCES

Armington, J. C. Discussant in symposium on visual perception in infants. Biennial meeting of Society for Research on Child Development, Philadelphia, Pennsylvania, March, 1973.

Armington, J. C., Corwin, T. R., & Marsetta, R. Simultaneously recorded retinal and cortical responses to patterned stimuli. *Journal of the Optical Society of America*, 1971, *61*, 1514–1526.

Aslin, R. N., & Salapatek, P. Saccadic localization of visual targets by the very young human infant. Paper presented at meetings of the Psychonomic Society, St. Louis, Missouri, October, 1973.

Barnet, A. B., Lodge, A., & Armington, J. C. Electroretinogram in newborn human infants. *Science*, 1965, *148*, 651–654.

Berlyne, D. E. The influence of the albedo and complexity of stimuli on visual fixation in the human infant. *British Journal of Psychology*, 1958, *56*, 315–318.

Blakemore, C., & Cooper, G. F. Development of the brain depends on the visual environment. *Nature*, 1970, *228*, 477–478.

Blakemore, C., Garner, E. T., & Sweet, J. A. The site of size constancy. *Perception*, 1972, *1*, 111–119.

Bond, E. K. Perception of form by the human infant. *Psychological Bulletin*, 1972, 77, 225–245.

Brennan, W. M., Ames, E. W., & Moore, R. W. Age differences in infants' attention to patterns of different complexity. *Science*, 1966, *151*, 354–356.

Bronson, G. The hierarchical organization of the central nervous system: implication for learning processes and critical periods in early development. *Behavioral Science*, 1965, *10*, 7–25.

Campbell, F. W., & Robson, J. G. Application of Fourier analysis to the visibility of gratings. *Journal of Physiology*, 1968, *197*, 551–566.

Clynes, M., & Kohn, M. S. Spatial visual evoked potentials as physiologic language elements for color and field structure. In W. Cobb & C. R. Morocutti (Eds.), *The evoked potentials*. New York: Elsevier, 1967. Pp. 82–96. Also, *Electroencephalography and Clinical Neurophysiology*, 1967, Supplement 26. Pp. 82–96.

Cogan, D. G. *Neurology of the visual system*. Springfield, Illinois: Thomas, 1966.

Cohen, L. Observing responses, visual preferences, and habituation to visual stimuli in infants. *Journal of Experimental Child Psychology*, 1969, *7*, 419–433.

Cohen, L. Attention-getting and attention-holding processes in infant visual preferences. *Child Development*, 1972, *43*, 869–879.

Conel, J. L. *The postnatal development of the human cerebral cortex. I. The cortex of the newborn*. Cambridge, Massachusetts: Harvard Univ. Press, 1939.

Conel, J. L. *The postnatal development of the human cerebral cortex. II. Cortex of the one-month infant*. Cambridge, Massachusetts: Harvard Univ. Press, 1941.

Conel, J. L. *The postnatal development of the human cerebral cortex. III. The cortex of the three-month infant*. Cambridge, Massachusetts: Harvard Univ. Press, 1947.

Cornsweet, T. N. *Visual perception*. New York: Academic Press, 1970.

Creutzfeldt, O. D., Watanabe, S., & Lux, H. D. Relations between EEG phenomena and potentials of single cortical cells. I. Evoked responses after thalamic and epicortical stimulation. II. Spontaneous and convulsoid activity. *Electroencephalography and Clinical Neurophysiology*, 1966, *20*, 1–18, 19–37.

DeHardt, D. C. Visual cliff behavior of rats as a function of pattern size. *Psychonomic Science*, 1969, *15*, 268–269.

Dixon, W. J. *BMD biomedical computer program*. Los Angeles: Univ. of California Press, 1971.

Donchin, E., & Lindsley, D. B. (Eds.). *Averaged evoked potentials*. Washington, D.C.: NASA SP-191, 1969.

Dustman, R. E., & Beck, E. C. Visually evoked potentials. *Science*, 1966, *151*, 1013–1015.

Dustman, R. E., & Beck, E. C. The effects of maturation and aging on the waveform of visually evoked potentials. *Electroencephalography and Clinical Neurophysiology*. 1969, *26*, 2–11.

Ellingson, R. J. Cortical electrical responses to visual stimulation in the human infant. *Electroencephalography and Clinical Neurophysiology*, 1960, *12*, 663–667.

Ellingson, R. J. Cerebral electrical responses to auditory and visual stimuli in the infant (human and subhuman studies). In P. Kellaway, & I. Petersen (Eds.), *Neurological and electroencephalographic correlative studies in infancy*. New York: Grune, 1964. Pp. 78–116.

Ellingson, R. J. The study of brain electrical activity in infants. In L. P. Lipsitt & C. C. Spiker (Eds.), *Advances in child development and behavior*, Vol. 3. New York: Academic Press, 1967. Pp. 53–97.

Ellingson, R. J. Variability of visual evoked responses in the human newborn. *Electroencephalography and Clinical Neurophysiology*, 1970, *29*, 10–19.

Elul, R. Brain waves: Intracellular recording and statistical analysis help clarify their physiological significance. *Data Acquisition and Processing in Biology and Medicine*, 1968, *5*, 93–115.

Fantz, R. L. Pattern vision in young infants. *Psychological Record*, 1958, *8*, 43–47.

Fantz, R. L. Visual perception and experience in early infancy: a look at the hidden side of behavior development. In H. W. Stevenson, E. H. Hess, & H. L. Rheingold (Eds.), *Early behavior: Comparative and developmental approaches.* New York: Wiley, 1967. Pp. 181–225.

Fantz, R. L., Ordy, J. M., & Udelf, M. S. Maturation of pattern vision in infants during the first six months. *Journal of Comparative and Physiological Psychology*, 1962, *55*, 907–917.

Ferris, G. S., Davis, G. D., Dorsen, M. M., & Hackett, E. R. Changes in latency and form of the photically induced average evoked response in human infants. *Electroencephalography and Clinical Neurophysiology*, 1967, *22*, 305–312.

Finn, J. D. Multivariate analysis of repeated measures data. *Multivariate Behavioral Research*, 1969, *4*, 391–413.

Fogarty, T. P., & Reuben, R. N. Light-evoked cortical and retinal responses in premature infants. *Archives of Ophthalmology*, 1969, *81*, 454–459.

Fox, M. W. *Integrative development of the brain and behavior in the dog.* Chicago: Univ. of Chicago Press, 1971.

Fox, S. S., & O'Brien, J. H. Duplication of evoked potential waveform by curve of probability of firing of single cell. *Science*, 1965, *147*, 888–890.

Fox, S. S., & Norman, R. J. Functional congruence: an index of neural homogeneity and a new measure of brain activity. *Science*, 1968, *159*, 1257–1259.

Gaito, J. Unequal intervals and unequal n in trend analyses. *Psychological Bulletin*, 1965, *63*, 125–127.

Ganz, L., & Fitch, M. The effect of visual deprivation on perceptual behavior. *Experimental Neurology*, 1968, *22*, 638–660.

Gibson, J. J. *The senses considered as perceptual systems.* Boston, Massachusetts: Houghton-Mifflin, 1966.

Greenberg, D. J. Accelerating visual compexity levels in the human infant. *Child Development*, 1971, *42*, 905–918.

Greenberg, D. J., & O'Donnell, W. J. Infancy and the optimal level of stimulation. *Child Development*, 1972, *43*, 639–645.

Gross, C. G., Rocha-Miranda, C. E., & Bender, D. B. Visual properties of neurons in the inferotemporal cortex of the *macaque. Journal of Neurophysiology*, 1972, *35*, 96–111.

Harter, M. R., & Suitt, C. D. Visually evoked cortical responses and pattern vision in the infant: A longitudinal study. *Psychonomic Science*, 1970, *18*, 235–237.

Harter, M. R., & White, C. T. Effects of contour sharpness and check-size on visually evoked cortical potentials. *Vision Research*, 1968, *8*, 701–711.

Harter, M. R., & White, C. T. Evoked cortical response to checkerboard patterns: effect of check-size as a function of visual acuity. *Electroencephalography and Clinical Neurophysiology*, 1970, *28*, 48–54.

Hershenson, M. Visual discrimination in the human infant. *Journal of Comparative and Physiological Psychology*, 1964, *58*, 270–276.

Hershenson, M. Development of the perception of form. *Psychological Bulletin*, 1967, *67*, 326–336.

Hershenson, M., Munsinger, H., & Kessen, W. Preference for shapes of intermediate variability in the newborn human. *Science*, 1965, *147*, 630–631.

Hirsch, H. V. B., & Spinelli, D. N. Visual experience modifies distribution of horizontally and vertically oriented receptive fields in cats. *Science*, 1970, *168*, 869–871.

Hoffmann, R. F. Developmental changes in human infant VEPs to patterned stimuli at different scalp locations and their relationship to visual attention. Unpublished Ph.D. dissertation. Univ. of Connecticut, 1973.

Hrbek, A., Hrbkova, M., & Lenard, H. G. Somato-sensory evoked responses in newborn infants during sleep and wakefulness. *Electroencephalography and Clinical Neurophysiology*, 1969, *26*, 597–603.

Hubel, D. H., & Wiesel, T. N. Receptive fields, binocular interaction and functional architecture in the cat's visual cortex. *Journal of Physiology*, 1962, *160*, 106–154.

Hubel, D. H., & Wiesel, T. N. Receptive fields of cells in striate cortex of very young, visually inexperienced kittens. *Journal of Neurophysiology*, 1963, *26*, 994–1002.

Hubel, D. H., & Wiesel, T. N. Binocular interaction in striate cortex of kittens reared with artificial squint. *Journal Neurophysiology*, 1965, *28*, 1041–1059. (a)

Hubel, D. H., & Wiesel, T. N. Receptive fields and functional architecture in two nonstriate areas (18 and 19) of the cat. *Journal of Neurophysiology*, 1965, *28*, 229–289. (b)

Hubel, D. H., & Wiesel, T. N. Receptive field architecture of monkey striate cortex. *Journal of Physiology*, 1968, *195*, 215–243.

Jacobson, M. *Developmental neurobiology.* New York: Holt, 1970.

John, E. R. *Mechanisms of memory.* New York: Academic Press, 1967.

John, E. R., & Thatcher, R. W. *Integrative neuroscience*, Vol. I. (In press.)

Jones-Molfese, V. J. Individual differences in neonatal preferences for planometric and stereometric visual patterns. *Child Development*, 1972, *43*, 1289–1296.

Jung, R., & Spillman, L. Receptive-field estimation and perceptual integration in human vision. In F. A. Young & D. B. Lindsley (Eds.), *Early experience and visual information processing in perceptual and reading disorders.* Washington, D. C.: National Academy of Sciences, 1970. Pp. 181–197.

Karmel, B. Z. Randomness, complexity, and visual preference behavior in the hooded rat and domestic chick. *Journal of Comparative and Physiological Psychology*, 1966, *61*, 487–489.

Karmel, B. Z. The effect of age, complexity, and amount of contour on pattern preferences in human infants. *Journal of Experimental Child Psychology*, 1969, *7*, 339–354. (a)

Karmel, B. Z. Complexity, amounts of contour, and visually dependent behavior in hooded rats, domestic chicks, and human infants. *Journal of Comparative and Physiological Psychology*, 1969, *69*, 649–657. (b)

Karmel, B. Z. Age, complexity and contour as determinants of attention in human infants. Participant symposium: Determinants of attention in infants. Society for Research in Child Development meetings, Santa Monica, California, March, 1969. (c)

Karmel, B. Z. Contour effects and pattern preferences in infants: a reply to Greenberg and O'Donnell. *Child Development*, 1974, *45*, 196–199.

Karmel, B. Z., Hoffmann, R. F., & Fegy, M. J. Processing of contour information by human infants evidenced by pattern-dependent evoked potentials. *Child Development*, 1974, *45*, 39–48.

Karmel, B. Z., Miller, P. N., Dettweiler, L., & Anderson, G. Texture density and normal development of visual depth avoidance. *Developmental Psychobiology*. 1970, *3*, 73–90.

Karmel, B. Z., White, C. T., Cleaves, W. T., & Steinsiek, K. J. A technique to investigate averaged evoked potential correlates of pattern perception in human infants. Paper presented at the meeting of the Eastern Psychological Association, Atlantic City, New Jersey, April, 1970.

Karmel, B. Z., & Walk, R. D. The development of depth perception in the cat. Paper presented at the Eastern Psychological Association meetings, Atlantic City, New Jersey, April, 1965.

Kessen, W., Salapatek, P., & Haith, M. The visual response of the human newborn to linear contour. *Journal of Experimental Child Psychology*, 1972, *13*, 9–20.

Kuffler, S. W. Discharge patterns and functional organization of mammalian retina. *Journal of Neurophysiology*, 1953, *16*, 37–68.

Lieb, J. P., & Karmel, B. Z. The processing of edge information in visual areas of the cortex as evidenced by evoked potentials. *Brain Research*, 1974, *76*, 503–519.

Lodge, A., Armington, J. C., Barnet, A. B., Shanks, B. L., & Newcomb, C. N. Newborn infants' electroretinograms and evoked electroencephalographic responses to orange and white light. *Child Development*, 1969, *40*, 267–293.

MacKay, D. M. Evoked brain potentials as indicators of sensory information processing. In F. O. Schmitt, T. Melnechuk, G. C. Quarton, & G. Adelman (Eds.), *Neurosciences research symposium summaries*. Vol. 4. Cambridge, Massachusetts: MIT Press, 1970. Pp. 397–489.

Maffei, L., & Fiorentini, A. The visual cortex as a spatial frequency analyzer. *Vision Research*, 1973, *13*, 1255–1267.

Maisel, E. B., & Karmel, B. Z. Failure to replicate the bull's-eye preference effect in infants. Paper presented at the meeting of the Society for Research in Child Development, Philadelphia, Pennsylvania, March, 1973.

Mann, I. *The development of the human eye*. London: British Medical Association, 1964.

McCall, R. B. Attention in the infant: avenue to the study of cognitive development. In Walcher, D. N. & Peters, D. L. (Eds.), *Early childhood: The development of self-regulatory mechanisms*. New York: Academic Press, 1971. Pp. 109–140.

McCall, R. B., & Appelbaum, M. Bias in the analysis of repeated-measures designs: some alternative approaches. *Child Development*, 1973, *44*, 401–415.

McCall, R. B., & Kagan, J. Parameters of attention in the infant. *Child Development*, 1967, *38*, 939–952.

McCall, R. B., & Melson, W. H. Complexity, contour and area as determinants of attention in infants. *Developmental Psychology*, 1970, *3*, 343–349.

McCarvill, S. L. *The effects of stimulus intensity on pattern preferences in infants*. Unpublished masters thesis, Univ. of Connecticut, 1973.

McCarvill, S. L., Brown, P. A., & Karmel, B. Z. Infants' looking preferences for temporal rates of change in visual stimuli. Paper presented to the Eastern Psychological Association meetings, New York, 1975.

McGraw, M. B. *The neuromuscular maturation of the human infant*. New York: Columbia Univ. Press, 1945.

McIlwain, J. T., & Buser, P. Receptive fields of single cells in the cat's superior colliculus. *Experimental Brain Research*, 1968, *5*, 314–325.

McIlwain, J. T., & Fields, H. L. Interactions of cortical and retinal projections on single neurons of the cat's superior colliculus. *Journal of Neurophysiology*, 1971, *34*, 763–772.

Miranda, S. B. Visual abilities and pattern preferences of premature infants and full-term neonates. *Journal of Experimental Child Psychology*, 1970, *10*, 189–205.

Peiper, A. *Cerebral function in infancy and childhood.* New York: Consultants Bureau, 1963. (Tr. Benedict & Hilde Nagler)

Perry, N. W., & Childers, D. G. *The human visual evoked response.* Springfield, Illinois: Thomas, 1969.

Pollen, D. A., Lee, J. R., & Taylor, J. H. How does the striate cortex begin the reconstruction of the visual world? *Science,* 1971, *173,* 74–77.

Regan, D. Some characteristics of average steady-state and transient responses evoked by modulated light. *Electroencephalography and Clinical Neurophysiology,* 1966, *20,* 238–248.

Regan, D. *Evoked potentials in psychology, sensory physiology, and clinical medicine.* New York: Wiley, 1972.

Reichardt, W. Autocorrelation, a principle for the evaluation of sensory information by the central nervous system. In W. A. Rosenblith (Ed.), *Sensory communication.* Cambridge, Massachusetts: MIT Press, 1961. Pp. 303–318.

Riesen, A. H. Stimulation as a requirement for growth and function in behavioral development. In D. W. Fiske & S. R. Maddi (Eds.), *Functions of varied experience.* Homewood, Illinois: Dorsey Press, 1961. Pp. 57–80.

Rose, G. H. Relationship of electrophysiological and behavioral indices of visual development in mammals. In M. B. Sterman, D. J. McGinty, & A. M. Adinolli (Eds.), *Brain development and behavior.* New York: Academic Press, 1971. Pp. 145–183.

Rose, G. H., & Lindsley, D. B. Development of visually evoked potentials in kittens: Specific and non-specific responses. *Journal of Neurophysiology,* 1968, *31,* 607–623.

Sackett, G. P. A neural mechanism underlying unlearned, critical period, and developmental aspects of visually controlled behavior. *Psychological Review,* 1963, *70,* 40–50.

Salapatek, P., & Kessen, W. Visual scanning of triangles by the human newborn. *Journal of Experimental Child Psychology,* 1966, *3,* 155–167.

Schapiro, S. Effects of neonatal hormone administration on the development of the nervous system. Paper presented at Biennial Meeting of Society for Research in Child Development, Santa Monica, California, March, 1969.

Schiller, P. H., & Koerner, F. Discharge characteristics of single units in the superior colliculus of the alert rhesus monkey. *Journal of Neurophysiology,* 1971, *34,* 920–936.

Sigman, M., & Parmelee, A. H. Visual preferences of four-month-old premature and full-term infants. *Child Development,* 1974, *45,* 959–965.

Simner, M. L. Age changes in preference for visual patterned stimulation in the newly hatched chick. *Proceedings of the 75th annual convention, American Psychological Association,* 1967, *2,* 107–108.

Spehlmann, R. The averaged electrical response to diffuse and to pattern light in the human. *Electroencephalography and Clinical Neurophysiology,* 1965, *19,* 560–569.

Spekreijse, H. *Analysis of EEG responses in man.* Ph.D. thesis, Univ. of Amsterdam. The Hague: Junk Publishers, 1966.

Sprague, J. M. Interaction of cortex and superior colliculus in mediation of visually guided behavior in the cat. *Science,* 1966, *153,* 1544–1547.

Stewart, D. L., & Riesen, A. H. Adult versus infant brain damage: behavioral and electrophysiological effects of striatectomy in adult and neonatal rabbits. In

G. Newton (Ed.), *Advances in psychobiology*, Vol. 1. New York: Academic Press, 1972. Pp. 171–211.

Thompson, R. F. Relations between evoked gross and unit activity in association cortex of waking cat. In R. Wahlen (Ed.), *The neural control of behavior*. New York: Academic Press, 1970. Pp. 55–62.

Van der Tweel, L. H., & Verduyn Lunel, H. F. E. Human visual responses to sinusoidally modulated light. *Electroencephalography and Clinical Neurophysiology*, 1965, *18*, 587–598.

Verzeano, M., Dill, R. C., Vallecalle, E., Groves, P., & Thomas, J. Evoked responses and neuronal activity in the lateral geniculate. *Experientia*, 1968, *24*, 696–698.

Walk, R. D. The study of visual depth and distance perception in animals. In D. S. Lehrman, R. A. Hinde, & E. Shaw (Eds.), *Advances in the study of animal behavior*, Vol. 1. New York: Academic Press, 1965. Pp. 99–154.

Walk, R. D., & Gibson, E. J. A comparative and analytical study of visual depth perception. *Psychological Monographs*, 1961, *75* (15), Whole No. 519.

Walk, R. D., & Walters, C. P. Texture and motion parallax interact in determining depth perception. Paper presented to the meeting of the Eastern Psychological Association, New York, April, 1971.

Warkentin, J. An experimental study of the ontogeny of vision in the rabbit. *Psychological Bulletin*, 1937, *34*, 542–543.

Weinmann, H., Creutzfeldt, O. P., & Heyde, G. Die entwicklung der visuellen reizantwort bei kindern. *Archiv für Psychiatrie und zeitschift für gesant Neurologie*, 1965, *207*, 323–341.

Wiesel, T. N., & Hubel, D. H. Comparison of extent of recovery from the effects of visual deprivation in kittens. *Journal of Neurophysiology*, 1965, *28*, 1060–1072.

Wozniak, A., Ham, S., Vanzini, P., & Garcia-Austt, E. Relationship between evoked potentials and unit activity in the visual system of the albino rat. *Acta Neurol. Latinamerica*, 1970, *16*, 184–191.

chapter 3: Pattern Perception in Early Infancy[1]

PHILIP SALAPATEK
University of Minnesota

I. Introduction

The human is a cognitive organism who directly senses only certain information from a highly structured world. Both the specific senses and the capacity to interpret their discharges are the result of a lengthy evolution. The full story of perceptual development is provided only when we understand the workings of an evolved mind presented with information by sensory systems idiosyncratically designed to extract only some information from a three-dimensional world of real objects and events. But all stories have beginnings, and much basic knowledge is culled from simple isolated preparations. In this chapter we consider only the relationship between mind and one sensory system—vision; we strip away

[1] Preparation of this manuscript, the collection and analysis of new data, and further analysis of existing data, were supported by the following funds: HD-01136 to the Institute of Child Development, University of Minnesota; HD-05027 and NSF P2BI389 to the Center for Research in Human Learning, University of Minnesota; the Grant Foundation; the Graduate School of the University of Minnesota; and NIH-RR-267 to the Health Computer Sciences Facility at the University of Minnesota.

much of mind and experience to begin with the visually naive organism; we collapse the third dimension to deal with contour[2] rather than object; we immobilize the stimulus to deal with contour and pattern rather than event; we deal with "simple" figure and contour to facilitate interpretation. We hope that the approach of the visually naive infant to meaningless, simple, stationary, two-dimensional visual contour, figure, and pattern will provide intelligible information regarding some of the most basic "givens" and early development of human visual perception.

II. THEORIES OF PERCEPTUAL LEARNING AND DEVELOPMENT

Although few major perceptual theorists have directly investigated infant perception, many have indicated that there are innate factors in visual perception, and most have discussed the nature of perceptual learning. We shall consider some of these theories with three foci in mind: (1) The extent to which the organization of perception is innately given; (2) the relative potency of focal versus peripheral processing of pattern; (3) the extent to which motor components enter into the definition of the visual stimulus.

A. Innate Organization in Perception

One finds every conceivable variation of innate capacity assigned to the human newborn by major perceptual theorists. The Gestalt

---

[2] For the purposes of this chapter the following working definitions are adopted:

Visual stimulus:	Any discharge in the retina discriminable by the subject.
Surface:	Any visual stimulus on which a determinate (in terms of accommodation and convergence) fixation point is possible.
Contour or feature:	Any perceptible brightness transition resulting from a steep gradient of light intensity.
Figure or shape:	A contour(s) defining a figure–ground relationship.
Form:	A three-dimensional figure.
Object:	A form with certain qualities, namely, tangibility and graspability.
Configuration or pattern:	Any arrangement of more than one contour, feature, figure, form, or object. Such an arrangement may result in a superordinate contour, figure, or form.

school proposes extensive innate organization in perception. D. O. Hebb and J. Hochberg, on the other hand, maintain that the spatial organization and identities of even simple figures and patterns must be laboriously learned. Most other theories lie determinately or indeterminately between these two extremes.

For the Gestalt school (Helson, 1933; Koehler, 1924, 1959; Koffka, 1935; Rubin, 1958; Wertheimer, 1923) figures are innately perceived as separated from ground. Innate tendencies toward figure–ground, primitive unity, and "good gestalt" or "configuration" sharpen and organize features and distinguish one figure from another, even when figures overlap. A variety of tendencies, for example, good continuation, similarity, proximity, and common fate, allow the innate perception of organizations of contours, figures, forms, and objects as patterns. For the newborn simple figures such as triangles, circles, and squares, whether formed by continuous contour or discrete elements, are perceived as totalities. The task of the infant is not to learn to discriminate, perceive, or organize such patterns, but to learn their significance (Koehler, 1959, p. 114): ". . . given specific entities, with their shapes, readily acquire meanings. But when this happens, these entities are given first, and the meanings attach themselves to such shaped things later." However, some modification of perception by experience is possible even in Gestalt theory (e.g., Zuckerman & Rock, 1957).

Hebb (1937, 1949, 1963, 1968, 1972) represents the opposite extreme,[3] a stance he has maintained in all essentials for more than 25 years. By and large the only perceptual organization granted the visually naive Hebbian newborn is the ability to segregate figure from ground and to assign a global coherence or primitive unity to the elements or contour features of this segregated entity. According to Hebb the human newborn confronted with a simple figure, for example a triangle, would perceive: (1) an "amorphous mass" on a ground, and (2) clearly only those pattern features lying in or near the fovea, or a slightly more extended central region of the retina, the macula. Pattern features stimulating the peripheral retina would not be clearly perceived or given much representation in the cortical areas (peristriate and temporal) believed by him to be involved in visual memory. Peripheral features would only excite

---

[3] However, it should be kept in mind that Hebb has clearly indicated (1949, pp. 17–37) much agreement with the Gestalt position regarding innate "figural unity"; his disagreement lies much more with their emphasis on the immediate perception of "figural identity."

visual sensory cortex (area 17) and cortical eye fields in the frontal lobes to influence the direction of the next macular or foveal fixation.

The relationships among central and peripheral vision, saccadic investigation, and perceptual learning will be discussed more fully in later sections. For our purposes here, it is only important to delineate Hebb's building blocks of perception beyond the immediate detection of "amorphous masses" in the visual field. In 1949 little in the way of receptive field mapping had been reported for the visual sensory system. Hebb (1949, pp. 80–84, 97) speculated that straight lines and angles might be the basic units of visual pattern sensation, with horizontal lines or edges perhaps unusually predominant. Any line portion or angle falling on the macula would result in distinctive sensory discharge in the striate cortex and would be given unique representation in a neural circuit (cell assembly) in cortical areas for memory (association cortex). Line or angle segments in the peripheral retina would be given little representation in association cortex. However, on the basis of their density and distribution *qua* angles and lines, they would excite visual motor cortex to determine the distance and direction of the next eye movement. These motor excitations toward eye movement would be stored as an indication of the spatial distribution of peripheral features of the stimulus. For Hebb, then, a simple figure is, at first, an "amorphous mass" with primitive unity. Any appreciation of its specific features and their arrangement is usually possible only by means of temporally contiguous motor and macular investigation of the edges and angles comprising the figure.

On the basis of stabilized retinal image experiments by Pritchard, Heron, and Hebb (1960), and on the basis of research on the neurophysiology of the visual system (Hubel & Wiesel, 1968), Hebb has twice since publication of his 1949 volume reiterated his view that the perception of simple figures and configurations is based on the sensorimotor integration of simple features or elements (Hebb, 1963, 1968). To date he has not attempted to integrate the full wealth of the literature on visual neurophysiology into his theorizing, but one may question whether this is crucial (as we shall do later in Section III-D-1).

Like the Gestalt school, Michotte (Michotte, Thines, & Crabbe, 1964) proposes innate perceptual tendencies to perceive simple figures as unified and continuous, particularly those undergoing occlusion. Bower (e.g., 1965, 1967a, 1974) shares this view and has attempted to demonstrate such perceptual tendencies in very young human infants. Although in theory the Gestalt–Michotte tendencies should hold for two- as well as for three-dimensional stimuli, Bower (1974) indicates that they may, in general, hold only in the three-dimensional case during early infancy.

For the Gibsons (E. J. Gibson, 1969; J. J. Gibson, 1950, 1951, 1966), especially J. J. Gibson, the naive human infant apparently perceives at least some of the structure that exists in stimulation from the visual world, structure such as surface texture, transitions in surface texture, and/or some of the distinctive features of objects. However, it is sometimes difficult to extract from Gibsonian theory what is learned and what is innate in two-dimensional perception. For J. J. Gibson the ability to perceive as different (but not necessarily to name the differences) *simple* two-dimensional figures on a ground, with appreciation of contour features and their arrangement, is apparently immediate without experience (J. J. Gibson, 1950, pp. 216–220). However, the perception of depth, e.g., depth at an edge, and the perception of the constancies may be innate and immediate, but may require three-dimensional information, e.g., motion or binocular parallax. Very relevant to the two-dimensional case is the Gibsonian notion of "distinctive features" or differentiation. Apparently, recognition, discrimination, and classification, at least of complex visual stimuli, is often accomplished by means of an investigatory-comparison process by the infant (or adult) whereby features and their arrangements within and among stimuli, initially unidentified, become perceived (E. J. Gibson, 1969; Gibson & Gibson, 1955). It would appear that the naive human infant may immediately perceive simple two-dimensional figures comprised of closed, external contour as organized and distinct. For complicated shapes, however, or shapes with internal features, perceptual learning may be necessary. This interpretation is reinforced by E. J. Gibson's treatment of the human infant's learning of faces (E. J. Gibson, 1969, pp. 347–356).

The ethologists (e.g., Hess, 1970; Lorenz, 1965; Tinbergen, 1948; Tinbergen & Perdeck, 1951) propose a good deal of innate organization in perception. Certain visual configurations are held to innately release certain responses (innate releasing mechanisms). For many such stimuli, however, perceptual learning may also be involved. For example, a number of stimulus elements, each innately but separately effective, may become organized through experience to release a response only when presented together in a certain arrangement (Klopfer, 1962). Bower (1966) has extended the perceptual learning aspect of this approach into human infancy. There has not been much success, however, in finding specific, innately "known" configurational releasers in the human infant, although some attempts have been made (Ahrens, 1954; Fantz, 1958, 1961, 1963; Hershenson, 1964; Spitz & Wolf, 1946).

Neisser is somewhat vague about the innate in visual perception, but appears to take an intermediate stance. He explicitly refuses to deal with the question of perceptual development (Neisser, 1967, p. 95). However, he slips from this resolve occasionally, as when he discusses whether feature detectors are learned or innate (pp. 77–85). His model proposes perceptual learning such that an increasing number of hierarchically organized operators may be brought to bear on a stimulus array. However, the "innate" operators are not clearly specified.

Some computer simulation theorists have specifically tried to deal with perceptual learning (e.g., Dodwell, 1964, 1970; see Uhr, 1963 for a general review). Perceptual learning in such systems may involve, for example, either the changing of the dominance of operators as in the case of an *n*-tuple system with storage (Roberts, 1960; Uhr & Vossler, 1961), or the selection of invariants and the grouping of temporally contiguous stimuli, as in Uttley's (1958) conditional probability store. Most simulation theories include both operators that detect local and those that detect global features of a two-dimensional figure (e.g., Deutsch, 1960; Dodwell, 1964; Sutherland, 1973). Thus, information about area, relationships among features, symmetry (Sutherland, 1973, p. 175), albedo, perimeter, total contour, number of contour transitions, and whether the figure is open or closed may be extracted, in addition to the presence of particular features such as an angle or a curved line. Computer simulation theorists have not been particularly successful in dealing with more elaborate processing, such as the perception of multiple, overlapping shapes, although there have been some successes (e.g., Guzman, 1968; Minksy & Pappert, 1969). Recent simulation has maintained the commitment of taking into account the neurophysiology as well as the psychophysics of the visual system (see Barlow, Narasimhan, & Rosenfeld, 1972 for an excellent review). However, this literature has not placed many specific constraints on the properties of learned versus unlearned operators in early human visual perception, nor has it devoted much thought to investigative processes in perceptual learning (Gyr, Brown, Willey, & Zivian, 1966), with some exceptions (e.g., King, 1971).

Russian motor copy theorists (Zaporozhets, 1965; Zaporozhets & Zinchenko, 1966; Zinchenko, 1967; see Pick, 1964 for a review) appear to approximate Hebb with respect to the innate in pattern perception. Although they have not specified innate figure and pattern operators as explicitly as Hebb, it would appear that they view perception as only minimally organized at birth. Figures appear to be segregated from ground at birth and have some coherence on the basis of primitive unity; and features are detected, especially if macularly fixated. But the organization of features into figure and pattern is usually accomplished only via sensorimotor investigation. Hochberg (1968, 1970, 1971a, b) shares a similar view, indicating further that even the perception of figure and ground in some instances may depend on visual investigation, rather than being immediately given.

B.   Focal and Peripheral Processing

The notion of more intensive processing of events in some circumscribed focal region of the visual field versus a more global, less acute, more automatic, or qualitatively dissimilar processing of events in peripheral regions has been and remains a popular concern in many theories of perceptual learning or development. It has been strangely neglected in other theories. The focal visual field has often been assumed to be almost isomorphic with the macular, foveal, or central visual field for an actively looking observer (e.g., Hebb, 1949; Hochberg, 1968, 1970; Sanders, 1963; Trevarthen, 1968). However, this is not necessary for all theories that distinguish between focal and peripheral processing (e.g., Neisser, 1967), since the senses and causes of "focal" are multiple. Hebb (1949) points to the markedly higher acuity values in the macula versus peripheral retina and to the inordinate representation of the macula in visual sensory cortex (among other things) in order to propose that *only* macular or near-central features in the visual field are acutely perceived and encoded; pattern features on the peripheral retina lead mainly toward motor tendencies to localize blurred peripheral features. Hochberg (1968, 1970) is close to this view, similarly positing that extramacular features are very poorly resolved by the sensory system. Perceptual learning of the specific features of an extended novel figure by an infant would necessarily involve for both Hebb and Hochberg successive exposure of the spatially extended figural features to the central retina.

A somewhat different, but not mutually exclusive, basis for "focal" processing is emphasized by Neisser (1967) and by other attentional theories, for example, those of Broadbent (1958, 1970, 1971), Sperling (1960, 1963, 1967), Atkinson and Shiffrin (1968), Norman (1970), Posner (1969), and Treisman (1969). Haber and Hershenson (1973), Moray (1970), and Mostofsky (1970) provide representative reviews of such theories. In whatever guise, attentional theories stress that "focal," conscious processing is typically directed toward only one region of the retina or visual field, or toward only one attribute or a limited number of attributes (e.g., color versus form, physical structure versus meaning) of a stimulus in a particular region of the visual field at a time. Consequently, thresholds for peripheral stimuli are elevated (e.g., Mackworth, 1965), or peripheral stimuli are processed by unconscious automatic mechanisms (e.g., the preattentive process proposed by Neisser).

Figure 3.1 is a flow chart constructed by Haber and Hershenson (1973, p. 162) to illustrate some of the stages of attentional or information-processing models in general, including their own. It is very instructive for our purposes in a number of respects. First, the information that enters brief visual or iconic storage is drawn from all areas of the retina, limited only by the structure of the retina and by receptive fields in the central nervous system. Second, to be

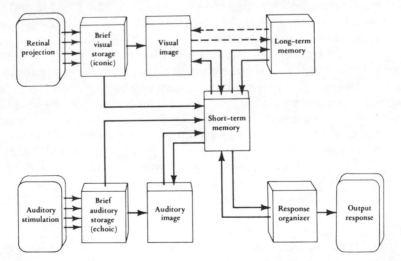

Figure 3.1   An information-processing model illustrating the more important stages, storages, processes, and channels. [From R. N. Haber & M. Hershenson, *The psychology of visual perception*, 1973. Reprinted by permission of Holt, Rinehart & Winston, Inc.]

transferred into long-term memory, iconic information is typically processed through short-term memory. This processing is apparently very much influenced by what is in long-term memory (allowing set and reconstruction; cf. Haber, 1966), is limited in the number of items that may be processed at any time, and apparently, in adults, very much involves some form of rehearsal probably making use of an acoustic code. Finally, Haber and Hershenson leave open the possibility that visual *images*, formed from the icon, may be transferred into long-term memory without being processed via short-term memory. We shall consider the implications for the infant of such models of visual processing in Section III-D-2. For the moment, however, it may be stressed that higher attentional and memorial processes, rather than purely sensory factors, appear to receive the most stress as determinants of pattern processing in information models.

The focal line of sight is typically coincident with the foveal line of sight, i.e., we normally look directly at what interests us most. However, it need not be so, especially in the adult who can voluntarily inhibit an eye movement to focally attend to an event on the peripheral retina. For example, an adult may deliberately look off target in order to maximize detection of a faint star in the night sky. Nevertheless, it should be noted that Neisser, like Hebb and Hochberg, indicates that learning of a novel configuration extended in space involves at least shifts of focal, if not macular, attention from feature to feature.

Most other theories of perceptual development either ignore or are rather nonspecific regarding focal or macular versus peripheral processing of pattern. One suspects that the Russians (e.g., Zaporozhets & Zinchenko, 1966), Piaget (1969; Piaget & Vinh-Bang, 1961), E. J. Gibson (1969), and Jeffrey (1968), among others, with their emphasis on investigative activity, subscribe to such a view. But whether it is a sensory, an attentional, or even a necessary aspect of perceptual learning is unclear. Others such as J. J. Gibson, T. G. R. Bower, and most computer simulation theorists tend to ignore the general issue.

C. Oculomotor Involvement in Perceptual Learning

The role of investigative or oculomotor activity in perceptual learning receives most stress in theories that assign particular importance to the notion of focal or macular attention; if there is a circumscribed region of the visual field that is more acute in pattern processing, either in terms of visual acuity, attention, or encoding, then the features of at least novel figures or patterns extended in space may have to be examined or processed sequentially if local details and their spatial arrangement are to be learned. However, the proposed relationship among perceptual investigation, perceptual learning, and eye movements varies widely among perceptual theories, even among those subscribing to some concept of focal attention. It is possible to find any one of the following alternatives, or some combination of them, stressed in any one theory of perceptual learning and/or development:

1. The global properties as well as the local features (and their arrangements) of figures and patterns distributed broadly across the retina are perceived and processed with equal facility without eye movements.

2. Whether because of the pronounced acuity of the fovea and its inordinate representation in visual cortex, or whether because of attentional focalizing, figures or patterns extending into the peripheral visual field must be investigated sequentially, either by means of changes in the line of sight or via attentional shifts in processing.

3. Shifts in line of sight, whether actual eye movements or unexecuted efferent commands to eye movements, are not only a typical but also a *necessary* accompaniment to the learning of novel spatially distributed patterns. (This is the case since it is the motor aspect of the eye movement system that "tags" peripheral features in terms of their direction and distance from the current line of sight and thus spatially relates features one to another. Somehow these motor tendencies are stored along with purely sensory aspects of the stimulus during perceptual learning.)

4. Eye movements or tendencies toward eye movements are not a *necessary accompaniment* to perceptual learning, although they may be a typical accompaniment. However, they are a *necessary consequence* of such learning.

Hebb is most explicit and most demanding regarding the necessary role of eye movements during the naive organism's learning of a novel visual stimulus. He maintains that the novel visual stimulus on the retinal surface is segregated into a figure (amorphous mass) on a ground on the basis of primitive unity. Only features falling on or near the macula are distinctively processed in visual cortex and stored in visual areas involved in memory (areas beyond area 17, e.g., areas 18, 19, and temporal cortex) to become "knowledge" of the stimulus. However, local stimulus features on the peripheral retina are not without their effect. Via unknown pathways peripheral events stimulate motor cortex (involving transmission from area 17 to the frontal eye fields), resulting in a motor tendency or specific excitation to execute a particular saccade. The choice of next macular fixation is primarily determined by peripheral stimulation, and the saccadic, peripheral localizing system that is aroused is *spatially accurate and probably innate.* Moreover, Hebb hypothesizes that the motor excitation regarding the size and direction of a saccade from one local feature to another is stored in memory in conjunction with the retinal information from each macular fixation. Because of the fixed spatial relationship among features of a particular figure, the probability of temporally contiguous fixations among features of the figure is high. Thus, since both sensory and motor excitations are stored during each eye movement and fixation, and since temporally contiguous excitations become associated in memory, the subject comes to expect or visualize other learned features when a given local known feature is being fixated. Further he expects features aroused in memory to be in a particular spatial distribution with respect to the feature on the macula, since storage included tendencies toward specific saccades toward peripheral features.

Hebb proposes in detail how such a process enters into visual imagery and memory, how part and whole of a configuration are alternately perceived, how eye fixations become more and more indeterminate on a stimulus as learning proceeds (because of the summed arousal of many stored motor excitations), how a brief glimpse of a known stimulus can result in recognition (because stored sensory and motor excitations are aroused), and how superordinate percepts (the constancies and generalizations) are formed through experience. However, for our purposes it is most important to note that, for Hebb, eye movement excitations and their stored representation are necessary for the initial perceptual *learning* of the spatial arrangement of the features, outline or internal, comprising a shape or form (Hebb, 1949, pp. 84–87).

Festinger (1971; Festinger & Canon, 1965; Festinger & Easton, 1974; Festinger, Burnham, Ono, & Bamber, 1967), the Russian investigators we have cited, Piaget (1952, pp. 62–76, 1962; see Cunningham, 1972, for a clear comparison of Hebb and Piaget), and Noton and Stark (1971) appear to share some of Hebb's demand for estimation and storage of the spatial distribution of a stimulus via some involvement of the oculomotor system.

Other theorists are either not as demanding (E. J. Gibson, 1969;

Hochberg, 1968) or not as explicit (J. J. Gibson, 1950, 1966; Neisser, 1967) regarding the *necessary* role of actual or intended eye movements and their stored representation during the learning of a simple figure by the *visually naive* human organism. All, however, would grant that there is usually some processing primacy of the fovea, and that eye movements typically accompany such learning. At least two would further argue that whether or not actual eye movements are necessary and actually occur during perceptual learning, at any rate, when learning is complete, eye movement tendencies, if not actual eye movements, are involved as part of the learned definition of the stimulus and are in evidence during recall and visual imagery (Neisser, 1967, pp. 153–154; Hochberg, 1970, p. 114):

> What I shall argue is that (a) the mature observer has a vocabulary of sequential visuomotor expectancies (e.g., "If I look along this edge to the left, I will see a corner concave to the right"), and that some of these expectancies . . . span a small period of time, and space, whereas others . . . span longer intervals of time and require multiple spatial fixations to encompass; (b) the perception of form over multiple fixations demands active looking . . . and it is the plan for such active looking-and-testing that is stored over successive fixations, not the myriad details that are glimpsed with each independent fixation; (c) . . . the structure or organization of visuomotor expectancies provides the basis for the selective perception of visual form [Hochberg, 1970, p. 114].

Hochberg, and perhaps Neisser and the Gibsons, may agree that eye movements typically accompany perceptual learning of spatially distributed stimuli, and that visuomotor expectancies eventually become part of the "definition" of the stimulus and are evidenced during recall and imagery. There is nothing in their theories, however, demanding that actual eye movements *must* be made *during* learning or that the efferent (or afferent) signals from eye movements are stored as part of the image.

III. LINES OF EVIDENCE PARTICULARLY RELEVANT TO INNATE ORGANIZATION, FOCAL PROCESSING, AND OCULOMOTOR INVOLVEMENT IN PERCEPTUAL LEARNING AND DEVELOPMENT

A variety of data have accumulated, especially in recent years, which bear at least indirectly on the issues we have raised. In this section we shall deal with data from animals and human adults.

Later we shall consider the relevance of these data for the visual perception of the human infant.

A. Innate Organization in Perception

1. ANIMAL STUDIES AND NEUROPHYSIOLOGICAL DATA

Single unit recordings from the visual cortex of a variety of organisms have indicated that the receptive fields of these cells are maximally responsive to particular spatial distributions of light on the retina. Representative recent reviews of this literature from both animals and humans are provided by Sekuler (1974), Brown (1973), McIlwain (1972), Leibowitz and Harvey (1973), Brooks and Jung (1973), recent volumes of the *Handbook of Sensory Physiology*, and the *Report of the U.S.–Australian Canberra Symposium on Vision*. These data make it clear that in most higher mammals investigated, cortical units may be maximally receptive to a particular orientation, spatial frequency or shape or feature or size, motion, or color of light falling on the retina. Further, the size of the receptive fields of cortical units generally increases from central to peripheral retina (Hubel & Wiesel, 1959, 1962, 1968).

In general it appears that many geniculate and cortical units for contour coding, although sluggish or immature, are present at or very shortly following birth (e.g., Hubel & Wiesel, 1963, 1965; Wiesel & Hubel, 1965a,b; but see Barlow & Pettigrew, 1971, for some reservations on this matter). However, a rapidly increasing accumulation of evidence indicates that: (1) both binocular and monocular units underlying detection of specific stimulus properties only develop or continue to develop on the basis of appropriate visual experience shortly following birth; (2) there is a direct relationship between development of these units and detection of the contour in question; (3) these effects vary with species. For example, kittens reared from birth until 5 months with exposure only to horizontal or vertical stripes provide (a) electrophysiological evidence of cortical units receptive to only horizontal or vertical stripes, respectively, and (b) appear behaviorally blind to vertical or horizontal contour, respectively (Blakemore & Cooper, 1970). Even within a single kitten both effects may be obtained by allowing only horizontal input to one eye and only vertical to the other (Hirsch & Spinnelli, 1970). Similarly, kittens raised with exposure only to spots of light develop mainly simple, atypical cortical cells for light spots, and few units whose receptive fields are maximally sensitive to extended contour (Pettigrew & Freeman, 1973). These experiments indicate that an early interaction of age by experience can affect the quality of cortical units developed, and that the development of such units has implications for perceptual discrimination. (But see Hirsch, 1972, for qualifications on this latter matter.) Finally, receptive field properties of the striate cortex of the rabbit, unlike those of the cat, do not appear to be similarly affected by early visual deprivation (Mize & Murphy, 1973), underscoring the need for careful generalization from species to species.

Binocular cortical units are also dependent on early visual experience. If early, appropriate binocular input is prevented, normal neurophysiological and psychophysical binocular processes are not later evidenced (Dews & Wiesel, 1970; Guillery, 1974; Guillery & Kaas, 1971; Hubel & Wiesel, 1970, 1971; Wiesel & Hubel, 1965a,b; von Noorden, Dowling, & Ferguson, 1970).

2. DATA FROM HUMAN ADULTS

There are sufficient psychophysical and electrophysiological data from humans to conclude that the human visual system processes pattern in a fashion similar to that suggested by the neurophysiological and psychophysical research on cortical and subcortical units in other mammals. The general references cited in Section III-A-1 provide relevant summaries.

Research conducted within an adaptation, or masking (e.g., Weisstein, 1969) framework has provided compelling support for the notion that *postretinal* visual processing is accomplished via contour-specific detectors. Campbell and Kulikowski (1972) demonstrated that a sinusoidal masking grating has its strongest masking effect the more similar it is in orientation to a sinusoidal grating being masked. McCollough (1965) demonstrated that such orientation-specific grating detectors may be color-coded. Andrews (1967a,b) indicated that such linear units are binocular, orientation-specific, most acute near the horizontal and vertical meridians, and hierarchically arranged with foveal receptive fields of about 9 min of arc. Other researchers have provided confirming evidence of an increase in size of receptive fields of cortical units with increasing distance from the fovea (e.g., Evans, 1967; Markoff & Sturr, 1971; Mayzner & Tresselt, 1969). It has also been recently suggested and debated whether cortical units specifically tuned for circular contour may be present, in addition to units maximally responsive to linear contour (Riggs, 1973, 1974; Stromeyer, 1974). Finally, there has been a considerable attempt to explain psychophysical data on pattern perception in terms of a limited number of channels, each maximally sensitive to a limited range of spatial frequencies, and/or, further, to describe such visual processing in terms of Fourier analysis (Blakemore & Campbell, 1969; Blakemore, Nachmias, & Sutton, 1970; Campbell et al., 1968; Campbell & Robson, 1968; Graham, 1972; Graham & Nachmias, 1971; Maffei & Fiorentini, 1972; Pantle & Sekuler, 1968; Pollen, Lee, & Taylor, 1971; Sachs, Nachmias, & Robson, 1971).

Electrophysiological, clinical, and "developmental" observations are generally compatible with the hypothesis that the human visual system processes pattern in a fashion similar to other higher mammals. Recordings of visually evoked cortical potentials reflect spatial frequency, orientation, and contrast parameters (Campbell & Kulikowski, 1972; Freeman, Mitchell, & Millodot, 1972; Freeman & Thibos, 1973; Marg & Adams, 1970; Marg, Adams, & Rutkin, 1968; Riggs, 1969; see also Chapter 2 by Karmel and Maisel in this volume, and a summary chapter by MacKay & Jeffreys, 1973). Bodis-Wollner (1972) has reported that patients with cerebral lesions show changes in their contrast sensitivity functions in ways consistent with a multiple channel spatial frequency model of visual processing. It has also been shown that astigmatic subjects exhibit neural deficits in response to certain stimulus orientations (Freeman et al., 1972; Freeman & Thibos, 1973; Mitchell, Freeman, Millodot, & Haegerstrom, 1973). Since astigmatic subjects were optically deprived of contour in particular orientations since infancy, and since the meridional amblyopia observed was strongly related to degree of astigmatism, these findings suggest that normal development of neural cells for the detection of contour in particular orientations may be dependent on early visual experience in humans as in other mammals. Fiorentini, Ghez, and Maffei (1972a,b) have demonstrated similar short-term neural adaptations in humans wearing dove prisms for 4–7 days. Recent observations of humans with a history of corrected or uncorrected deprivation of binocular vision (for example, corneal opacities, cataracts, or strabismus) are providing increasingly convincing evidence that neural units underlying binocular vision are dependent on early visual experience (Aslin & Banks, 1975; von Noorden, 1972; Taylor, 1974). Finally, there has been a recent systematic attempt to describe the contrast sensitivity function of the young human infant

(Atkinson, Braddick, & Braddick, 1974). More studies of this kind will soon allow a more exact comparison of infant and adult visual processing.

Studies employing stabilized retinal images similarly suggest that cortical units maximally responsive to specific distributions of contour on the retina may exist in humans (see Zusne, 1970, pp. 29–34, and Heckenmueller, 1965, for reviews of this literature). Apparently, there are marked consistencies in the manner in which fading and reappearance of fragments and wholes of meaningful and meaningless stabilized patterns occur. One must be cautious in interpreting this literature, however, since there is considerable controversy as to whether artifactual slippage of the "stabilized" image with respect to the retina may be in large part the cause of the effects obtained (Cornsweet, 1970, p. 408; Cosgrove, Schmidt, Fulgham, & Brown, 1972, pp. 401–402; Haber & Hershenson, 1973, pp. 182–183).

There remains far from good agreement on how best to characterize the visual processing systems of higher mammals, including man. For example, it is unknown to what extent the system is serial and hierarchical versus parallel. The "top" of the system is not clear, i.e., there may be other levels or types of cortical units to be discovered beyond the most complex ones described. It is not even clear how to best describe a cell's receptive field, given that many forms of input can excite it and many interactions with other fields are possible. Whether to speak of the system as consisting of a fixed number of spatial frequency channels, or whether to consider it, in addition, a feature (e.g., orientation) detecting system is unsettled. Finally, many of these characterizations may hold differently for threshold versus suprathreshold stimuli; Sekuler (1974) discusses such issues with remarkable clarity. However, for our purposes we shall consider the human visual system as performing a pattern analysis in a fashion generally similar to that described to this point in other higher mammals.

3. BLIND HUMANS RESTORED TO SIGHT

The literature on the immediate perception, discrimination, recognition, and identification of shapes by human congenitally blind (presumably) patients who have been later restored to sight sheds little conclusive light on the "givens" of shape perception. Von Senden (1960) and Gregory and Wallace (1963) summarize such cases. The von Senden report is a compendium of published cataract removal cases from approximately 1020 A.D. to the date of his original report (1932). It appears from these case histories that the perception of figure–ground or figural unity is immediately possible following cataract removal. Although there is some indication that same–different judgments between two objects presented simultaneously side by side was immediately possible for some patients, the patients appeared to have considerable difficulty in pointing out what the differences were. Further, identification (naming) of single objects appeared to develop very slowly, i.e., over weeks or months. Many of the von Senden histories, however, are sketchy and, consequently, it is difficult to draw firm conclusions regarding immediate capacities upon cataract removal. Even Hebb and J. J. Gibson differ in the conclusions they draw from the reports (J. J. Gibson, 1950, pp. 28–37; Hebb, 1949, pp. 216–220).

The Gregory and Wallace history is of a single individual, blind from approximately 10 months of age, and restored to sight at approximately 50 years of age. It is a very well-documented and well-designed study. Within a few days or weeks the patient was able to tell time from a wall clock, identify a wide variety of objects and shapes, for example, upper case letters and numerals, and even draw certain objects, for example, a bus. But he had great difficulty in recognizing lower case letters, and in learning to read. Close examination of his immediate abilities indicates that he was generally visually proficient with objects or their replicas that he had handled extensively while blind, e.g., he had handled a clock without a cover, three-dimensional capital letters and numerals, parts of a bus, etc. Apparently, tactual experience with shape plus an adult mental age enabled a great deal of transfer from touch to vision. However, we cannot but concur strongly with Zusne (1970, p. 376) who concludes:

> The case of S.B. is the best documented clinical case of vision gained in adulthood, and it does not confirm the slow identification learning rates reported by von Senden. It also throws doubt on the usefulness of adult clinical cases in making inferences about form perception in human infants. While some aspects of the initial stages of form perception may be similar, the differences between an immature and a mature nervous system, an intact and a damaged visual system, and, most important of all, between a totally inexperienced individual and an adult who has had all the experiences of adulthood with the exception of visual ones, are too great to allow anything but the simplest kind of analogy to be drawn.

B. Focal and Peripheral Processing

1. STRUCTURAL AND PSYCHOPHYSICAL CONSIDERATIONS

a. *The ocular media.*   Most structures in the human visual system appear to promote greatest acuity in the fovea or central retina. Figure 3.2 provides a schematic diagram of the most external structure of the visual system, the human eye. Selective absorption of light by the ocular media (the cornea, aqueous and vitreous humors, and the crystalline lens) render these media a cutoff filter for light, especially for short wavelengths. The cornea and lens appear to be most responsible for this light loss, with selective absorption apparently increasing with age (see Ruddock, 1972, for a recent review; also Chapter 1 by Maurer in this volume).

In the ideal case both the cornea and the crystalline lens refract

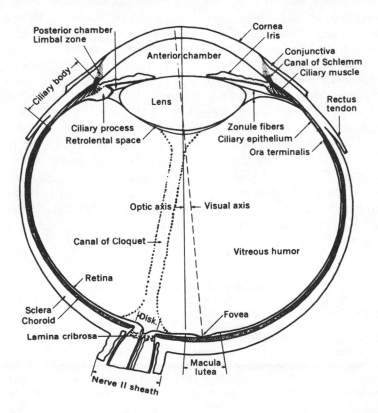

Figure 3.2   Horizontal section of the right human eyeball. [From Walls, 1942.]

light to converge emmetropically on the retina. The cornea (actually the aphakic eye) provides most (approximately +43 D) of the refractive power of the eye, while the crystalline lens provides approximately +19.1 D. The amplitude of accommodation of the lens is approximately 14 D at 10 years of age and decreases steadily with age to become a range of only 1–0 D by age 60 (Hamasaki, Ong, & Marg, 1956; Weale, 1962).

The effective lens of the reduced eye is both thick and imperfect. Thus, even when the lens of the normal eye is appropriately accommodated for a point source falling on the fovea, i.e., only 4°–5° from the optic axis, spherical and chromatic aberration, diffraction, scatter, coma, and astigmatism make the image on the fovea a blur circle rather than a point.[4] However, although there is some evidence that correction of some of these errors can improve acuity, the visual system is capable of sharpening and tolerating a reasonable amount of such blur, for example ± 0.25 D. Therefore, for stimuli that are well above threshold (such as we are generally discussing in this chapter), these errors are not serious for foveally fixated targets (Davson, 1972, pp. 618–621).

On the other hand, for peripheral targets in the visual field that are *not* close to the optic axis, e.g., that are 20° or more from the fovea, far more serious refractive errors occur even if they are at the same distance from the eye. This is because the marginal rays from a peripheral point source are not brought to a single point of focus on the retina because of the oblique, asymmetrical manner in which they meet and are refracted by the optical system. Therefore, in addition to being degraded by the same factors as blur the images of points near the optic axis, peripheral targets are greatly and variably degraded by the optical errors of coma, astigmatism, and distortion. These errors are both theoretically (Le Grand, 1967) and refractometrically (Ferree, Rand, & Hardy, 1931) considerable enough to affect acuity increasingly for increasingly peripheral targets, for example, for the peripheral features of figures extending beyond 20° into the peripheral visual field. Moreover, they vary widely from individual to individual, and within individuals nonuniformly with eccentricity (H. Leibowitz, personal communication).

In theory, then, refractive properties of the ocular media may place constraints on peripheral acuity, quite apart from retinal and

---

[4] The reader may consult Davson (1972, Section V, pp. 527–626) and Cornsweet (1970, pp. 56–57, *passim*) for recent, more explicit explanations of the optical errors here discussed, and for details regarding their implications for visual acuity.

postretinal structures in the visual system. There is some suggestion that this is the psychophysical case. Leibowitz, Johnson, and
Isabelle (1972) employed retinoscopy to determine refractive error
to eccentricities up to 80°. They then determined threshold for the
detection of peripheral motion both with and without correction for
the refractive errors found. Figure 3.3 illustrates motion detection
thresholds under each condition. It may be seen that, prior to
correction, there existed large individual differences in peripheral
refractive error and in threshold for the detection of peripheral
motion and a sharp increase in threshold for motion from central to
peripheral vision. Following lens correction of peripheral refractive
error, individual differences and peripheral motion thresholds decreased dramatically.[5] Leibowitz *et al.* (1972) suggest that motion
detection in the periphery is largely dioptrically rather than reti-

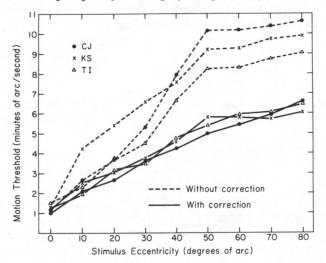

Figure 3.3.   Motion thresholds as a function of stimulus eccentricity with and
without correction for peripheral refractive error. [From H. W. Leibowitz, C. A.
Johnson, & E. Isabelle, Peripheral motion detection and refractive error. *Science,*
1972, *177,* 1207. Copyright 1972 by the American Association for the Advancement
of Science.]

    [5] Lamont and Millodot (1973) originally criticized these findings, claiming that the
Leibowitz *et al.* (1972) refractive error values for the periphery were at variance with
values predicted by LeGrand (1967) and Ferree, Rand, and Hardy (1931), and too low
to produce the psychophysical effects obtained in some cases. Lamont and Millodot
suggested that either the retinoscopic technique, or training effects, produced the
Leibowitz *et al.* results. Recently, however, Leibowitz and Millodot have conducted a
collaborative study, and have obtained results entirely congruent with the original
Leibowitz *et al.* (1972) findings (Leibowitz, personal communication).

nally limited, i.e., that the peripheral *retina* is structurally capable of better detection of motion than psychophysically indicated, but that the optical properties of the eye anterior to the retinal receptors degrade peripheral vision. This apparently is not true, however, for the resolution of static pattern. The acuity threshold for a stationary Landolt C, or for a stationary square wave grating, is much lower in the fovea than in the periphery, and correction of peripheral refractive error does not appreciably decrease threshold in the peripheral field.[6]

The implication of the findings with moving targets is that processing of motion by the peripheral retina is more acute than the optics of the ocular media, perhaps accomplished via subcortical centers (e.g., perhaps the superior colliculus), and usually better in the fovea because of the optical properties of the cornea and lens. Thresholds for fine pattern detail, on the other hand, are lower for central than for peripheral vision apparently because of the structure of retinal and postretinal receptive fields rather than because of limiting central and peripheral optical properties of the ocular media, *given the normal positioning of the fine-grained fovea close to the optical axis of the eye.*

b. *The retina and central visual system.*   From the retina upwards there is little question that the visual system is designed to resolve fine pattern detail more acutely in the central retina, or macula, than in the periphery. Receptors for light are distributed over the entire retina, but they are denser and more slender in the macula than in the periphery (Figure 3.4). Cones, primarily concerned with the detection of color and contour under photopic conditions, are much more numerous in the macula (Figure 3.5). Rods, primarily concerned with the detection of brightness (intensity), are more numerous extrafoveally. In the region of the macula it may be seen (in Figure 3.4) that neural layers of the retina, through which light must pass *before* striking rods and cones, are displaced and thinner allowing more optimal optical transmission to foveal cones. Macular pigmentation in the foveal retinal layers may also sharpen acuity by acting as a selective filter and decreasing chromatic aberration (Reading & Weale, 1974). The Stiles-Crawford effect (Crawford, 1972; Stiles & Crawford, 1933) is observed by which the effective-

---

[6] These findings were originally obtained by H. Leibowitz, and confirmed in a second collaborative experiment with M. Millodot (Leibowitz, personal communication).

ness of quanta of light striking the fovea at an angle is attenuated, probably because of a funneling property of the cones or cone pigments (O'Brien, 1951; Cornsweet, 1970, pp. 140–145). Finally, cortical receptive field size increases toward the periphery of the retina in man as in other foveated mammals (Andrews, 1967; Evans, 1967; Hubel & Wiesel, 1968; Mayzner & Tresselt, 1969), and the macula is disproportionately represented (on the basis of its retinal size relative to that of the peripheral retina) in the visual cortex, both anatomically and electrophysiologically (see Riggs & Wooten, 1972, and Whitteridge, 1973, for fuller details on this magnification).

The following psychophysics are in accord with the anatomical features of the visual system. In Figure 3.6 human sensitivity to an

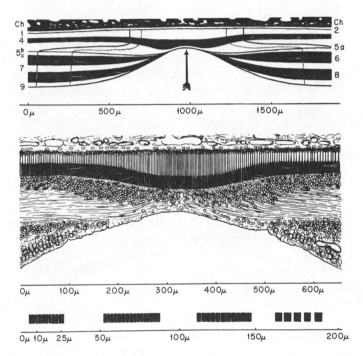

Figure 3.4   Sketch of the central fovea in the human eye. Upper sketch indicates semidiagrammatically, in a vertical section, the shape of the central fovea and the arrangement and thickness of layers. The middle sketch shows the actual structural composition of the deepest portion of the foveal pit. Note the length and thinness of the central cones. Lower sketch shows the relative size and number of cones, from the center of the fovea (left), the slope and edge of the outer fovea, and the periphery of the central area (right). The accompanying scales indicate actual dimensions in microns. [From S. Polyak, *The vertebrate visual system*, Chicago: University of Chicago Press. © 1957 by the University of Chicago Press.]

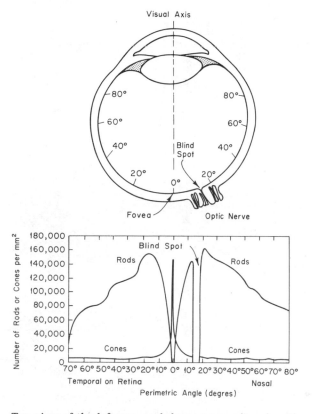

Figure 3.5   Top view of the left eye, and the corresponding densities of rods and cones across the retina. [Adapted from Pirenne, 1967.]

increase in target luminance is plotted as a function of target size and retinal locus for both scotopic (upper plot, a) and photopic (lower plot, b) conditions. Especially to be noted is that under conditions of complete dark adaptation the peripheral retina is much more sensitive to the introduction of a luminance increment regardless of target size. Under photopic conditions (lower plot, d) the fovea is slightly more sensitive to luminance increments than the periphery, but the overall sensitivity of the entire retina to a luminance increment is very poor, i.e., the luminance increment (ΔL) required for detection is vastly greater under photopic than under scotopic conditions. Visual acuity, on the other hand, is much better in the fovea than in the periphery under all conditions. In Figure 3.7, visual acuity, the size of targets necessary for discrimination (ordinate), or the luminance increment of targets from

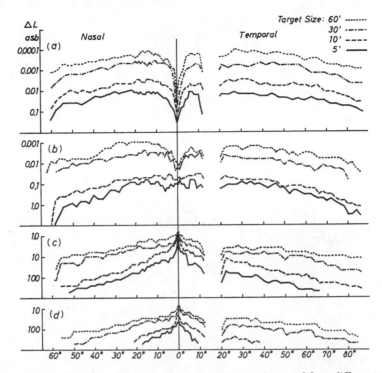

Figure 3.6   Profile perimetry with various target sizes and four different states of adaptation. Abscissa: retinal locus. Ordinate: target luminance ΔL in apostilb (asb). Parameter: target size. (a) Complete dark adaptation. (b) State of adaptation corresponding to .0063 asb background luminance. (c) State of adaptation corresponding to 6.3 asb background luminance. (d) State of adaptation corresponding to 630 asb background luminance. [From Aulhorn & Harms, 1972.]

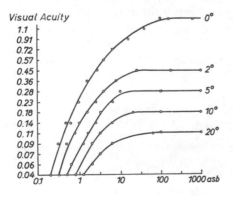

Figure 3.7   Visual acuity in five different retinal regions. Abscissa: test-type luminance ΔL. Ordinate: visual acuity for square circle test. Parameter: investigated retinal region. Background luminance: 10 asb. [From Aulhorn & Harms, 1972.]

background necessary for discrimination (abscissa, ΔL), is indicated for five retinal loci. It is clear that for both measures visual acuity is markedly more sensitive for foveal (0°) than for peripheral, e.g., 20°, vision. Consequently, some investigators (e.g., Alpern, 1962, pp. 4–5; Hebb, 1949, pp. 85–86; Hochberg, 1970, p. 111) have suggested that we view the real well-illuminated world (particularly if unknown) as through a very small window (approximately 3°) of acute vision surrounded by a peripheral visual field in which pattern is largely a blur.

However, it should be made clear that many contour or surface transitions some distance from the fovea are well within acuity limits. For example, a line 5 min wide can be detected 16° from the fovea (Alpern, 1962, p. 4). There should be no difficulty because of acuity alone in accurately detecting a solid figure as large as 25° or more in extent. And, indeed, adults recognize or identify figures entirely in peripheral vision (Collier, 1931; Crannel & Christensen, 1955; Day, 1957; Ferree & Rand, 1931, 1932; Ferree, Rand, & Monroe, 1930; Geissler, 1926; Graefe, 1964; Grindley, 1931; Kleitman & Blier, 1928; Munn & Geil, 1931; Salaman, 1929; Whitmer, 1933). In general these studies indicate that the type of form (e.g., triangle, circle, diamond, square, rectangle, hexagon, or octagon), the size of the form, the contrast of the form, the age of the subject (the younger the better, but no infants or very young children were tested), training, and the duration of presentation affect the extent of the form field, i.e., the eccentric angle at which the form is identified. However, it should be noted that Grindley (1931, pp. 46–47), after demonstrating form discrimination far in the periphery for some large figures at long (e.g., 200-msec) exposures, partially summarizes his findings by stating:

> The present experiments show that peripheral form perception is very much influenced by the observer's past experience of experiments of this kind, by his expectation of the kind of figure likely to be shown, and by the direction of his attention. It seems likely that similar effects occur in other kinds of peripheral perception under difficult conditions; and that even in experiments on such subjects as the peripheral perception of color, movement, or flicker, great care should be taken to control, as far as possible, these psychological factors.

It would appear that pattern perception is possible peripherally, but is far less acute than in central vision, and may be very much constructed on the basis of set, reconstruction, and experience (Haber, 1966; Sanders, 1963). Further, it should be noted that the very young infant cannot use set and reconstruction for the identification of patterns presented peripherally, a point to which we shall later return (Section III-D).

c. *Two visual systems.* The increasing literature on cortical versus subcortical contributions to pattern processing among species has led to a number of paradigms seeking to explain central versus peripheral processing within an evolutionary or comparative framework (Bronson, 1974; Diamond & Hall, 1969; Held, 1968; Humphrey, 1970, 1972; Humphrey & Weiskrantz, 1967; Schneider, 1969; Trevarthen, 1968, in press). Investigations in this area have stressed increasing cortical involvement in pattern discrimination and eye movements, in conjunction with the evolution of foveation. In this section we shall consider foveal and peripheral processing at cortical and subcortical levels; in later sections we shall consider the regulations of eye movements by such centers.

Some have proposed that in the course of vertebrate evolution a *primary visual system*, deeply involving the lateral geniculate, visual cortex, and other cortical areas, has evolved in higher vertebrates, including man, to analyze, encode, recognize, or identify pattern, and to allow the voluntary regulation of eye movements. The *primary visual system* appears particularly to serve the fovea. A more phylogenetically primitive visual system, the *second visual system*, most heavily involving the midbrain superior colliculus, the homologue of the primitive optic tectum, remains in higher vertebrates. The *second visual system* supplies information regarding the location of stimuli, interacts with the *primary visual system* in controlling eye movements, and may be as much or more functional for peripheral as for foveal targets.

Figure 3.8 provides a schematic flow chart of the *primary* and *second visual systems* in man, and the interaction of their neural components, as outlined recently by Bronson (1974). The schematic representation should not be construed as a full description of all visual centers and their directional interactions, but rather as a reduced, simplified picture of some major components and their interactions. According to Bronson the *primary visual system* analyzes and encodes pattern, as well as regulating voluntary eye movements and steady fixation. Retinal stimulation, primarily from the central retina, is analyzed for pattern features by means of a basically hierarchical, receptive field organization in the lateral geniculate and visual cortex. Features such as size, shape, orientation, and direction of movement, regardless of retinal locus, are ultimately extracted. Pattern features are organized and encoded in

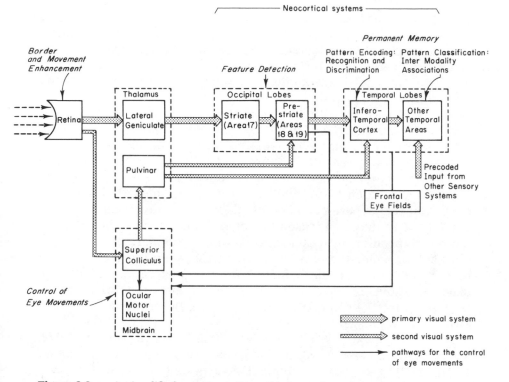

Figure 3.8   A simplified representation of information processing in the human visual system. [Adapted from G. W. Bronson, The postnatal growth of visual capacity. *Child Development*, 1974, *45*, 873–890. © 1974 by The Society for Research in Child Development.]

the inferotemporal cortex, allowing subsequent "recognition"; other temporal areas are involved in classification of pattern with respect to contiguous events occurring in other modalities.

The main structures of the *second visual system* are the superior colliculus and the other motor nuclei of the midbrain. Bronson points out that, at least in higher primates, this system is inadequate for the analysis of visual shapes or patterns. It is most sensitive to the location of stimuli falling on the peripheral retina and according to arguments advanced by Bronson could possibly mediate saccadic localization of peripheral stimuli and optokinetic nystagmus without involving neocortical areas. Under normal conditions, however, the information from the *primary visual system* and other cortical areas would participate with the *second visual system* in the regulation of many eye movements.

Other investigators have elaborated on this dualistic view of visual processing in higher vertebrates. Held (1968, 1969) has proposed two modes of visual processing to account for dissociation of form analyzing versus spatial orienting systems following visual deprivation, visual rearrangement via prisms, and split-brain, destriate, and colliculectomized preparations. Humphrey and Weiskrantz (1967; Humphrey, 1970, 1972) have demonstrated that destriate monkeys (with subsequent degeneration of the lateral geniculate) are capable of avoiding obstacles in space, of reaching for and manipulating even small objects, and, in general, of displaying an awareness of figure–ground relationships, although exhibiting *no recognition* of visual stimuli. These investigators maintain that such visual abilities are largely mediated subcortically via the superior colliculus. Numerous investigators have demonstrated that, in addition to visual localization, or the discrimination of position in visual space, or the regulation of visually initiated or guided motor responses, the superior colliculus or tectum in many species (including primates) is implicated in discriminations of flux, contour density, and simple shape or brightness (see Gordon, 1972, and Sprague, Berlucchi & Rizzolatti, 1973, p. 73 ff. for general reviews).

Trevarthen (1968, in press; Levy, Trevarthen, & Sperry, 1972; Trevarthen & Sperry, 1973) has advanced an extensive evolutionary argument for two visual systems. He suggests that "vision involves two parallel processes; one *ambient*, determining space at large around the body, the other *focal* which examines detail in small areas of space [1968, p. 299]." He marshals evidence, including a number of his own experiments with split-brain primates, to argue that the ambient system is mainly midbrain, present in both diurnal and nocturnal animals under scotopic conditions (although cones participate under photopic conditions), mainly involved in the regulation of movements and orientation of the total organism in space, and best at discriminating those transformations an object undergoes during movement of the object or observer in space, e.g., larger versus smaller, expanding versus receding, moving versus stationary, dim versus bright, five-pointed versus six-pointed star. He further suggests that retinal receptive fields for the ambient system are probably represented by tectal units whose receptive fields are homogeneously representative of all areas of the retina (i.e., the fovea is not favored). Tectal receptive fields are also fairly large (a degree or two) relative to the size of the foveal receptive fields of cortical units.

Trevarthen argues that the focal system has evolved to the

greatest degree in those primates who are diurnal, and who have adopted foveation, a body posture, and manual dexterity to allow the visual-manipulatory inspection of the fine details of objects. The focal system processes information from a circumscribed central region in space near the organism, i.e., points close to the subject within approximately 20° of the fovea. During such processing head and body posture are usually held constant, and the new, highly evolved saccadic system, regulated by the cortex, "intelligently" samples (i.e., brings to the fovea) points within the circumscribed focal field. The focal and ambient systems continually interact as inspection, search, prehension, locomotion, and eye movements occur. This interaction involves a continual trade-off between fine and gross inspection. Finally, fine pattern acuity, analysis, and memory are accomplished via the inordinate representation of the focal (foveal) area in the visual cortex. Behavioral schemata, visual explorations, and fixations of the focal system similarly involve the cortex, in this case the anterior forebrain visual mechanisms (the frontal eye fields and the adjacent lateral frontal cortex).

The material relating to the concept of two visual systems appears to indicate that in higher vertebrates: (*1*) The fovea is inordinately represented in the visual cortex, and the peripheral retina in the superior colliculus; (*2*) receptive fields for pattern are smaller for cortical than for superior colliculus units, and lead to finer visual acuity at least in the central retina; (*3*) the visual cortex is primarily concerned with a fine analysis of pattern features and the colliculus with a loose analysis of pattern density, flux, spatial location, movement, and simple shape; (*4*) cortical mechanisms are mainly concerned with pattern identification, voluntary eye and other motor movements, and the storage of pattern and movements; subcortical mechanisms are mainly concerned with regulation of reflex movements.

It would be very convenient to accept such straightforward cortical-midbrain distinctions if it were not for other data and some excellent reviews (Doty, 1973, pp. 496–520; Schneider, 1969; Sekuler, 1974; Sprague, Berlucchi, & Rizzolatti, 1973) that urge caution against simple dichotomizing. Schneider, for example, emphasizes the importance of varying both stimuli and responses when using visual cortical versus tectal lesions to determine locus of function. For example, hamsters with cortical lesions make many untrained head-raising responses to overhead visual movements or sudden sounds, but very few freezing responses. Animals with tectal lesions, on the other hand, show many more freezing responses to such stimuli. Schneider also points out the dangers of overgeneralization among species and overinterpretation within species. For example, in the tree shrew ablation of the striate cortex alone does not disrupt pattern discrimination, apparently because, unlike the case in many other mammals, there exists a superior colliculus–thalamic–circumstriate cortical route that is capable of pattern processing (Diamond & Hall, 1969). Sprague *et al.* (1973) similarly emphasize the complexity of pathways and centers, between and within species, that are implicated in visual processing.

There are further difficulties in ascribing locus of function. Some result from interactive effects of neural centers. For example, Sprague (1966) found that unilateral removal of most of the posterior neocortex in cats resulted in lasting hemianopia in orienting unless the opposite superior colliculus was also subsequently removed. Apparently the visual cortex provides massive input to the tectum and, if removed, inhibition of normal tectal function occurs. Further, contralateral ablation of the superior colliculus apparently relieves the inhibition resulting from cortical ablation, in the ipsilateral colliculus. Without this sequential technique of ablation, one might underrate tectal function.

Schneider also criticizes evidence suggesting that tectal lesions result in "a severe loss in visual attention." He points out that although orienting is deficient in hamsters following tectal lesions, freezing to a visual stimulus is not. He also cites evidence indicating that attentional deficits in monkeys with tectal lesions may only exist in the peripheral visual field rather than in the entire visual field as in hamsters.

Additional studies, well summarized by Gordon (1972) and by Sekuler (1974, pp. 202–204), further point out the structural and functional complexity of the colliculus versus cortex. For example, the duplication of retinotopic maps in midbrain and cortical structures is hard to explain. Superior colliculus cells do not appear to be as finely tuned to stimulus characteristics, such as direction of movement or stimulus orientation, as are cortical cells. It is possible that shifting of attention rather than coding of exact location of the eye movement target is accomplished by the colliculus. Finally, collicular cells may be more responsive to movement outward from the center of the visual field, and may be driven either by visual or by auditory stimuli.

These complexities, however, while suggesting caution, do not negate the notion of two distinct visual systems as earlier outlined. Although it is unclear whether it is best to speak of the differences between the two visual systems in man as cortical versus subcortical, pattern identification versus localization of pattern, evolved versus primitive, voluntary versus reflex, or foveal versus peripheral, it would appear that there exists some truth in all such dichotomies. But we do not know, with certainty, whether either system can function independently to perform the same function that each does jointly, and whether such dichotomies are strong in man. We might speculate as to whether the cortically immature human newborn relies more on the *second* than on the *primary visual system*, as Bronson (1974) has explicitly proposed.

2. ATTENTIONAL FACTORS IN FOCAL AND PERIPHERAL PROCESSING

An additional reason for emphasizing a distinction between focal and peripheral processing in the visual field has to do with more central processes such as attention and memory than with more sensory processes involving optics and receptive fields. Information processing models have been introduced in Section II-B and schematized in Figure 3.1. The literature within this area is extensive and the best characterization and locus of the processes involved are far from resolved. Since our primary concern in this chapter lies with infant perceptual learning and development, we shall examine and emphasize only those aspects of attentional theories we feel are most pertinent to very early infancy.

Apparently it is impossible or extremely difficult for the human adult to consciously and actively process more than a very limited amount of new information through more than one channel at a time. Channels may be defined as different sensory modalities, as different regions within the same modality (e.g., different retinal locations), or as different attributes of a stimulus within the same modality and region (e.g., color versus form). In addition, in vision (as in other modalities), if attention is being directed toward one event in the visual field, for example, one region, then probability of detection of other information in the visual field is lowered, i.e., the size of the effective visual field decreases (Easterbrook, 1959; Mackworth, 1965). Finally, focal attention can be directed only successively to discrete events spatially distributed across the visual field (e.g., Sperling, 1960, 1963, 1967).

Neisser (1967) has extended such attentional theorizing by means of his constructs of focal versus preattentive process. Focal processing occurs when conscious, voluntary attention is directed toward the visual field. Preattentive processing occurs when unconscious, involuntary "attention" is directed toward events in the visual field. Focal attention involves the serial application of visual operators for processing, and most often occurs during new learning or nonrepetitive tasks. Preattentive processing may involve the parallel application of visual operators on information widely distributed across the visual field, and most often occurs during the performance of highly practiced tasks and perhaps during some innate processing. However, the operators for both focal or peripheral processing may be learned or innate, simple or complex.

Notice that Neisser's account of focal versus preattentive processing includes no reference to the distribution of focal versus preattentive processing across the retinal (visual) field. Presumably, focal attention could be directed toward any region of the retinal field, although it may be a circumscribed region as Mackworth (1965), for example, suggests. What, then, leads Hochberg (1968, p. 111) to equate Neisser's focal attention with macular processing? Probably the fact that in the human there are extremely strong involuntary tendencies to position on the fovea all stimulus events that are intended for focal processing. In the normal case it is most difficult to maintain one fixation point, while directing full attention (focal processing) toward another point in the visual field.

Finally, preattentive processing is *not* to be confused with subcortical processing nor is focal to be confused with cortical processing. Preattentive processing may involve complex, highly learned operators; focal processing may make use of unlearned, primitive operators. The distinction between the two forms of processing appears to lie not so much in the complexity of the operators used for visual processing, but rather in the attentional and memorial processes brought to bear on the information being processed.

C. Oculomotor Involvement in the Perception of Spatially Extended Figures

As indicated in Section II-C theories differ greatly on the role they assign to eye movement systems in perception. Disagreement exists as to (1) whether actual or intended eye movements are necessary for perception or perceptual learning, (2) whether eye movement systems serve merely to allow peripheral features to be localized on the macula for acute processing or whether they provide information regarding the spatial distribution of spatial features, and (3) whether input from eye movement systems is stored during original learning or whether activity in the eye movement system is a consequence of perceptual learning.

In order to both simplify the discussion of this topic and to remain within the limits originally set for this chapter, we shall immediately clarify the scope of some of the data and issues on eye movements to be considered. We are primarily concerned with data regarding the ability of the eye movement system to estimate the distance and direction of stationary peripheral targets *relative to the line of sight*. We are further interested in the extent to which the perception of the positions of multiple stationary targets, relative to each other, are dependent on the interaction of the eye movement system with these targets. We shall not consider the subject's perception of the *absolute* position of objects, relative either to himself or to some fixed referent in the world, e.g., gravity or the horizon. We shall also not consider the perception or estimation of the absolute or relative positions of moving objects. Finally, we shall not consider the perception of the position of objects widely extended in three-dimensional space. The topics not under consideration are cogently dealt with in other sources (e.g., Bower, 1974; Festinger & Easton, 1974; Gyr, 1972; Rock, 1966; and, in Volume II of this work, Chapter 1 by Yonas & Pick and Chapter 2 by Bower).

We are interested in how the subject perceives spatial arrangement on a plane surface and in any evidence that the eye movement system participates in this perception. But since we are dealing with the young infant who has very little voluntary intercoordination of different sensorimotor systems, we shall limit our discussion to oculomotor contributions to perception. Thus, we are interested in how accurately the eye movement system localizes peripheral targets, but not for our purposes in how accurately an "unrelated" system, e.g., the hand, or reaching, localizes a visible target. Similarly, we are interested in the extent to which distortion of retinal input, e.g., prismatic, affects perception, but not primarily in how it affects spatial behavior in other systems, e.g., reaching or walking. (The reader should consult Bower, 1974; Dodwell, 1970; Harris, 1965; Held & Freedman, 1963; Pick & Hay, 1964; and Rock, 1966, for examples and discussions of intercoordination among effector systems under conditions of altered vision.)

As Matin (1972, p. 333) points out:

Perhaps the most elementary fact of visual space perception is that the spatial order of stimulus points in the environment remains correctly preserved in perception. Around this central fact has developed the general viewpoint that the visual perception of direction is mediated in the visual neurosensory pathway by a system of local signs that topographically maps locations of retinal stimuli into values of perceived direction. In essence this viewpoint assumes that a foveally fixated point is perceived as lying in what may be called the principal visual direction; an object whose image strikes any other retinal point is then perceived at a distance to the left, right, above, or below this principal direction in accordance with the retinal signal, i.e., the direction and distance values of the stimulated retinal point relative to the fovea . . . .

In accordance with Matin we shall define the "local sign" of a particular retinal point as the perceived visual direction associated with stimulation of that point, "quite apart from any considerations regarding the neuroanatomical, genetic or developmental basis of such a mapping or its modifiability." Stated this generally, there is little question that local signs function in adult visual discrimination and memory. For example, the relative positions of two or more targets can be discriminated to within seconds of arc (in the fovea) on a wide variety of tasks, e.g., vernier offset, relative widths of two rectangles, or the alignment of three dots (see Matin, 1972, for a review of such tasks). Second, the specific retinal size of a familiar object must logically be stored in memory (Rock, 1966, pp. 145 ff). For example, without eye or head movement a familiar object, e.g., a half-sized playing card, viewed monocularly in a dark room, may be perceived as a full-sized card at twice the distance from the observer. This could only occur if information for specific retinal size is tagged in memory with information for specific distance. Finally, many motor systems in adults, e.g., eye movements and reaching, appear to be highly dependent on visual local signs.

One might view the substrate for local signs as purely sensory. For example, cortical units for the detection of contour (as discussed in Section III-A) may provide the basic and sole information for the relative spatial ordering of targets falling on the retina, i.e., for local sign.[7] On the other hand, some investigators (e.g., Fes-

---

[7] It is also possible that the neurosensory and motor fields of the superior colliculus could serve as the substrate for local sign. There is little question that the superior colliculus is implicated in some way in the detection of the visual direction of visual targets, and in the regulation of saccadic eye movements toward particular targets in space (see Section III-B-1-c). This indicates that at least striate cortical units (and probably geniculate units) are not required for localization, although the accuracy of such localization in the foveal region would undoubtedly be poorer since tectal receptive fields do not apparently become as small as the smallest fields of cortical units. However, it should be recalled from Section III-B-1-c that identification of pattern or shape does not appear to be readily accomplished subcortically. It would

tinger, 1971; Hebb, 1949, 1968; see also Section II-C) have argued that during the perceptual learning of a spatially extended figure or pattern, eye-movement systems are necessarily involved in the spatial ordering of separated features. To understand this position it is necessary to briefly examine the nature of eye movement systems in man.

Four oculomotor systems[8] in man allow both eyes to capture and/or track a target in three-dimensional space in spite of head and body movements (Robinson, 1968; see also Alpern, 1962, 1971; Bach-Y-Rita, Collins, & Hyde, 1971, *passim*; Streiff, 1972, *passim*). All systems interact during normal viewing although there is evidence that the respective systems are controlled by separate neurological centers and may be manipulated independently (Robinson, 1968). The *vestibular eye movement system* (or coordinate compensatory system) moves the eyes to compensate for head movement, allowing the same fixation point to be maintained in the visual field. The *smooth pursuit system* matches eye movement direction and velocity to the direction and velocity of a moving target to allow the smooth visual pursuit of a wide variety of moving targets. The *vergence system* moves the eyes in opposite directions (convergence or divergence) so that the visual axes of both eyes converge on the same point in space, allowing fusion and stereopsis. Finally, the *saccadic system* moves the eyes conjugately and ballistically from one point in the visual field to another (usually from a point falling on the fovea to a point initially on the peripheral retina). If these shifts are large, e.g., 20°, head movements are jointly programmed with eye movements to shift the line of sight (Gresty, 1974; Sanders, 1963).

The *vestibular* and *vergence* systems will not be considered in detail in this chapter; the arguments to be advanced here are valid if a monocular subject with a stationary head is alone considered. However, it should be remembered that under binocular conditions with freedom to move the head, deficiencies in the *vestibular, vergence,* or head movement system would affect eye movement accuracy and perhaps perceptual information relevant to local sign, both in infant and in adult. The *smooth pursuit system* will also not

---

appear, then, that apart from simple localization of a target in space, learning the spatial organization of specific features of a pattern or shape probably requires analysis by cortical units for pattern.

[8] Other eye movement systems regulating very small, or image-enhancing eye movements, such as drift, oscillations, refixations, and microsaccades, will not be dealt with here.

be treated for two reasons: (*1*) This chapter is limited to the perception of stationary displays, and (*2*) it appears that this system provides at best only limited spatial information (Festinger & Easton, 1974; Mack & Herman, 1972).

The *saccadic system* has received the most attention as a possible source of information regarding the spatial distribution of targets. Some of its most outstanding features are the following: First, it has a very short latency of response to a peripheral target, as brief as 120 to 350 msec depending on stimulus conditions (Bartz, 1962; Komoda, Festinger, Phillips, Duckman, & Young, 1973; Leushina, 1965; Saslow, 1967; Wheeless, Boynton, & Cohen, 1966; White, Eason, & Bartlett, 1962). Second, saccadic eye movements accelerate very rapidly to very high velocities, e.g., a peak velocity of about 400° per sec for a 10° movement, and up to about 800° per sec or more for longer movements (Alpern, 1971). Third, saccades may be executed voluntarily, i.e., at will in the absence of a visual target, in the dark, or even by the congenitally blind; one can also decide not to execute a movement to a peripheral target, although there may be involuntary tendencies to saccade to sudden salient peripheral targets. Fourth, saccades are remarkably accurate in bringing a peripheral target to the fovea (Bartz, 1967; Becker & Fuchs, 1969; Rashbass, 1961; Weber & Daroff, 1971). (In general, the first saccade following introduction of a peripheral target brings the line of sight to within 90% of the distance to the target. For targets beyond 10° from the fovea the first movement is generally 90% to target and an undershoot; a small, corrective saccade of very short latency then brings the target onto the fovea.) Fifth, the *saccadic system* is largely a sampled system (Westheimer, 1954). [In general, the distance and direction of an eye movement to a peripheral target are irrevocably preprogrammed some 80 msec *prior* to the actual movement; beyond that point no further information, e.g., target movement, can alter the form of the eye movement executed (Wheeless *et al.*, 1966).]

If the saccadic system is to play a role in perceptual learning and memory, beyond that of moving peripheral features to the fovea, then distance and direction information from the saccadic system activated during the presentation of a stimulus must be accurate and available to the subject in some form for perceptual use and storage. Theoretically, this information could originate in either or both of two ways: First, sensory receptors located in the eye muscles [e.g., spindle (stretch), or tendon receptors] could provide "inflow" information regarding eye position. Second, motor cells in the central nervous system, underlying the appropriate efferent commands for ballistic eye movements, could provide "outflow" information regarding local sign even prior to an eye movement. At this time "outflow" rather than "inflow" appears to provide the most accurate and useful information to the conscious perceiver regarding actual or potential changes in eye position or the spatial distribution of a stimulus (Brindley & Merton, 1960; Festinger, 1971; Festinger & Easton, 1974; Festinger *et al.*, 1967; Held, 1961; Mach, 1885; Skavenski, Haddad, & Steinman, 1972).[9] Motor units that may underlie "outflow" information have been recently described (e.g., Evarts, 1973; Evarts, Bizzi, Burke, DeLong, & Thach, 1971; Streiff, 1972, *passim*).

There are a number of puzzles yet to be solved with regard to the *saccadic system* and its relationship to perception. For example, it is not yet clear how the system can program an accurate saccade between two points separated by a fixed angular distance, when head position is varied. Clearly, a different efferent signal is required to move the eye the same angular distance if the initial position of the eye in the socket is different. And yet "inflow" information regarding position of the eye in the socket and, therefore, starting position is supposedly poor. Further, if information regarding eye position in the socket is unavailable to conscious perception, then it is unclear how efferent signals regarding the distance of a target from the line of sight are interpreted by the conscious perceiver. Each eye position would result in a different efferent command to rotate the eyes the same angular distance.

Regardless of the difficulties previously mentioned, it appears that the *saccadic system* knows direction and distance accurately in advance of an eye movement, and it may be that at least some of this information is available to conscious perception. Therefore, one may question whether *actual* eye movements are necessary for the perception or perceptual learning of large simple shapes and patterns, given that spatial information may be available from either or both neurosensory or sensorimotor centers prior to actual eye movements. In this regard it is unequivocally clear from a wide

---

[9] But the reader should consult Matin (1972, pp. 368–369) for a recent and excellent critique of this generalization. It should also be kept in mind that we are here concerned with sources of information from the sensory or motor systems of the eye that are actually available as a basis for local sign, i.e., for the *perceived* direction of stimuli. One might conceive of "inflow" information subserving accurate eye movement localization and control, but never becoming available to the conscious perceiver.

variety of sources that *actual* eye movements and multiple fixations are not required for the perception, and even perceptual learning, of many simple displays by the normal child and adult. This is true at least and especially if the figures are familiar and foveally located, or moved so that separated features fall successively on the fovea. Literally hundreds, probably thousands, of studies employing the tachistoscope have indicated that familiar and unfamiliar stimuli presented to the central retina for durations less than 200–250 msec, i.e., too short for multiple fixations, are readily recognized or learned (citations of many such studies may be found in Haber & Hershenson, 1973; Mostofsky, 1970; Neisser, 1967; Zusne, 1970). In adults presentations as brief as several milliseconds can result in the recognition or, if repeated, the perceptual learning of visual stimuli (e.g., Haber & Hershenson, 1965). Even if the "icons" of such presentations are persistent beyond the duration of exposure, and, in the extreme case, an eidetic image, actual eye movements could not shift the macula with respect to the original stimulus but probably some serial internal shift of focal attention must be involved in processing (see Sections II-B and III-B-2). Gestalt principles of perceptual grouping apparently occur under conditions of brief tachistoscopic presentation (Mooney, 1957, 1958, 1959). Recognition and identification of stimuli extended or positioned well beyond the macular or central retinal region are possible without actual eye movements (see Section III-B-1-b). Similar perception without eye movements is possible even in children as young as 4–5 years of age although somewhat longer stimulus exposure times may be required (Haith, Morrison, Sheingold, & Mindes, 1970; Liss & Haith, 1970).

Strong demonstrations of perceptual learning of extended figures without eye movements are provided by Hochberg (1968) and Farley (1974). In these studies adult subjects viewed only a portion of a two-dimensional shape through a peephole. Either the experimenter or the subject manipulated the shape behind the occluder so as to successively expose contour features to the subject's view in the peephole. Subjects were capable of learning characteristics of the overall shape. It should be noted that under these conditions *actual* retinal stimulation from peripheral features, leading to localizing tendencies, could not have served as the mechanism by which knowledge of spatial distribution (direction and distance) was accomplished; peripheral features were never in the field of vision at the same time as the fixated feature.

Other lines of evidence cast strong doubt on the necessary role of eye movements as a source of data regarding the spatial distribution of the features of a shape. Zusne and Michels (1964) found no consistent relationship between the subjects' postexposure eye movements during recall and eye movements during exposure to, and learning of, random two-dimensional shapes. Noton and Stark (1971) and Locher and Nodine (1974), examining adults, and Whiteside (1974), developmentally, report some relationship between "scanpaths" formed during the learning of punctate patterns and random shapes, and later identification of these patterns. However, it is unclear whether the "scanpaths" were necessary for spatially ordering the stimulus, or merely served the function of bringing each feature of the extended patterns to the fovea for clear viewing.

The foregoing studies indicate that *actual* eye movements are not necessarily required for the learning or recognition of many spatially extended forms by children and adults. In Section III-D we shall consider whether this is the likely case for infants. In Section VI-C we shall examine whether the eye movement system is in any way (actual or intended) implicated in the spatial ordering and the perceptual learning of stimuli.

D. The Human Infant as a Special Case

Up to this point we have attempted to present theories of perceptual development and learning, and animal, childhood, and adult data within the framework of innate organization, focal-peripheral, and oculomotor foci in order to emphasize certain fundamentals in infant perception. Here we shall consider the direct relevance of these data and foci for the newborn human.

1. THE INFANT: INNATE ORGANIZATION IN PERCEPTION

As indicated in Section III-A there is every reason to conclude that in man there exist cortical units whose receptive fields are maximally sensitive to contour of a particular size, shape, orientation, or spatial frequency. It further appears that in many species some of these units may be present, if immature, at birth, but development or continued development of some may be very dependent on early experience. We might, then, very well expect the newborn and young human infant to provide some evidence of pattern detection based on similar units. And not surprisingly there is ample evidence that the human newborn detects contour. This evidence is both electrophysiological (see Chapter 1 by Maurer and Chapter 2 by Karmel & Maisel, in this volume) and behavioral (see Chapter 4 by Fantz, Fagan, & Miranda, and Chapter 2 by Karmel & Maisel in this volume; also see Sections IV and V in this chapter).

However, two *caveats* are in order. First, the entire cortex and specifically those sensory areas of the cortex demonstrably containing cortical units (e.g., the striate cortex) appear to exhibit massive developmental changes in cell size, length of axons, and arborizations (among many other parameters) over the first few months following birth (Conel, 1939, 1941, 1947, Larroche, 1966; Yakovlev & LeCours, 1967). Figure 3.9 illustrates development in the striate cortex over the first 3 months. Whether in the human these changes have qualitative effects on visual discrimination is yet to be determined.

Second, regardless of the exact nature of cortical unit organization in the infant visual system, but granted that differences in the discharge of cortical units ultimately underlie a differential response to two stimuli, the ultimate processes involved in visual perception must lie beyond the relatively stable units of the visual cortex. We all learn to detect and remember differences, unnoticed at first, among stimuli repeatedly presented. Presumably the same preliminary feature analysis, i.e., discharge of cortical units, occurs on each presentation. But also, presumably, processes beyond this level, such as attention and memory, allow selective analysis and encoding of this sensory discharge. At this time we have no exact idea where the neurological substrate for relatively invariant sensory analysis ends and that for encoding, investigation, or "mind" begins. However, the ultimate solution of "innate in perceptual organization" lies as much in the status of mind and memory during infancy as in the status of early cortical units for pattern. Dodwell (1970) provides an excellent discussion of the distinctions here made.

It should be kept in mind however that even if the newborn possesses little capacity for encoding, it is entirely possible that visual discriminations may be possible in the sense that neurosensory units may be innately tied to reflex responses. For example, a defensive response to a geometrically expanding object or to depth at an edge, or visual orientation toward a face, to contour density, or to circular contour, could be innate, reflexive, and never require

Newborn   3- Month-Old

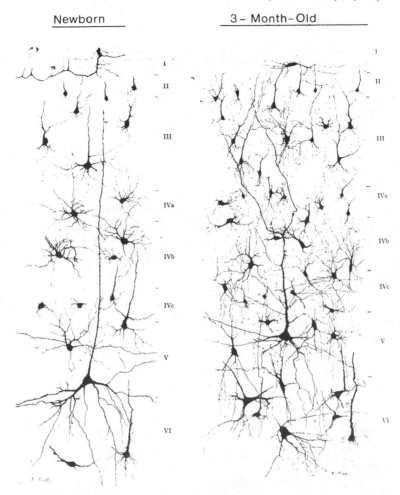

Figure 3.9   Drawings from Golgi-Cox preparations of the area striata, OC, of lobus occipitalis. Left: Section from newborn. Right: Section from 3-month-old. [Adapted from J. L. Conel, *The postnatal development of the cerebral cortex* Vol. 1, Vol. 3. Cambridge, Massachusetts: Harvard University Press. © 1939, 1947 by Harvard University Press.]

encoding. Alternatively, we must recognize that the human newborn, even if found to possess adultlike cortical units for pattern analysis, may perceive little that is unique or organized in even a simple stimulus, for example, the difference between a regular versus a scrambled array of elements.

2. THE INFANT: FOCAL AND PERIPHERAL PROCESSING

There are data to indicate that the very young human infant may exhibit a curious blend of central or focal versus peripheral processing in the sense in which we earlier used these terms (Sections II-B and III-B). A number of factors may tend to weaken the processing strength of the fovea relative to the peripheral retina.[10] First, the lens of the infant apparently differs from the adult lens in spectral absorbance (Cooper & Robson, 1969; Hosoya, 1929) and is apparently fixed in refraction (Haynes, White, & Held, 1965; White, 1971, pp. 65–70). The nature of these differences would tend to make visual acuity generally poorer during early infancy. Macular pigmentation differs in the infant as compared to the adult (Stiles & Burch, 1959). Although there is some debate (Yamada & Ishekawa, 1965), it appears quite clear that the final shape and arrangement of foveal cones only develop over the first several months following birth (Mann, 1964). The factors mentioned would degrade foveal acuity relative to the periphery, and relative to adult foveal acuity. Further, a reasonable argument has been made (Keibel, 1912; Kestenbaum, 1963; Knighton, 1939; Slater & Findlay, 1972) that the fovea of the newborn is approximately 8°–10° temporally displaced from the optic axis, as compared to the average 4°–5° displacement of the adult fovea. If this is the case then one might expect more blurring of the retinal image on the infant fovea because of peripheral refractive errors, since the fovea would now become a more peripheral point with respect to the optic axis of the infant's eye (see Section III-B-1-a).

Beyond the retina some argument has been made that subcortical visual centers, especially the colliculus, mainly concerned with localization of peripheral features, are considerably more mature at birth than cortical visual centers concerned with pattern analysis, encoding, identification, and voluntary shifts of attention (Bronson, 1974). One might expect to find in the newborn and very young infant, then, an organism with poor foveal acuity, reflexively localizing peripheral pattern features on the basis of primitive pattern properties. Selective attention to pattern features, based on inhibition of tendencies toward peripheral localization and based on stored representation, may only slowly develop.

---

[10] The reader should consult Chapter 1 by Maurer (in this volume) and Haith (in press) for further details on much of the material to be mentioned here.

3. THE INFANT: OCULOMOTOR INVOLVEMENT
   IN PERCEPTUAL LEARNING

As discussed earlier (Section III-C), if the oculomotor system is to play a role in the perceptual learning of the spatial arrangement of the features of a visual display and/or if output from the eye movement system is to be stored as part of the definition of a stimulus, then the system must provide consistent, reasonably exact information regarding the location of peripheral features relative to the line of sight. At this time we have no data regarding the accuracy of the newborn and infant saccadic system. The best available evidence indicates that at least some directional specificity is present from birth (Dayton & Jones, 1964; Dayton, Jones, Aiu, Rawson, Steele, & Rose, 1964; Dayton, Jones, Steele, & Rose, 1964; Harris & Macfarlane, 1974; Kessen, Salapatek, & Haith, 1972; Salapatek & Kessen, 1966, 1973; Tronick, 1972; Tronick & Clanton, 1971). We shall later (Section IV-A) provide some new data on this matter.

Earlier (Section III-C), however, we provided evidence indicating that both children and adults are capable of perceptual recognition and learning of a wide variety of shapes without eye movements, even when the shapes are presented for very brief durations or extrafoveally. May we assume, then, that the very young infant can perceive simple form "in a glance," rather than by means of laboriously investigating and piecing together features through scanning? The question is an open one. Very young infants are unlike children and adults in at least two respects: (1) They have had very limited visual experience, and (2) they have very limited cognitive ability. Therefore, they are unable to apply internally guided and symbolically mediated strategies of hypothesizing, verification, and investigation, making use of partial detection of features and based on years of stored experience with objects (visual or nonvisual), in order to recognize or learn a visual stimulus. Children and adults in tachistoscopic or peripheral vision experiments, on the other hand, guess about what they have seen or are likely to see. Their visual field is also *conceptually* mapped by means of spatial reference systems on the basis of which immediate directional classification of retinal events is possible. Similarly, subjects in the Hochberg and Farley studies cited in Section III were apparently capable of immediately grasping the fact that features of a single, larger structure were being continuously but successively exposed to view through a peephole. Further, they were capable of building increasingly elaborate mental representations of the hidden structure and verifying and correcting these representations on the basis of feedback. These are unlikely feats for the young infant.

Finally, the patient examined by Gregory and Wallace apparently recognized or identified visual objects immediately following cataract removal by cleverly transferring his tactual knowledge of objects to the visual realm. Mind and experience in any modality will influence perceptual discrimination and learning in a deprived modality, rendering the deprivation experiment inadequate as a tool for the study of infant perception. The infant, himself, must be examined, and for the "mindless" infant laborious investigation of even simple forms may be necessary for perceptual learning (since peripheral "guessing" may be minimal). This may be true even if spatial information from eye movement systems is not directly used and stored in perception, if only to make peripheral features more acute.

IV. INFANT RESEARCH RELEVANT TO THE ISSUES RAISED

It is clear that we must directly examine the developing perceptual capabilities of the human infant if we are to solve the issues posed by theories of visual development. Specifically, we should like to consider (1) the accuracy of the *saccadic system* during the early months, and (2) the evidence for early shape and pattern discrimination by both the central and the peripheral retina. In a concluding section we should like to draw those generalizations regarding innate organization, focal and peripheral processing, and sensorimotor involvement that seem most warranted at the present time. Finally, since there exist a number of reviews of the literature on early pattern perception (Bond, 1972; Gibson, 1969; Haith, in press; Hershenson, 1967, 1970; Kessen, Haith, & Salapatek, 1970; Spears & Hohle, 1967; Thomas, 1973), we shall selectively sample this literature to make our points, focusing heavily on our own research.

A. Early Development of the Saccadic System

Casual observation indicates that the newborn exhibits saccadic eye movements. More sophisticated studies employing electrooculography (EOG) or corneal photography similarly leave little doubt that saccadic eye movements occur from term, as part of optokinetic nystagmus, during REM (rapid eye movements), during visual pursuit, during scanning of stationary figures, and even in premature and damaged infants (Aserinsky & Kleitman, 1955; Dayton & Jones, 1964; Dayton *et al.*, 1964a, b; Dreyfus-Brisac, 1968; Dreyfus-Brisac & Monod, 1970; Dreyfus-Brisac, Monod, Parmelee, Prechtl, & Schulte, 1970; Kessen *et al.*, 1972; Kris, 1967; Parmelee, Wenner, Akiyama, Stern, & Fleischer, 1967; Prechtl, 1969; Prechtl & Lenard, 1967; Roffwarg, Muzio, & Dement, 1966; Salapatek, 1968, 1969; Salapatek & Kessen, 1966, 1973; Schulman, 1973; Stern, Parmelee, Akiyama, Schultz, & Wenner, 1969). Visual preference and scanning studies, taken as a whole, have also made it clear that some form of directional localization of peripheral targets is present even at birth (see the general references cited in Section IV). In many studies of newborn visual preference the dependent variable was direction or duration of *first* fixation when two patterns were presented simultaneously. The systematic choices often exhibited imply some degree of appropriate saccadic localization of peripheral targets; it is most unlikely that one of two targets in the field was consistently selected on the basis of an initial random walk of the line of sight.

However, while it is abundantly clear that the very young infant executes saccades and localizes peripheral targets in a nonrandom fashion there are very few studies that have provided any exact answers to the following questions during infancy: (1) How quickly can a saccade be initiated when a peripheral target is introduced? (2) Are the first and subsequent saccades toward a peripheral target directionally appropriate? (3) Are saccades toward a peripheral target as distance-accurate for the infant as for the adult? (4) Is the saccadic system equally efficient in all meridians of the visual field? (5) Do the speed, accuracy, and form of the foregoing parameters improve with age following birth?

It is possible, but unlikely, that perfect calibration of the saccadic system is present at birth or matures without visual experience and feedback. This would require that each retinal locus be innately linked to motor centers and effector organs that could program and execute a saccade of appropriate direction and magnitude so as to move the line of sight to the retinal locus stimulated by a target in the visual field. If such an innate system were to remain invariant across development, it would be necessary that one or another of the following conjunctions be true: (1) The relative angular positions of peripheral points on the retina with respect to the fovea remain unchanged during development; the mass of the eyeball and the strength of the extraocular muscles remain invariant during development; the actual rotation of the eyes required per unit angular distance remain constant across age; among other things; or (2) an appropriate conjunction of changing maturational values on the foregoing and any other relevant parameters effectively hold constant retinal locus–saccadic response parameters across age; or (3) the saccadic programming centers maturationally change input–output values to take into account maturing sensory and motor characteristics of the eye; or (4) saccadic programming values remain constant across age, at adult value, and, therefore, infant saccades to peripheral targets be grossly in error because of peripheral immaturity.

The foregoing alternatives are neither mutually exclusive nor exhaustive, but they do serve to point out some of the difficulties involved in an innate, immutable system for saccadic localization. Nevertheless it appears to be the case that in some species at least some components of the eye mature in a conjunctive fashion that does tend to preserve specificity of locus of retinal cells. For example, in the rabbit developmental changes in the cornea and crystalline lens offset an increase in the axial length of the eye to create a dynamic equilibrium of refractive state from 8 to 100 weeks of age (Ludlam & Twarowski, 1973).

In the human case the eyes exhibit marked structural change following birth. Retinal cell loci shift relative to the optic axis (Mann, 1964). The resting position of the eyes becomes more convergent and perhaps the force required for vergence becomes less (Mann, 1964). There are large increases in eyeball mass (Todd, Beecher, Williams, & Todd, 1940). The diameter of the eyeball increases and this may be accompanied by differential alteration in the dimensions of the various refractive surfaces of the eye (Wilmer & Scammon, 1950). There are large changes in the size and strength of the oculomotor muscles. Finally, it is undoubtedly true that pre- and postnatal environmental factors affecting components of the eye could distort an innate and immutable system for saccadic localization.

The foregoing considerations make it at least maladaptive, if not unlikely, that localizing saccades are genetically and immutably tied to specific peripheral retinal cells in humans, even if retino–cortical or retino–collicular projections are (see Section III). Moreover, it has been recently demonstrated that at least the distance component of the adult saccadic system may quickly be recalibrated with some flexibility (Matin, 1972; McLaughlin, 1967; Pola, 1974). In these studies it was generally found that if a peripheral target 10° distant was repeatedly made to step closer, e.g., to move from 10° to 8° from the initial line of sight after the subject had programmed and while he was executing a saccade toward it, the subject quickly began to program and execute a shorter saccade to the target. We (R. N. Aslin, P. Salapatek, H. L. Pick, & A. Yonas, unpublished data) have recently replicated this effect in our own laboratory, also with adults. Given this demonstrated malleability in human programming of saccades one might expect only gross innate saccadic localization by human infants, with increasing developmental accuracy as calibration to the changing structure of the eye occurs on the basis of visual feedback.[11]

Only a limited number of studies have more or less systematically investigated the saccadic localization of targets introduced into the peripheral visual field of the very young infant. Tronick and Clanton (1971) recorded looking, by means of electrooculography (EOG), and head movement responses of three 4- to 5-week-old, two 8- to 10-week-old, and two 14- to 15-week-old infants presented with three 2-inch × 2-inch × 2-inch targets, each 18 inches from the subject, one at midline and the others 30° displaced to the right and left. All targets were constantly in the field, but efforts were made to encourage looking among targets by "activating" (jiggling or rotating the targets) occasionally. The authors reported four clear looking patterns in all infants studied: (1) a *Shift* pattern consisting of a fairly large, high velocity single saccadic shift of the eyes integrated with a fairly rapid head movement in the same direction; (2) a *Search* pattern consisting of a slow displacement of the head during which occurred a series of eye fixations and saccades in the same direction producing a steplike saccadic series across a large distance in the visual field; (3) a *Focal* pattern in which the head remained stable for a brief period of time, but the eyes exhibited a series of small saccades and fixations; and (4) a *Compensation* pattern in which the line of sight was maintained as the eyes and head slowly displaced in opposite directions. The major difference among age groups was quantitative and not qualitative; younger infants did not change gaze as often and exhibited shorter saccades.

---

[11] It should be pointed out, however, that for some reason as yet unclear no research has succeeded in demonstrating a lengthening of saccades toward targets repeatedly displaced outward during eye movement localizations.

Many of the results of the Tronick and Clanton study are in general agreement with other studies on infant eye movements. The presence of coordinate, compensatory movements during early infancy is generally accepted. The existence of a limited or *Focal* scan and few shifts of gaze, especially at younger ages, has been reported by many investigators (e.g., Ames & Silfen, 1965; Mundy-Castle & Anglin, 1969; Salapatek, 1968, 1969; Salapatek & Kessen, 1966; Stechler & Latz, 1966; see Section IV-B in this chapter). However, the *Shift* and *Search* patterns described by Tronick and Clanton are more relevant to this section on saccadic localization and yet more difficult to interpret within the context of their study. The authors seem to have concluded that a *Shift* pattern was essentially a single ballistic saccadic eye and head movement that shifted the subject's line of sight from one object in the field to a second object approximately 30° distant. Their steplike *Search* pattern appears to have been interpreted as a series of head and eye movements in the same direction, but with no peripheral object governing localization from initiation of the series. But the investigators were never able to calibrate the EOG signal to indicate line-of-sight in the visual field because of limited observation time, and because of drift and nonlinearity in the EOG records. As a result it was impossible to identify in the *Shift* and *Search* patterns the initial and terminal positions of the line of sight in the visual field, or the latencies or magnitudes of saccades involved in *Shift* and *Search*. In short, we do not know whether *Shift* was in fact an accurate shift from one target to another, or whether *Search* was aimless or in fact a *Shift* from one target to another.

A second study by Tronick (1972) speaks a little more directly to these issues. Eight infants, initially 2–3 weeks of age, were observed longitudinally each week for 9 weeks. During each observation each infant was presented with a midline 2-inch × 1½-inch × ½-inch brightly colored block 18 inches from the eyes, that could be rotated about its short axis. When an observer judged that the subject was looking at the block, a second block was introduced 10° to the left or right of midline. The observer then judged over a 15-sec period whether, and with what latency, the subject exhibited "a definite shift in gaze to the peripheral object and a brief fixation of it." If the subject shifted when the peripheral object was introduced at 10° the procedure was repeated at 10° steps toward the periphery until he no longer shifted to the peripheral target.

Tronick reported that between 2 and 6 weeks of age infants shifted their gaze toward a peripheral target only when it was within 15°–20° of midline. Between 6 and 10 weeks of age infants responded to targets as far as 40° in the periphery. Shifts toward the peripheral target were most marked either when the peripheral target was rotating and the central target was stationary or when both were stationary. There did not appear to be any systematic latency differences in shift to peripheral targets at varying distances (with no movement trials excluded, the mean shift time was approximately 5 sec), although across all stimulus conditions latency to shift decreased with age. The author attributed his findings to a growth in the size of the infant's effective visual field across the first 10 weeks of life.

The Tronick study clearly indicates that infants as young as 2–3 weeks of age are capable of shifting their gaze toward a peripheral target within approximately 5 sec, if the peripheral target is introduced within approximately 15° or 20° of midline. However, there are some weaknesses in the study that render it less than satisfactory toward clarifying the exact form of saccadic localization. In the first place, the definition and method of recording saccadic shifts were not adequate to indicate whether such shifts were single, ballistic, and accurate, or whether, for example, the infant executed a series of saccades before reaching the peripheral target. Second, the central target remained in the center of the field following the introduction of the peripheral target. Thus Tronick investigated the developing sensitivity of the infant to a peripheral target, given that he was actively looking at a central target. The sensitivity of the infant to a peripheral target might have been much greater if no central target had been present in the field.

Harris and Macfarlane (1974) have recently examined the visual response of newborn and 7-week-old infants to a peripheral stimulus with a central stimulus either present or absent following introduction of the peripheral target. In a first experiment 16 newborns were presented with peripheral targets in 5° steps from midline along the horizontal meridian while two observers judged for each position whether the infant "oriented toward the peripheral light following its onset." Trial duration was 5 sec and each trial began with the introduction at midline of a target identical to the peripheral target. The results indicated that, similar to the youngest infants in the Tronick study, newborns responded to a peripheral target only 15° or less from midline, *if the central target remained in the field following introduction of the peripheral target.* On the other hand, when the central target was extinguished, and *replaced* by the peripheral target, the newborn oriented significantly to peripheral targets displaced as much as 25° from midline.

In a second study in which the borders of the visual targets were better delineated, Harris and Macfarlane examined the localization of peripheral targets by 12 newborns and 12 infants approximately 50 days of age, following the procedures of Study 1. As in Study 1 newborns responded to more distant peripheral targets when the central target disappeared (mean response distance = approximately 26.5°) than when it remained on (mean response distance = approximately 15°). These figures are almost identical to those of Study 1. Older infants (50 days old) similarly oriented toward more distant targets when the central target disappeared (mean response distance = approximately 34°) than when the central target remained on (mean response distance = approximately 15°). However, although there was increased sensitivity across age to peripheral targets at further distances in the replacement condition, there was no significant age improvement in response to peripheral targets at further distances when the central target remained on. This result is consistent with Tronick's study in which orientation toward a stationary peripheral target, when the central target remained on, occurred across 2–7 weeks of age only for targets 20° or less from midline. Infants responded to slightly more distant targets in the Tronick study probably because the stimulus targets were considerably larger and perhaps more detectable than in the Harris and Macfarlane study. The duration of a trial was also 15 sec in the Tronick study, but only 5 sec in the Harris and Macfarlane study, perhaps allowing more long latency responses to be counted. But both studies are in agreement that little growth in the effective visual field occurs during the first 7 weeks if a central target remains on when a peripheral target is introduced.

In the Harris and Macfarlane study, as in the Tronick study, orientation or shift in gaze toward a peripheral target was judged by the eye of the observer(s). Although the reliabilities for this measure were sufficiently high so as to leave little doubt that such shifts occurred where indicated, the nature of the measure, as mentioned earlier, tells us little regarding the exact latency, form, and accuracy of the localizing saccade(s).

In an attempt to describe more accurately the latency, form, and accuracy of the infant's saccadic localization of peripheral targets R. N. Aslin and I (1975) employed both EOG and direct observation. Twenty-four 1-month-old and the same number of

2-month-old infants were each repeatedly presented with peripheral targets displaced at 10° steps from center along one of four axes of the visual field (Figure 3.10). Targets were bright annuli approximately 4° in diameter, projected on a dark screen, and viewed by the subject as a virtual image 35 cm distant in a mirror (Figure 3.11).

Each infant in each axis group repeatedly received four types of trials in random order: (1) *Replacement* trials: A Central Fixation Stimulus was introduced in the center of the field. When an observer judged that the subject was fixating it, it was turned off and instantaneously replaced by an identical peripheral target at one of the target distances along the subject's axis. (2) *Addition* trials: These were identical to *Replacement* trials except that the Central Fixation Stimulus remained on following introduction of the peripheral target. (3) *Center–Off* control trials: When the subject fixated the Central Fixation Stimulus it was turned off, but no peripheral target was introduced. (4) *Center–On* control trials: When the subject fixated the Central Fixation Stimulus no peripheral target was introduced, but the Central Fixation Stimulus remained on.

In addition to the judgment of direction and shifts in gaze in all axes conditions by the two independent observers behind the mirror, EOG recordings were obtained from all infants in the horizontal and diagonal axis conditions. These were recorded AC (alternating current) with a time constant of .6 sec.

Observers' records[12] were first analyzed to see if the subjects executed directionally appropriate *first* eye movements toward the peripherally introduced targets. Figure 3.12 presents the mean probability of executing a directionally appropriate first saccade for each target condition. First, it may be seen that *Replacement* means were consistently higher than *Addition* means toward peripheral targets at all distances and along all axes. This is the effect that Harris and Macfarlane observed. However, it should also be noted that respective mean ratios for *Replacement* and for *Addition* control trials *(Center–Off* and *Center–On)* were similarly different along each axis: During *Center–Off* trials infants shifted their gaze from center much more than when the Central Fixation Stimulus

---

[12] Only trials on which both observers agreed on their judgment of direction of first fixation were included in all analyses. Observer agreement was approximately 84% under all conditions.

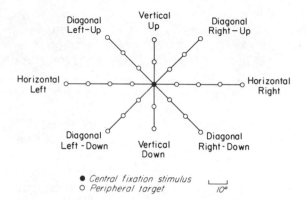

Diagonal Left–Up   Vertical Up   Diagonal Right–Up

Horizontal Left   Horizontal Right

Diagonal Left-Down   Vertical Down   Diagonal Right-Down

● Central fixation stimulus
○ Peripheral target
10°

Figure 3.10 Schematic representation of the axes along which peripheral targets were presented. [From Aslin & Salapatek, 1975.]

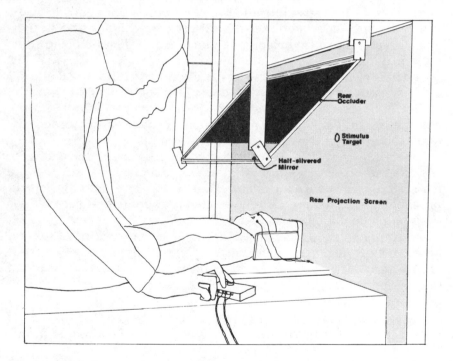

Rear Occluder

Stimulus Target

Half-silvered Mirror

Rear Projection Screen

Figure 3.11 Infant eye movement recording apparatus. [From Aslin & Salapatek, 1975.]

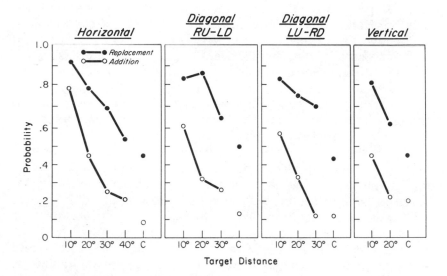

Figure 3.12   Mean probabilities of making a directionally appropriate first eye movement to peripheral targets, as a function of target distance, for the four axis groups. C = *Control* trial means. Filled circles = *Replacement* trials; open circles = *Addition* trials. RU = right–up vector; LD = left–down vector; LU = left–up vector; RD = right–down vector. [From Aslin & Salapatek, 1975.]

remained on and no peripheral target was introduced (*Center–On* trials).[13]

Infants responded significantly more to near than to far targets. Individual comparisons indicated that infants made significantly more directionally appropriate first saccades on experimental than on control trials to targets displaced 10°, 20°, and 30° along the horizontal and diagonal axes, although only to 10° targets along the vertical axis. Infants in our study responded to targets further along the horizontal axes than infants in the studies by Tronick and by Harris and Macfarlane, especially for the *Addition* condition. This may have been because our first eye movement measure was more sensitive than their measures, and our N larger.

Finally, no effects of age were obtained. This is somewhat at odds with the findings of Harris and Macfarlane for the *Replacement* condition, at odds with those of Tronick for the *Addition* condition,

[13] A more exact measure of successful localization of target would have undoubtedly resulted in a stronger *Replacement* × *Addition* × *Control* interaction.

and similar to those of Harris and Macfarlane for the *Addition* condition. However, it should be noted that the first expansion of the effective visual field reported by Tronick and by Harris and Macfarlane occurred at about 7 weeks of age; our oldest subjects were only at the lower borderline of age at which expansion of the effective visual field has been reported.

The remaining analyses were based on EOG records collected from each infant along only the horizontal and diagonal axes.[14] A directionally appropriate first saccade, if it occurred, was executed more immediately toward the peripheral target when the central target disappeared *(Replacement)* than when it remained on *(Addition)*, and more immediately toward less distant peripheral targets. Figures 3.13a and 3.13b provide percentage histograms of latencies, in 500-msec intervals, to initiate a directionally appropriate first saccade across the 10-sec trial duration. On *Replacement* trials an appropriate eye movement was generally initiated within 2 sec, and more quickly by 2-month-olds than by 1-month-olds. A significant number of first saccades were also initiated within 500 msec on 10° *Replacement* trials by both 1- and 2-month-olds, and on 20° trials by 2-month-olds. These data indicate that even at this young age the infant is capable of responding very quickly and in a directionally appropriate fashion to a peripheral target.

On *Addition* trials EOG data were sparse because of the combination of our stringent response criterion and the lower probability of a directionally appropriate first saccade. However, an appropriate saccade was generally initiated within 2 sec following the onset of a 10° target and very often within 500 msec, especially by 2-month-olds. Significantly shorter latencies to first movement were shown by 2-month-olds than by 1-month-olds on 10° trials.

To our minds the most interesting finding to emerge from the Aslin and Salapatek study was the form of saccadic localization as indicated by the EOG records. Infants, unlike adults,[15] typically

[14] Only trials on which both observers and the EOG record were in agreement regarding occurrence and direction of movement were included in all analyses.

[15] Infants executed hypermetric single saccades on only approximately 16% of scorable EOG trials. Adults placed in the apparatus and instructed to "Look at the light that comes on" exhibited only single saccades to target on 192 of 192 trials. However, it should be remembered that our recording technique was sensitive only to eye movements of approximately 2° or more. Therefore, the very small undershoots and overshoots for near targets and the typical small undershoots for distant targets, along with subsequent corrective saccades, reported for adults (Weber & Daroff, 1971), would not have been detected by our apparatus.

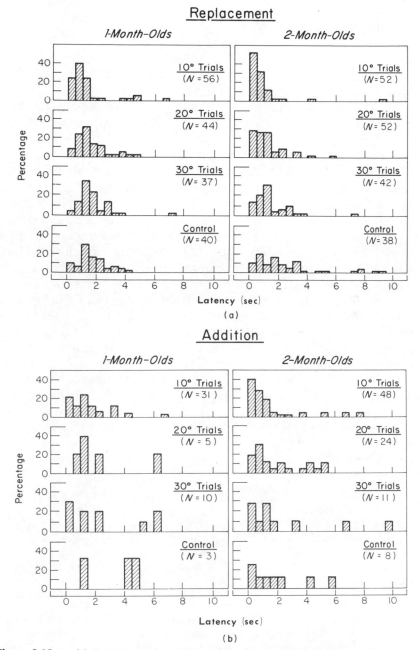

Figure 3.13 (a) Percentage histogram of EOG latencies, in 500-msec intervals, to initiate a directionally appropriate first eye movement on *Replacement* trials for 1- and 2-month-olds. N = Number of trials on which each distribution is based. (b) Percentage histogram of EOG latencies, in 500-msec intervals, to initiate a directionally appropriate first eye movement on *Addition* trials for 1- and 2-month-olds. N = Number of trials on which each distribution is based. [From Aslin & Salapatek, 1975.]

localized peripheral targets by means of a series of discrete, hypometric, directionally appropriate saccades, rather than by a single, distance-appropriate and directionally appropriate saccade. Figure 3.14 provides examples of infant single (a), double (b), triple (c), quadruple (d), and adult (f) saccadic localizations of a peripheral target. Figure 3.15 provides the relative incidence of each type of saccadic localization across all infants by *age* and *distance*. Infants generally localized a 10° target by means of a single or double saccade. Beyond 10° single saccades occurred infrequently and most localizations were accomplished by a multiple saccade.

For the human adult there is a reasonably linear relationship between angular rotation of the eye and magnitude of EOG potential for approximately ±15°–20° excursions of the eye from center orbit (Alpern, 1962). Horizontal linearity also appeared to be true for our infant sample out to but not beyond 20° of the Central Fixation Stimulus (Figure 3.16). The total change in EOG amplitude in localizing targets at 20°, summed across all subjects and trials, was twice the EOG amplitude change when 10° targets were localized. Therefore, we were able to examine in some detail the amplitudes of saccades executed during localization. By comparing the EOG amplitudes of the second, third, and fourth saccades within each multiple saccade with respect to the first saccade of each series, we found that the sizes of all potentials in a series were approximately equal for localizations of targets at both 10° and 20°

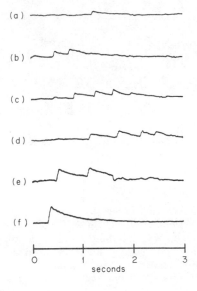

Figure 3.14 Examples of infant and adult EOG records: (a) A single saccade to target at 10°. (b) A double saccade to a target at 20°. (c) A triple saccade to a target at 30°. (d) A quadruple saccade to a target at 40°. (e) A double saccade to a target at 30° followed by a return movement. (f) An adult record of a single saccade to a target at 30°. Time marks represent seconds after target onset. [From Aslin & Salapatek, 1975.]

(Figure 3.17). That is, infants appeared to be localizing a target, when executing a multiple saccade, by means of series of eye movements, with each step in the series approximately the same in amplitude.

We next examined the total summed potentials across all steps in

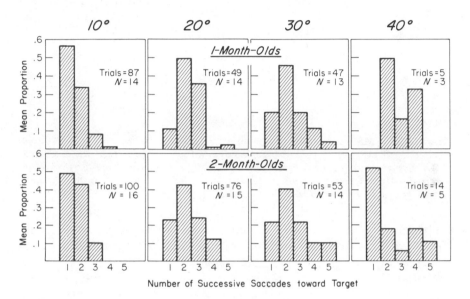

Figure 3.15 Mean proportions of single and multiple saccades as a function of target distance for 1- and 2-month-olds. N = Number of infants contributing to each distribution. [From Aslin & Salapatek, 1975.]

Figure 3.16 Mean EOG amplitude of all single and multiple saccades per trial (total eye rotation). The mean EOG amplitude for each target distance is expressed as the percent increase over the mean EOG amplitude on 10° trials. The unbroken diagonal line is the expected value of EOG amplitude as a function of target distance if the two are related in a linear fashion. [From Aslin & Salapatek, 1975.]

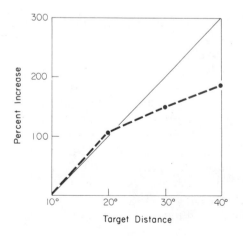

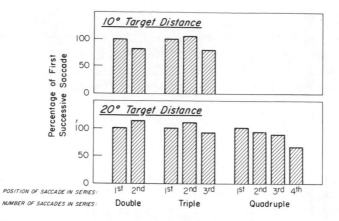

Figure 3.17   Mean amplitude of second, third, and fourth saccades in a multiple saccade localization expressed as a percentage of the first saccade of the localizing series. Every available trial for which a directionally appropriate first saccade occurred and for which a scorable EOG record existed, contributed to the averages plotted. [Adapted from Aslin & Salapatek, 1975.]

each multiple saccade type for localizations of targets at 10° and 20°. Two facts became apparent (Table 3.1). First, within a given target distance, i.e., for targets at 10° or at 20°, the summed potential for a double saccade was considerably greater than (approximately twice as great as) the potential for a single saccade to a target at the same distance, and both were less than the summed potential for a triple saccade to the same peripheral target. Second, the potential for a single saccade to a target at 20° was approximately twice the potential for a single saccade to a target at 10°. Similarly, the summed potential for a double saccade to a target at 20° was considerably greater than (approximately 1.5 times as great as) that for a double saccade to a 10° target. Assuming linearity between EOG potential and eye rotation across ±20°, this pattern of results suggested that: (1) Infants moved their eyes approximately twice as far, on the average, in localizing a target at 20° as they did at 10°. (2) Infants moved their eyes approximately twice as far in localizing a target at a given distance if they made a double versus a single saccade. (3) For any given target distance, a saccade, whether a single saccade or a step in a multiple saccade, was relatively fixed in magnitude, and the magnitude of the saccadic step increased, apparently linearly, with distance.

Perhaps most puzzling in these data was the finding that at a

TABLE 3.1   MEAN AMPLITUDE OF SUMMED EOG POTENTIALS
(TOTAL EYE ROTATION) TO TARGETS AT DIFFERENT
DISTANCES RELATIVE TO THE MEAN EOG POTENTIAL
OF SINGLE SACCADES TO TARGETS AT 10° [a,b]

Type of saccade	10° distance	N[c]	20° distance	N[c]
Single	1.00	26	2.06	16
Double	1.99	26	2.97	25
Triple	2.76	11	3.55	21
Quadruple	—	—	4.81	9

[a] From Aslin and Salapatek, 1975.
[b] The value of the EOG potential for single saccades to a target at 10° is arbitrarily set at 1.00.
[c] N = number of infants contributing to each mean. Each infant contributed his mean summed potential across trials to the means tabled.

given target distance the infant could localize the peripheral target by means of a single saccade of a certain amplitude, or by means of two saccades summing to twice the amplitude of the single saccade. This suggested that on some trials the eyes rotated twice as far from center to, say, a target 10° displaced, as they did on others. This may in fact have been true. Central and peripheral targets were each approximately 4° in diameter. Therefore, the line of sight of an infant executing a multiple saccade to a peripheral target may have initially been on the side of the central target away from the peripheral target, and the terminal line of sight following localization may have been on the side of the peripheral target most distant from the central target. Thus, localization of a 10° target by means of a single saccade may only have occurred when the infant shifted his line of sight the shortest possible distance between the contours of central and peripheral targets, i.e., 6°; a multiple saccade may have been executed when the line of sight was shifted between the most separated contours of central and peripheral targets, i.e., 14°. A similar analysis may be made of multiple saccades to targets 20° displaced from center.

If the preceding reasoning is correct, then it appears that the young infant may generally execute an approximately normometric saccade toward a target approximately 10° or less from his line of sight. For more distant targets a series of saccades, each approximately equal in magnitude, but whose saccadic step unit is related to distance, appears to be executed. This latter possibility is particularly perplexing. If the infant is capable of modifying the amplitude of the *first* saccade of either a single or multiple saccade to a peripheral target on the basis of the angular distance of the target from the initial line of sight, then clearly he is capable of estimating the angular displacement of a peripheral target accurately and *prior* to movement. However, if the saccadic system executes an eye movement only a fixed percentage of the distance to target, then one would expect the amplitude of saccades later in a multiple saccade series to become smaller since the remaining angular distance to target becomes progressively shorter. The fact that second and third saccades in a multiple saccade did not become smaller in any obvious fashion (Figure 3.17) suggests that the entire series of movements in a multiple saccade series may be programmed in advance of the first movement of the series. To test this, one might remove the peripheral target during the first saccade, and examine whether the same number and form of multiple saccades occur as to a peripheral target that remains on.

Finally, the pervasive finding that most infant saccades are grossly hypometric might be the result of the accurate programming but poor execution of head movements at this young age. If, for example, the infant programmed both an appropriate head movement and eye movement in the same direction in order to localize a peripheral target beyond 10°, but for motoric reasons associated with immaturity the head movement was not executed, then his line of sight would fall short of target, and a second or third eye movement might be required for localization. In the adult, head movements of high velocity are programmed with eye movements during localization (e.g., Gresty, 1974), especially for targets beyond 10°.

Studies on infant saccadic localization are consistent with the following generalizations:

1. *Directional Responsivity:* Very shortly following birth and during early infancy the infant is capable of moving his eyes nonrandomly to the side of the visual field in which a peripheral target is introduced. At present it is unknown how much more directionally accurate than this the system is.
2. *Extent of Responsivity:* Directionally appropriate localization may occur to a target as far as ±25° to 30° distant along the horizontal meridian shortly following birth. By 1 month directionally appropriate movements occur to targets as far as ±30° along the diagonal and ±10° along the vertical axes of the visual field. We have no comparable data for the newborn on vertical and diagonal localization.
3. *Conditions of Responsivity:* From birth on, peripheral re-

sponsivity is lowered if a central fixated target is in the field.

4. *Accuracy of Localization:* At 1 and 2 months of age the first saccade to a peripheral target further than 10° is generally grossly hypometric, but distance-related (i.e., approximately 50% of target distance). This indicates that infants of this age can program first saccades related appropriately to target distance, but with a constant percentage error of undershoot.

5. *Form of Saccadic Localization:* For the moment it appears that infant saccadic localization of targets further than 10° generally consists of a series of saccades of approximately equal magnitude. This suggests that infants in the Tronick and in the Harris and Macfarlane studies probably shifted the eyes more than once toward peripheral targets. This explains rather exactly the difference between reported latencies to *reach* target in their studies (approximately 5–7 sec) and latency to *first* directionally appropriate eye movement in our study (approximately 2–3 sec). Finally, it appears that in the Tronick and Clanton study *Search* patterns of eye movements observed may well have been multiple localizing saccades between two targets 30° apart. *Shift* patterns, on the other hand, may have been single saccadic localizations of a peripheral target by a line of sight within 10° of target. Unfortunately, Tronick and Clanton were unable to calibrate in any way the infant's line of sight to allow this discrimination.

B. Investigation of Pattern by the Very Young Infant

1. BRIEF SUMMARY OF EARLIER RESEARCH ON INFANT VISUAL INVESTIGATION, DISCRIMINATION, AND MEMORY

Since there are a number of extensive and critical reviews of research on early infant perception (Gibson, 1969; Haith, in press; Hershenson, 1967, 1970; Kessen, Haith, & Salapatek, 1970; Spears & Hohle, 1967; Thomas, 1973; Chapter 4 by Fantz, Fagan, & Miranda and Chapter 2 by Karmel & Maisel in this volume; see especially Bond, 1972), we shall summarize here only research and conclusions particularly germane to this section.

Prior to 1 to 2 months of age the data on infant selection, discrimination, and memory of two-dimensional visual figures and patterns are generally consistent with the following generalizations:

(1) There is little evidence of selection or discrimination among features, figures, or patterns if they are equated in brightness and contour density (number or size). (2) There is little evidence of memory for features, figures, or patterns. (3) "Attention," the line of sight, or visual scanning tends to center on a single or limited number of features of a figure or pattern. Coupled with data regarding the early development of visual accommodation, visual acuity, and receptive field size, visual preferences and discriminations before 1 to 2 months (and perhaps preferences for meaningless material beyond 2 months) might at this point be best explained by sensory–reflex mechanisms similar to those proposed by Karmel (Chapter 2 in this volume). The infant may discriminate and fixate that portion of the visual field that results in the most sensory discharge in cortical or subcortical units for contour, i.e., that contains the greatest amount of contour density sufficiently above acuity threshold.

Beyond 1 to 2 months, however, it is clearly the case, from numerous studies summarized in the reviews cited, that the infant is capable through either experience or maturation, or both, of escaping the lure of contour density in some instances, of focusing on qualitatively distinct features, figures, or patterns, and of storing visual material (see Chapter 5 by Cohen & Gelber, and Chapter 4 by Fantz, Fagan, & Miranda in this volume).

2. Visual Scanning of Simple Outline Figures

In earlier studies it was found that the newborn generally, although not invariably, fixates a single feature of a simple outline or solid shape (Nelson & Kessen, 1969; Salapatek, 1968; Salapatek & Kessen, 1966). In a more recent study in which newborns were presented with a simple shape repeatedly, we found that while some newborns consistently exhibited single feature selection, others were capable of both single and extensive feature scanning (Salapatek & Kessen, 1973). It was unclear, however, because of the limited age range, whether maturation, experience, some interaction of the two, state, or other individual differences were responsible for the between-subject differences in scanning observed. Figure 3.18 illustrates typical single feature selection and extensive scanning by the newborn.

It seemed that a reasonable strategy for determining which form of newborn scan was developmentally more advanced was to examine the scanning of slightly older infants on similar simple

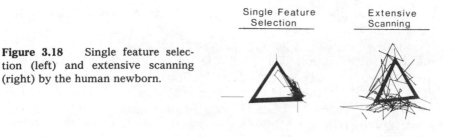

Single Feature
Selection

Extensive
Scanning

Figure 3.18 Single feature selection (left) and extensive scanning (right) by the human newborn.

figures. It also seemed important to study the scanning of infants beyond 6 to 8 weeks of age to examine whether visual scanning changed when infants become generally capable of discrimination and memory of figures. We (Salapatek & Miller, unpublished study)[16] presented each of 10 infants between 4 and 6 weeks of age (1-month-olds) and 11 infants between 8 and 10 weeks of age (2-month-olds) with five outline figures, each for 50 sec, in random order. Stimuli were two-dimensional white outline figures, with contours approximately .5 cm wide (approximately 55 min), and approximately 15 cm (approximately 30°) in horizontal and vertical extent. The figures were mounted on a black screen and centered approximately 25 cm above the bridge of the infant's nose. An infrared T.V. camera mounted behind the stimulus directly above the subject's right eye continually transferred to videotape a picture of the subject's right eye and corneal reflections of infrared lights behind the screen (Haith, 1969).

Prior to the presentation of the first figure, between presentations of each figure, and following the presentation of the final figure, infants were presented with a homogeneous black panel for 50 sec. Between changes of stimulus panels, which took approximately 5 or 6 sec, the infant's eyes were occluded. During most stimulus presentations a pacifier was used to maintain the infant's head in a centered position.

The first result noted was that both 1- and 2-month-old infants, unlike the newborn, would not look at a blank panel for 50 sec. On only 23 of 126 presentations of the blank panel did infants direct their eyes upward into a photographable position. On the remaining trials they fussed, cried, or fell asleep. In contrast, infants looked

[16] These data were originally presented in an oral address to a Symposium on Pattern Perception at the meetings of the American Association for the Advancement of Science, Boston, December, 1969. However, at that time only schematic drawings of infant scanning, and not the exact computer plots to be here presented were available (Salapatek, 1969).

upward on all 105 experimental trials; infants were clearly attracted by all figures.

Figure 3.19 parts a and b provides schematic plots of visual scanning based upon observers viewing the videotape replay of each infant eye and the corneal reflections of the infrared lights in the field on the eye.[17] It is clear from inspection of these plots that 1-month-olds typically fixated only a single feature of all figures and 2-month-olds tended to show a more extensive scan.

To verify this technique of scoring, and in order to more exactly examine the form of scanning, an attempt was made to film each videotape replay at the rate of 3.8 frames per sec,[18] and to replot the scans using the more exact digitizing technique described by us earlier (Salapatek, 1968; Salapatek & Kessen, 1966). Figure 3.20 parts a and b provides the exact visual scans of those infants for whom the videotape records of at least four of the five figures presented could be transferred to film with sufficient fidelity to allow reliable digitizing. For each subject two plots are provided for each stimulus viewed. The first, "uncorrected" (U), is the scan obtained by estimating the line of sight merely on the basis of the deviation of the center of the pupil from the nearest reference light in the field. Inspection of the first plot (U) for each subject and stimulus, in conjunction with the schematic plots in Figure 3.19 parts a and b indicates that there is reasonable agreement[19] between schematics and exact plots with respect to the features of the figures selected for inspection, i.e., 1-month-olds tend to select only a single feature of all stimuli and 2-month-olds scan somewhat more extensively, although less so with exact than with schematic measurement.

Examination of the first plot (U) for each trial in Figure 3.20 parts a and b also indicates that infants appeared to look more to the right of the center of the field than to the left, and generally to the right of

[17] Scorers were provided with a sheet of paper on which the spatial distribution of invisible reference lights mounted in the visual field was depicted. This distribution of reference lights appeared as a corneal reflection on the infant's eye on the videotape record. Scorers were simply asked to view the videotape replay of each trial and to draw the excursion of the center of the pupil with respect to the reference lights during each trial. At least two scorers judged each trial. Later, the stimulus that had been in the infant's visual field was added to the schematic drawing of pupil center excursion, on the basis of the position of the stimulus in the field with respect to the reference lights.

[18] This framing rate captures virtually every fixation.

[19] Although some very poor matches between schematic and exact plot are clearly evident in some cases.

1 - Month - Olds

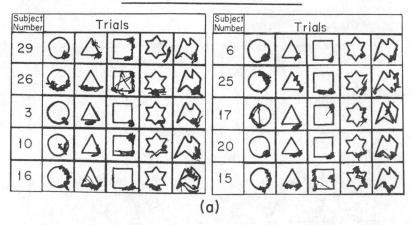

(a)

2 - Month - Olds

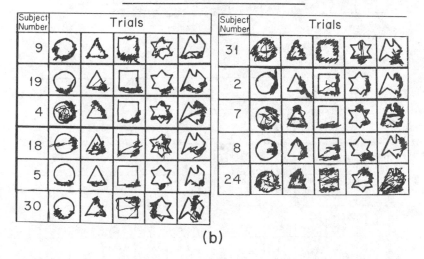

(b)

Figure 3.19 (a) Schematic plots of visual scanning of five outline shapes by 1-month-olds in the Salapatek and Miller study. Plots are displayed in regular order by subject, although randomly presented in the experiment. Plots of scanning are hand drawn by scorers viewing videotape replay of the infant's eye and corneal reflections of reference lights in the stimulus field. (b) Schematic plots of visual scanning of five outline shapes by 2-month-olds in the Salapatek and Miller study. Plots were derived as in part (a).

1 – Month – Olds

(a)

2 – Month – Olds

(b)

figure contour. At least a partial explanation for this is undoubtedly artifact resulting from the fact that the right eye was photographed. Slater and Findlay (1972) have attributed this phenomenon to systematic errors of ipsilateral divergence inherent in the corneal photographic–center-of-pupil technique; for anatomical and optical reasons it should be particularly pronounced at birth. Other investigators have suggested that the phenomenon may be the result of a failure of binocular convergence (e.g., Ling, 1942; Wickelgren, 1967; see Chapter 1 by Maurer in this volume). We (Salapatek, Haith, Maurer, & Kessen, 1973) have indicated that the error is variable even among adults, and that, therefore, it is difficult to correct in infants by using an average correction factor.

Nevertheless, we have replotted the "uncorrected" scans in Figure 3.20 parts a and b, but with the horizontal correction suggested by Slater and Findlay applied to the x-coordinate of each eye fixation on each plot. These are the second plots, (C), for each subject and stimulus. It should be remembered that the correction employed was based on newborn data and therefore may be inappropriate in magnitude for 1- and 2-month-olds. However, as is readily apparent from comparison of corrected and uncorrected plots, it appears to be generally in the correct direction and of surprisingly appropriate magnitude for most infants, given expected maturation. The correction factor did tend to center scanning in the visual field, and to move fixations toward the contour of the figure in most instances. However, conclusions regarding feature selection remain essentially unchanged.

The foregoing study on spontaneous scanning is highly consistent with the literature on visual discrimination and perception during the first 2 months. In the first place, it appears that the typical scan during the first month involves capture by a single feature or limited set of features. By contrast, the infant of 2 months tends to scan more broadly, at a time when infants are reported to be beginning to exhibit memory and appreciation of figures and pat-

Figure 3.20   (a) Visual scanning of five outline shapes by 1-month-olds in the Salapatek and Miller study. On each plot successive locations of eye position, separated by 3.8 sec, across at least 50 sec of viewing, are joined. The first plot, U, for each shape is based on an uncorrected estimation of line-of-sight essentially following the procedure of Salapatek and Kessen (1966). The x-coordinate for each fixation on the second plot for each shape, C, is corrected for error in the corneal photographic technique as recommended by Slater and Findlay (1972). (b) Visual scanning of five outline shapes by 2-month-olds in the Salapatek and Miller study. Plots were derived as in part (a). (The boxes in row 29 labelled with the superscript 1 represent unscorable data.)

terns. Although a greater number of infants should be observed, one is tempted to speculate that the shift to more extensive scanning at 8 to 10 weeks may be the result of cortical maturation of encoding centers. This maturation may allow the infant to habituate to a feature in central vision, and thus to become more receptive to peripheral stimulation, resulting in a shift in gaze. The foregoing data are also very much in agreement with the localization data reviewed earlier (see Section IV-A). Apparently, the effective visual field begins to expand at about 2 months of age, although it is constant in extent before then. Slow encoding, in conjunction with poor receptivity to additional peripheral stimuli, might also explain why 1-month-olds in this study, when presented with figures containing features in close proximity (e.g., the random shape), scanned no more extensively than when presented figures with features widely distributed spatially (e.g., a triangle or square).

3. VISUAL SCANNING OF COMPOUND FIGURES

Mothers often remark that their infants did not typically "look them in the eyes" or did not "recognize" them until the first or second month. The data concerning the developing infant's investigation and discrimination of faces suggests there may be some truth to these remarks. First, it does seem to be the case that a strong preference for curvature (eyes?) emerges at about 2 months of age. Second, effective and sufficient stimuli for eliciting smiling appear at first to be partial internal cues associated with the face, e.g., moving eye spots. Third, the arrangement and elaboration of features as necessary and sufficient for the infant's definition of a face appear to be progressively required between 2 and 5 months (see E. J. Gibson, 1969, pp. 347–356, for a review of studies on the infant's perception of faces). Finally, the actual data regarding infant scanning of faces lends support to the claims of mothers.

In an unpublished study (Maurer & Salapatek, 1975) 12 infants 1 month old and 12 at the age of 2 months repeatedly viewed their mothers and also strange males and females in a mirror apparatus (Haith, 1969). One eye of each infant was photographed via infrared television corneal photography. Each infant viewed the virtual image of his centered, motionless mother or of a stranger at a distance of approximately 48 cm. Each face was presented three times for at least 75 sec. Successive eye fixations on each face were later determined by judging pupil center deviation from the corneal reflections of reference lights in the field during videotape replays, as described in Section IV-B-2.

We found that 1-month-olds tended to inspect the external contour of the face, usually devoting long periods of time to a particular area, e.g., hairline, chin, ear. Two-month-olds, on the other hand, invariably inspected one, or several, internal features of the face, e.g., eyes, mouth. Figure 3.21 provides schematic visual scanning of a strange female face by a typical 1-month-old and a typical 2-month-old.

Bergman, Haith, and Mann (1971) have reported similar findings. Employing corneal photography they found a shift at approximately 7 weeks from scanning of the external border of a real face to scanning of internal features. Donnee (1973) similarly reports data indicating a shift from scanning of external contour of a photograph of a face and of a compound two-dimensional figure at 4–5 weeks of age to scanning of internal features of both stimuli at approximately 7 weeks (but not at 10 weeks).

On balance there does appear to be some shift in visual selection from external toward internal features of a face during the first 2 months. If this is the case, then it becomes of interest to ask: (*1*) Is

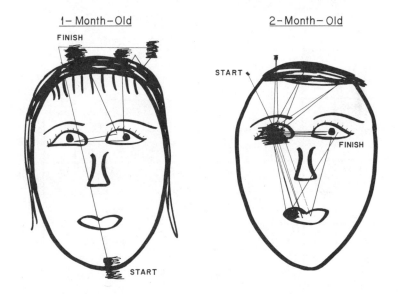

Figure 3.21   Schematic plots of visual scanning of a real head by a representative 1- and 2-month-old in the Maurer and Salapatek study. Plots were derived as in Figure 3.19a.

1 – Month – Olds

(a)

2 – Month – Olds

(b)

this shift peculiar to faces, or is it reflective of a more basic, more general investigative approach toward all compound stimuli during this age range? (2) If the 2-month-old begins to direct his full focal and foveal attention toward limited, internal, perhaps defining features of compound stimuli, does this mean that he does not notice or extract shape information from nonattended features, i.e., from peripheral vision? In this section, we shall present data bearing on the first question. In the next section we shall approach the second.

In order to examine the generality of the apparent developmental shift in attention from external to internal features during the first 2 months, Jill Moscovich and I (Salapatek & Moscovich, unpublished study)[20] presented 18 infants 1 month old and 15 infants 2 months old with the stimuli illustrated in Figure 3.22 parts a and b. Construction of stimuli, apparatus, manner of presentation of stimuli, and recording and analysis of eye fixations were identical to those earlier described in the Salapatek and Miller study of scanning of outline figures (Section IV-B-2). In this study, however, the midline of each geometric pattern was displaced 2.54 cm (approximately 5°–6°) to the left of the bridge of the infant's nose. This was done to position the internal element(s) and the right external contour equidistant from the centered right eye and hence to decrease the probability of spatially weighing fixation in favor of the internal element.

Figure 3.22 parts a and b provides schematic plots of visual scanning for each stimulus trial. It may readily be seen that: (1) One-month-olds generally looked at only a limited portion of the external contour of a large simple or compound square.[21] (2) Two-month-olds generally selected the internal features of com-

[20] See footnote 16.
[21] Especially to be noted is the scanning of the single, large outline square. A limited contour segment, usually an angle, was typically fixated by 1-month-olds, substantiating our earlier results with newborns (Salapatek & Kessen, 1966).

Figure 3.22   (a) Schematic plots of visual scanning of five simple and compound outline shapes by 1-month-olds in the Salapatek and Moscovich study. Plots are displayed in regular order by subject, although randomly presented in the experiment. Plots of scanning are hand drawn by scorers viewing videotape replay of the infant's eye and corneal reflections of reference lights in the stimulus field. (b) Schematic plots of visual scanning of five simple and compound outline shapes by 2-month-olds in the Salapatek and Moscovich study. Plots were derived as in part (a).

pound stimuli for inspection. (3) Both age groups reliably fixated the internal element(s) when presented without a frame, clearly indicating that the internal elements were well above acuity threshold.

Figure 3.23 parts a and b provides the exact "uncorrected" (U), and "corrected" (C), visual scanning plots for those complete videotape records that could be photographed and digitized for a subject on at least four of five trials. As in the Salapatek and Miller study these plots (1) objectively verify the most outstanding findings regarding feature selection provided by the schematic plots, (2) appear representative of the schematic plots, and (3) verify the apparent general usefulness of the Slater and Findlay correction factor (note especially trials on which a single small square was presented).

The pattern of results in the Salapatek and Moscovich study is clearly consistent with the data on scanning of faces earlier described. But does it indicate that the shift to selection of internal features is a general property of the visual perception of the 2-month-old, and, if so, why might this be? It is not possible to answer this question unequivocally at the moment, but several alternatives may be proposed. In the first place, one might argue that the compound stimuli presented were, in fact, essentially perceived as faces, i.e., a face for the 2-month-old may be essentially a frame of any shape with a small number of distinctive internal elements of any shape and arrangement. Therefore, 2-month-olds may have been motivated to look at the "eyes" (internal squares) as they do on a regular face at that age. This explanation is possible but does not explain the scanning of 1-month-olds. Why should they generally confine their attention to only a limited segment of the external contour of a compound figure? Random selection should have led to at least some selection of internal elements, especially for those compound stimuli in which two internal elements were present and therefore considerable contour internally concentrated.

There is a more general, more basic alternative which may underlie the qualitative shift in investigation of both faces and compound figures during the first 2 months. It is possible that maturation of the visual system results in a shift from a subcortical to a more cortical–foveal processing of pattern. As indicated earlier (Section III-B-1) there exists some evidence and a good deal of theorizing regarding the pattern processing capabilities of the primitive tectal system (second visual system) versus the neocortical, foveated visual system (primary visual system). In connection

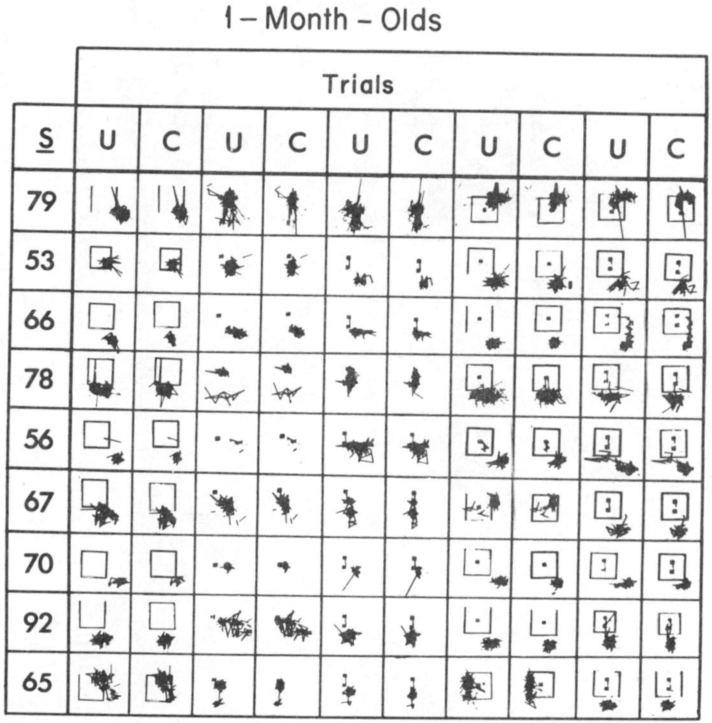

1 – Month – Olds

Trials

Figure 3.23 (a) Visual scanning of five simple and compound outline shapes by 1-month-olds in the Salapatek and Moscovich study. On each plot successive locations of eye position, separated by 3.8 sec, across at least 50 sec of viewing, are joined. The first plot for each shape, U, is based on an uncorrected estimation of line-of-sight essentially following the procedure of Salapatek and Kessen (1966). The x-coordinate for each fixation on the second plot for each shape, C, is corrected for error in the corneal reflection technique as recommended by Slater and Findlay (1972).

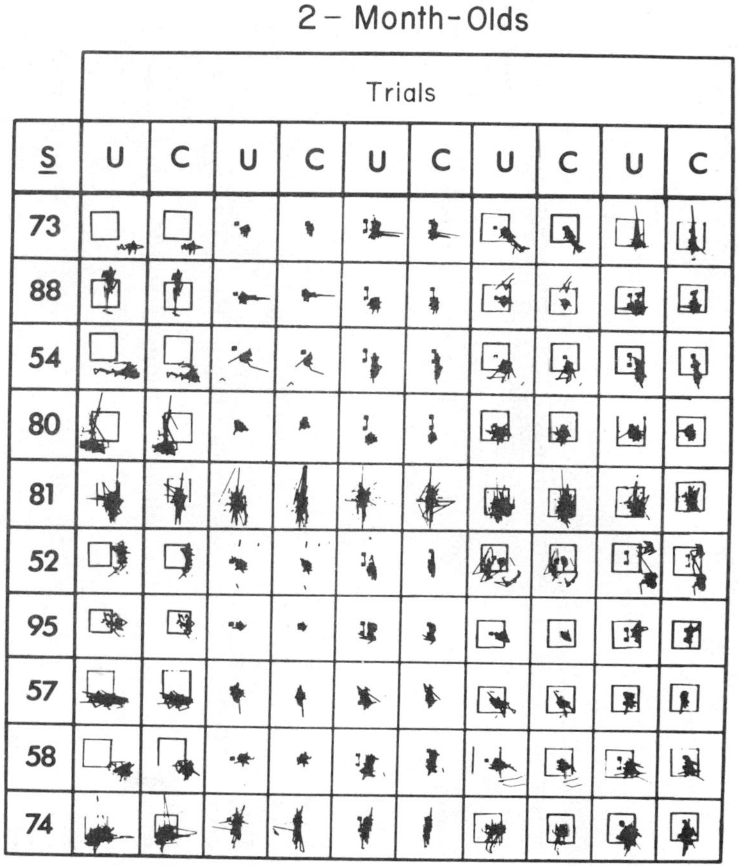

2 – Month – Olds

Trials

Figure 3.23 (b) Visual scanning of five simple and compound outline shapes by 2-month-olds in the Salapatek and Moscovich study. Plots were derived as in part (a).

with this and of particular interest toward explaining our results are observations made over the past several years by N. K. Humphrey and L. Weiskrantz regarding the visual and sensorimotor capabilities of two monkeys from whom most of the striate cortex had been removed, with subsequent degeneration of the lateral geniculate nucleus (Humphrey, 1970, 1972; Humphrey & Weiskrantz, 1967). Over several years following the operation one or the other of the destriate monkeys became capable of the following abilities: (1) simple visual discriminations involving differences in the total amount of contour or brightness among figures, (2) saccadic and praxic localization of static and moving large and small objects in space, and (3) visually guided locomotion and the avoidance of obstacles.

On the other hand the investigators report that there was never recovery of shape discrimination based on the recognition of features. A carrot, the experimenter's face, a circle, and a square were never discriminated or recognized despite repeated encounters or training attempts. The authors characterized the destriate monkeys as essentially capable of perceiving only "figure–ground" relationships.

One of the monkeys became extremely adept at picking up bits of chocolate or currants (Humphrey, 1972, p. 683):

> When a room became available I set up an indoor arena in which she could freely move around. The game was for her to pick up small bits of chocolate or currants from the white floor. She soon learned, for instance, to run straight to a tiny currant as much as eight feet distant from her, and the average time she took to pick up all of 25 currants scattered over an area of 50 square feet was only 55 seconds. To find out how she would manage when there were obstacles in the way I placed in the area a number of solid black objects, baffles and bits of board lying flat on the floor. Although at first she sometimes bumped into them within a few days she could move among them as deftly as a monkey with almost perfect vision. . . .

Recently Humphrey (personal communication) has mentioned another property of the destriate system that is of unusual interest here. As indicated, one of the monkeys was remarkably adept at securing single or scattered currants. However, if instead of being strewn discretely in open space, the currants were placed within a frame, so that they remained in full view, she lost all ability to secure them. It was as if she did not see them. One could hardly question, however, either (1) that she was motivated to secure them, or (2) that she was able to see and secure the embedded currants if presented without the frame. Apparently she could perceive only extended surfaces and discrete objects, i.e., figure–ground relationships with external contour or surface transitions defining the objects. Relationships involving form within form, or figure within figure, or patterns involving different arrangement of features were probably reduced to a single figure or form, perhaps more or less bright or textured. This phenomenon appears to parallel our findings regarding the early visual investigation of compound figures and in many ways is in line with early visual preference and discrimination data in human infants.[22] Indeed, Karmel (Chapter 2 in this volume), on the basis of infant pattern preferences and measurement of visually evoked potentials, has suggested, as has Bronson (1974), a subcortical system underlying vision prior to 2 months, followed by the increasing involvement of the cortex.

4. VISUAL SCANNING AND MEMORY FOR FIGURES

We cannot and do not foveally examine every feature of every figure, form, or pattern we perceive. As indicated earlier (Sections III-B and III-C) receptive fields for contour extend throughout the retina, peripheral acuity is adequate for many contour transitions presented outside the fovea, adults recognize shapes far outside the fovea, and a brief, random fixation allows perception of many figures and patterns. However, we have also indicated that factors such as mental age and visual experience may interact heavily with the perception of peripheral or briefly presented stimuli (Section III-D). And we have also presented some evidence that the neocortical visual system is primarily geared toward foveal feature detection (Section III). The foregoing considerations seemed to us to warrant an examination of the ability of the very young infant to detect shape presented on the peripheral retina.

[22] In a recent personal communication, A. Milewski reports that he has conducted visual habituation studies with 1- and 4-month-old infants at Brown University. Following habituation of sucking that produced presentation of compound figures similar but not identical to those employed in the Salapatek and Moscovich study, 4-month-old infants exhibited dishabituation to changes in shape of either external, internal, *or* both external and internal elements of the compound figures. On the other hand, 1-month-olds exhibited dishabituation only when either the shape of the external contour or the shape of both the external and the internal contour were changed. Infants 1-month-old did *not* exhibit dishabituation when the shape of the internal element alone was changed. These findings are entirely consistent with the view that the very young infant does not attend to or process the internal shape in a compound figure.

In the study described in Section IV-B-3 we found that 2-month-olds fixated the internal element of a compound stimulus for extended periods of time, many infants almost exclusively. It appeared to us, therefore, that a natural experiment existed for the investigation of shape processing by the peripheral retina. We could ask the question whether or not following extended exclusive fixation of an internal element, the infant had registered anything regarding the presence or shape of the external frame which surrounded his fixation point some distance out on the peripheral retina.

In 1967 T. Bower performed a series of experiments indicating that infants of 2 months of age (and older) "expected" an object that had been slowly occluded to continue to exist for at least 5 sec. His subjects showed "surprise" if the occluded object had vanished if the occluder was removed within 5 sec following occlusion. We (Salapatek & Maurer, unpublished study)[23] decided to allow 2-month-olds to fixate the internal feature of a compound stimulus for a prolonged period of time and then to occlude the stimulus for 5 sec. We reasoned that the infants should be "surprised" if the compound stimulus were reexposed with alterations in shape, if they had processed and stored the unaltered shape during initial exposure. We further hoped that their surprise would be evidenced by the directing of fixation toward the region of the stimulus that had been altered.

Each of 26 infants 8–11 weeks old were presented with nine pairs of stimuli in random sequence (Figure 3.24). The presentations of each pair of stimuli were separated by an interval of approximately 10 sec, presumably beyond the span of short-term visual memory in the 2-month-old. The first member of each pair of stimuli was presented for 15 sec. A straight edge occluder then slowly (approximately 5° per sec) covered the stimulus and then retracted to reveal the second stimulus. The total time of occlusion was approximately 5 sec. The second member of each stimulus pair represented a transformation of the first; either the internal element (foveally attended), or the external shape (processed only by the peripheral retina) was deleted or transformed in shape. In addition, there were a number of control conditions (Figure 3.24). The second stimulus was presented for approximately 15 sec. All stimuli were presented

[23] All data here described were presented as part of a presentation at the meetings of the Society for Research in Child Development, Philadelphia, March, 1973 (Salapatek, 1973).

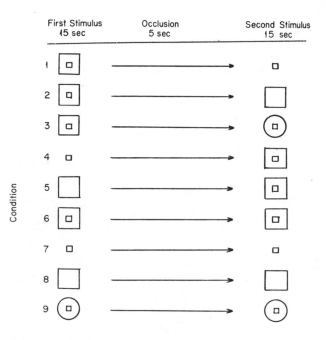

First Stimulus Occlusion Second Stimulus
15 sec 5 sec 15 sec

Condition

Figure 3.24 Stimuli and stimulus transformations in the Salapatek and Maurer memory study.

approximately 50 cm above the infants' eyes in a mirror. External shapes were approximately 15° to a side or in diameter; the embedded internal square was approximately 3° to a side. All stimulus elements were formed of contours approximately 45 min in width, and all were white outline shapes on a gray background. Throughout the course of the experiment the fixations and eye movements of each infant were determined by means of infrared television corneal photography (Haith, 1969).

We expected that if an infant noticed that a particular feature had been altered or transformed from the first to the second member of a stimulus pair, the infant would show more eye fixations in the area of this transformed or deleted feature following occlusion as compared with control trials on which the first and second member of a pair were the same. Analysis of the results indicated that this was *not* the case. Two independent scorers viewed the videotape replay of the subjects' eyes (as in the experiment reported in Section IV-B-2) and assessed for each stimulus presentation whether the subject looked predominantly at the central element (whether present or not), the external shape (whether present or not), or at both about equally. Of 468 stimulus presentations, 8 were unscorable because of a poor videotaped record. Of the remaining 460, both observers agreed in their judgment 377 times (82% agreement). Only data from trials on which there was scorer agreement are included in all subsequent analyses.

Table 3.2 provides the trials of predominantly central, predominantly external, and both central and external looking for each type of stimulus. It may be seen, in accord with our earlier findings (Section IV-B-3), that a central internal element attracted much more looking in the 2-month-old than the external contour of a compound figure. However, it should be noted that 2-month-olds looked at the contour of either a small central element or a large outline shape when either was presented singly.

Table 3.3 indicates the direction of predominant looking for all experimental stimulus pairs. We could find only 157 of 228 (69%) such pairs on which both scorers agreed on their judgments on both stimuli, and where there was a single region of predominant looking on each stimulus. It may readily be seen that there was little indication of any strong shift of attention toward altered or deleted elements, although our N was not overly large.

No one is particularly impressed by a negative result. The null hypothesis is not open to proof and one must consider a number of alternatives as possible explanations for the effect not obtained. First, it is possible that the infants did not perceive the alterations and deletions introduced. This might have been because they were in fact incapable of such discriminations under any condition. For peripheral changes this may well have been true, since no data of

TABLE 3.2   NUMBER OF TRIALS ON WHICH PREDOMINANTLY CENTRAL, PREDOMINANTLY EXTERNAL, AND BOTH CENTRAL AND EXTERNAL LOOKING OCCURRED FOR EACH STIMULUS

Predominant looking	Stimulus				Total
	□ (small central)	□	□ (large)	(□)	
C[a]	112	72	10	59	253
E[b]	28	9	59	4	100
CE[c]	8	0	0	1	9
Other	2	6	5	2	15
Total	150	87	74	66	377

[a] C = Central.
[b] E = External.
[c] CE = Both central and external.

TABLE 3.3 TOTAL NUMBER OF TRIALS FOR EACH TYPE OF SHIFT IN DIRECTION OF PREDOMINANT LOOKING AS A FUNCTION OF EACH TYPE OF STIMULUS TRANSFORMATION

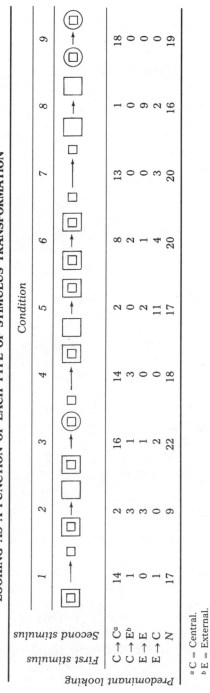

Predominant looking			Condition								
First stimulus / Second stimulus			1	2	3	4	5	6	7	8	9
	C → C[a]		14	2	16	14	2	8	13	1	18
	C → E[b]		1	3	1	3	0	2	0	0	0
	E → E		0	3	1	0	2	1	0	9	0
	E → C		1	0	2	0	11	4	3	2	0
	N		17	9	22	18	17	20	20	16	19

[a] C = Central.
[b] E = External.

211

any kind exist to indicate whether the 2-month-old can discriminate a circle from a square without foveal inspection. However, the deletion condition is more of a problem: Probably 2-month-old infants can discriminate between something, anything, versus nothing, foveally or peripherally. This negative result suggests that no strong expectation was built up by the occlusion manipulation or that our measure of eye fixation did not reflect any expectation that might have developed. The 15-sec measure of predominant looking may have masked a series of quick glances at the locus of alteration or deletion immediately following retraction of the occluder. However, the retracting occluder made this measure difficult to obtain since the infants tended to track its edge. Finally, it may have been the case that infants were not motivated to encode the peripheral stimulus. If their attention was very strongly drawn to the internal element, the external shape may not have been noticed.

It appears that stronger tests of peripheral processing using the visual scanning paradigm but with different procedures for ensuring expectancy, such as habituation or conditioning, are called for before one concludes that the processing of shape in the periphery is impossible for the young infant. The A. Milewski study referred to in footnote 22 is such an experiment. It strongly suggests encoding of only the external form, presumably foveally examined, at 1 month. Combined with a visual scanning measure, the habituation paradigm should allow a test of whether *only* directly inspected features are encoded during early infancy.

Finally, the Salapatek and Maurer study does have some positive merit in that it very strongly replicated the earlier findings presented in Section IV-B-3 regarding the tendency of the 2-month-old to inspect primarily the internal detail of compound stimuli.

5. ATTENTION TO PATTERN

The very young infant gives little indication of visual memory for shape or pattern. Therefore, to study such basic questions as whether the infant under 1 month can tell the difference between two simple figures, e.g., an X and an O, it is generally not useful to employ conditioning or habituation techniques. For this reason investigators in recent years have extensively employed the visual preference technique to assess the visual discriminative capacities of the very young infant. This technique, unfortunately, has a serious drawback: if the infant prefers to look at one pattern versus another pattern, then discrimination between these patterns, on some basis at least, is established. However, if no preference is found, nothing is learned regarding innate or very early pattern or shape discrimination since the patterns may have been discriminable, but neither preferred. And, again unfortunately, apart from possible circular over linear, and vertical over horizontal, preferences (and, therefore, discrimination), virtually all early pattern preferences may be explained as a preference by the infant for the pattern with the most contour density, provided the contour is somewhere above acuity threshold. That is, the infant in the first month or thereabouts tends to look at that stimulus which has the clearest and the most contour per unit area. This summary, while brief, is generally in line with recent reviews of the field (e.g., Bond, 1972), with our own reading and research, and with the general views of Fantz *et al.* (Chapter 4) and Karmel and Maisel (Chapter 2) in this volume.

The visual system of many mammals requires early and varied patterned stimulation for normal neurophysiological development and this appears also true for humans (Section III-A). Therefore, it would probably be adaptive for the very young infant to orient toward the region of maximum contour density rather than strongly select only particular features or contourless surfaces. If this is the case, however, visual preferences will reveal very little regarding the innate or very early perception of simple pattern or shape, since all preferences will be based on stimulus differences in brightness or contour density. But, as we have indicated in the introductory theoretical review, it is questions regarding the innate or very early perception of pattern and shape that are most important in differentiating perceptual theories. For example: Can a newborn tell an X from an O when their brightness and total contour are equated? Or between a horizontal (—) and a vertical (|) line?

We cannot easily motivate very young infants to reveal such discriminations by means of discriminative training; they are unlikely to reveal such discriminations in habituation paradigms; and they exhibit few visual preferences for simple figures equated for contour density and brightness. Therefore, we must seek some other motivational system, not heavily dependent on memory, to encourage the very young infant to reveal any capacities he possesses for distinguishing simple shapes and pattern.

Over the past few years we have investigated a new paradigm that might overcome some of the foregoing difficulties. We have attempted to see whether the infant can distinguish simple shapes by motivating him to look at one shape rather than another on the basis of what we felt were strong, perhaps innate, tendencies to look at figure rather than ground, at strong contour transitions, however formed, and at discrepancies in surface texture or patterning. For example, when presented with arrays of the following kind, the adult immediately notices and spontaneously looks at the discrepant elements:

```
X X X X X X X          O O O O O O O
X X X O O X X          O O O X X O O
X X X O O X X          O O O X X O O
X X X X X X X          O O O O O O O
```

It makes some, but not a critical, difference which specific shape serves as the embedded element and which one serves as the background or embedding element. In each case detection and visual regard of the discrepant element indicates that: (1) We often attend to discrepancies in patterning rather than to particular shapes. (2) We discriminate between Xs and Os (in this case on the basis of shape, since there is a reasonable equation of brightness, contour density, and size between the two shapes). The basis for the saliency of embedded elements was, however, proposed a long time ago. It is the formation of a strong figure–ground relationship, contour, or pattern discrepancy on the basis of Gestalt principles such as proximity, similarity, good continuation, and goodness of form.

We felt that this paradigm might be particularly effective in revealing discriminative abilities in the very young infant since the effectiveness of the paradigm apparently does not depend on memory, or on visual preferences for particular matrix elements. In an attempt to see whether human infants under 2 months of age would behave in a fashion similar to adults we (Salapatek & Maurer)[24] conducted the following study (Matrix Study 1) as a first approximation. Infants, 8–11 weeks of age, were each presented a random series of matrices (Figure 3.25). Each matrix contained a discrepant element embedded in either the left or the right half of the matrix. In each case the background elements were 35 squares arranged in a 7 (horizontal) by 5 (vertical) matrix.

[24] These data were presented as part of a presentation at the meetings of the Society for Research in Child Development, Philadelphia, March, 1973 (Salapatek, 1973).

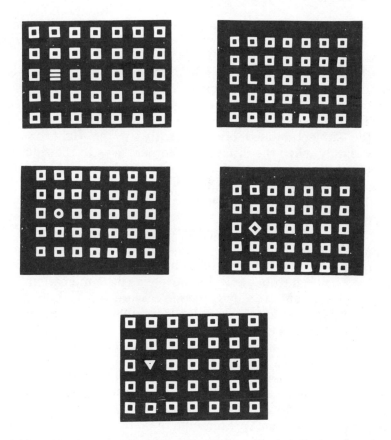

Figure 3.25   Matrices presented to infants in Matrix Study 1. Each matrix element was approximately 3° square.

Embedded elements were an assortment of figures designed to vary in shape, brightness, and contour density from the background squares. The matrices were presented at a distance of approximately 50 cm from the infant's eyes in a mirror, as in the Aslin and Salapatek study (Section IV-A). Each element in the matrix was approximately 2°–3° square with contours approximately 45 min wide, and light gray on a dark gray background. Control matrices, that is, matrices consisting simply of 35 squares and no embedded elements, were also presented to each infant. Twenty-seven infants between 8 and 11 weeks of age were each presented with at least 12 matrices: a random series of each of the five embedded elements, presented once to the right and once to the left in the matrix, and two control matrices. Each matrix was presented for 30 sec while the infant's eye fixations were recorded by means of infrared television corneal photography.

The videotape record for each infant for each matrix presentation was scored by two blind independent observers as to whether the subject looked predominantly to the right, to the left, or centrally on the matrix during each trial.[25] Each trial was classified as either a HIT (the subject looked predominantly to the right or the left appropriately when the discrepant element was to the right or left, respectively), a MISS (the subject looked predominantly to the right or left inappropriately when the discrepant element was to the left or right, respectively), or a TIE (the subject looked predominantly centrally). Since all subjects received each discrepant element an equal number of times to the left and to the right, the expected number of HITS and MISSES was equal regardless of any side preferences individual infants may have exhibited.

As may be seen from Table 3.4 there was little indication that any discrepant element was detected. We were led to conclude that infants of 8–11 weeks of age were incapable of discriminating the embedded elements from squares, and/or that infants of this age do not spontaneously attend to a pattern discrepancy in the same fashion as do adults, and/or that our measure of direction of eye fixation across a 30-sec trial was too insensitive.

To verify that an older subject would spontaneously look at a discrepant element in a homogeneous array of elements, we (Salapatek & Saltzman) presented a child of 3½ years with the same

TABLE 3.4   NUMBER (TRIALS) OF HITS, MISSES, AND TIES AS A
FUNCTION OF TYPE OF EMBEDDED ELEMENT
IN MATRIX STUDY 1

| | Embedded element | | | | | |
	☰	▽	◇	Γ	O	Σ
HITS	3	8	6	7	9	33
MISSES	11	10	11	5	8	45
TIES	13	11	10	19	13	66
						144

[25] The videotapes from 47 of the total 312 matrix presentations were judged unscorable by both scorers because of poor picture quality. Of the remaining 265 trials scorers agreed in their ratings on 169 (64%). Twenty-five of these trials were control trials and are not included in the current analysis.

square matrices presented to the 2-month-old infants, as well as with some square matrices containing different embedded elements (Matrix Study 2). Square matrices, each containing one of the following embedded elements, were randomly presented to the child, with the discrepant element randomly embedded in the right or left side of the square matrix:

$$\Xi, \bigcirc, \triangledown, \lrcorner, \diamondsuit, \bigcirc, |||, \mathsf{N}, |\,|, \mathsf{M}, \triangledown, \diamondsuit, \square, \mathsf{M}, |\,|.$$

The child was placed in the infant apparatus and merely instructed to "Look at the pictures, right at them." An observer behind the mirror noted on each matrix presentation (1) the direction of first fixation, and (2) the predominant direction of fixation during the matrix presentation. On 11 of 15 trials first fixation was toward the discrepant element; on two trials direction of first fixation was indeterminate (*one was the control matrix*); on one trial first fixation remained central; and on only one trial was first fixation toward the "wrong" side of the matrix. The results: 11 HITS, 1 MISS, and 3 TIES. However, beyond the first fixation the child did not necessarily stare at the discrepant element for the greater percentage of the 30-sec trial; she did so on only 4 trials; on all other trials, she soon scanned extensively or completely away from the mirror.

We next re-presented the matrices, but with the instruction to "Look at or point to the one that is different, the one that is funny." She correctly indicated the location in the matrix of the discrepant element on 12 of 15 presentations, found an additional one with urging ("Look for the circle"), and missed only 2 entirely (the ◇ and the control slide).

The slides were then presented again without instructions. First fixation was directed toward the discrepant element on 13 of 15 trials; only the ◇ was missed; the final slide was the control. Apparently a 3-year-old only has difficulty discriminating diamonds from squares, a well-known finding at this age.

The data from the single 3-year-old indicated that she would spontaneously look at a single discrepant element in an array of homogeneous elements. For our purposes, it is worth reemphasizing that: (1) This detection was immediate and probably based on peripheral vision since the first eye movement was appropriate and the starting point of the line of sight was variable. (2) Interest in (fixation on) the discrepant element did not extend beyond a lengthy

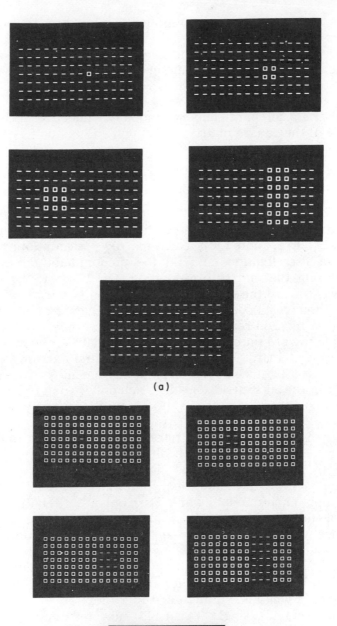

(a)

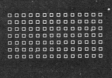

(b)

first fixation. (3) The spontaneous tendency was to look at a shape discrepancy, and not merely to look toward the region of highest local brightness or contour density.

We next reexamined the 2-month-old's detection of discrepant elements in matrices of homogeneous elements (Matrix Study 3). We presented 31 infants between 8 and 11 weeks of age with matrices of line elements in which either one, a 2×2 matrix, a 3×3 matrix, or a three-element wide column of squares was embedded in the line matrix, with the inner edge of the embedded elements offset approximately 10° to either the right or the left of midline above the subject's nose (Figure 3.26a). Each matrix element was outline in shape, approximately 4°–5° wide or high, with approximately 4°–5° spacing between elements. All matrices were presented in the mirror apparatus at a viewing distance of approximately 33 cm from the subjects' eyes. The matrices were designed to draw the infants' attention to the discrepant element(s) on the basis of local brightness and contour density as well as on the basis of shape. Moreover, they were presented closer to the subject than in Matrix Study 1, reported to be optimal for acuity at this age (Haynes *et al.*, 1965). Finally, they were designed to indicate whether infants of 2 months would attend to *any* discrepant element(s) in a homogeneous *multielement* matrix.

A second set of matrices presented was more subtle (Figure 3.26b). These matrices were the pattern reversal of the first set and were designed to show that not only would the 2-month-old look at a discrepant element(s) in a multielement matrix, but also that the detection of local *maximum* contour and brightness does not fully motivate this effect.

Each infant was randomly presented each matrix, with a presentation of each embedded element on both the left and the right sides of the visual field. In addition six control matrices (three homogeneous square and three homogeneous line matrices) were presented randomly with the experimental matrices. Each of the 31 subjects viewed each of the foregoing matrices at least twice.

Prior to the presentation of each matrix the infant's line of sight was brought to the center of the visual field by the introduction of a

Figure 3.26   (a) Line matrices with embedded squares presented to infants in Matrix Study 3. Each matrix element was approximately 5° high and/or wide near field center. (b) Square matrices with embedded lines presented to infants in Matrix Study 3. Each matrix element was approximately 5° high and/or wide near field center.

small circular target. When an observer behind the mirror judged that the infant was looking at the center of the field, a matrix was introduced and the central circular target simultaneously removed. Two blind, independent observers behind the mirror then judged whether the infant's first fixation moved to the left or to the right in the stimulus field.[26] Following this they continued to judge the direction of the infant's fixation for the duration of the presentation. By introducing the initial central target we hoped to correct a flaw of Matrix Study 1, that is, direction of first fixation rather than total looking time might best reveal attention to a discrepant element, as was the case with the 3-year-old subject. Each matrix was presented for 10 sec at which time the central target was reintroduced and the next trial began.

A first analysis was made of the direction of each subject's first fixation on each type of matrix as in Matrix Study 1. Since each infant received more than a single presentation of each embedded matrix element(s) and its control matrix, each subject's first fixations on each type of matrix were summed to give the following HIT–MISS ratio:[27]

$$\frac{\text{Total number of HITS}}{\text{Total number of HITS plus total number of MISSES}}$$

The HIT–MISS ratio was computed for control as well as for experimental matrix trials. For each subject each control matrix viewed was randomly assigned a dummy value, "right" or "left," with the constraint that he receive the same number of "right" and "left" control matrices. The infant's direction of first fixation was then scored as a HIT or MISS for each control matrix, as it had been for experimental matrices, to provide a HIT–MISS ratio for each of the two types of control matrices.

Table 3.5 indicates for each experimental condition in Matrix Study 3 the number of infants whose experimental HIT–MISS ratio exceeded $(E > C)$, equaled $(E = C)$, or was smaller than $(E < C)$

---

[26] Observers agreed on their judgment of direction of first fixation on approximately 84% of matrix trials in this and other matrix studies to be reported here. Only trials on which there was scorer agreement are included in all analyses. Scorer agreement did not vary by stimulus condition.

[27] Ties (nonmovements) were not included in this ratio, since they occurred only approximately once per 100 trials.

TABLE 3.5   NUMBER OF INFANTS WHOSE EXPERIMENTAL HIT–MISS
RATIO EXCEEDED ($E > C$), EQUALED ($E = C$), OR
WAS LESS THAN ($E < C$) THEIR CONTROL HIT–MISS
RATIO, FOR EACH TYPE OF MATRIX PRESENTED
IN MATRIX STUDY 3

Size of embedded matrix:	1×1		2×2		3×3		*Column*	
Type of embedding:	− in □	□ in −	− in □	□ in −	− in □	□ in −	− in □	□ in −
$E > C$	12	16	16	17	10	21	7	22
$E = C$	2	1	4	1	3	1	6	5
$E < C$	17	14	11	13	18	9	18	4

their appropriate control HIT–MISS ratio. It may be seen that 2-month-old infants gave no evidence of directionally selective first eye movements when either a single or a 2×2 matrix of elements (squares or lines) was embedded in a background of homogeneous elements. This result, or lack of result, is in complete accord with the findings of Matrix Study 1. On the other hand, if the discrepant embedded elements were either a 3×3 matrix or a column of discrepant elements, then clear evidence of selective first fixation was obtained: Infants looked *toward* the embedded square matrices, and *away from* the embedded line matrices. However, since squares served as the background for embedded line matrices, one might best summarize the results as indicating that infants looked toward the side with most squares, given that the right versus left square-to-line ratio reached a certain critical value.

Matrix Study 3 was originally designed to obtain evidence of simple form discrimination by 2-month-olds by not relying on memory or visual preference for shape. We had hoped to take advantage of what we had hypothesized to be an age-unrelated tendency to spontaneously look at a pattern discrepancy, or at a strong contour or figure–ground relationship based on "basic" principles of perceptual grouping. Matrix Study 3 failed entirely in this regard. Even where there was clear evidence of discrimination of lines from squares (3×3 and Column conditions), first fixation was always directed toward the side of the visual field containing most squares. This is apparently at variance with the tendency of the human child and adult to initially and spontaneously attend to the pattern discrepancy or figure in a figure–ground relationship, largely regardless of the shapes, brightnesses, or contour densities of the elements used to form the discrepancy.

On the more positive side the fact that infants in Matrix Study 3 reliably directed first fixation toward the side of the visual field containing squares indicates that they were capable of detecting pattern elements (squares) when they were embedded in a field of other pattern elements. Therefore, failure to move toward embedded lines may not be explained solely on the basis of perceptual confusion resulting from a multielement display. Moreover, selection of squares was very immediate and undoubtedly involved mainly extrafoveal processing since embedded elements were offset from midline by 10°, since each trial began with the infant's line of sight at midline, and since *direction* of *first* fixation was the dependent variable.

What stimulus properties determined the selection of squares over lines in Matrix Study 3? Three obvious variables come immediately to mind, the three that were deliberately placed in the design to maximize the discrepancy effect. First, matrix areas containing more squares than lines were brighter since elements were light gray. Second, the difference in contour density between squares and horizontal lines was very large: approximately 4 to 1 per unit element in favor of squares. Therefore, infants may have simply directed their first fixations toward the side of the matrix containing most contour. Finally, the matrix elements differed in shape. It is possible that squares were preferred over horizontal line segments with no effect of, or in interaction with, brightness and contour density.

To explore some of these alternatives in an initial way Matrix Study 4 was conducted. Thirty-five infants between 8 and 11 weeks of age were each presented with multiple instances of each of the matrices shown in Figure 3.27 parts a and b. Procedure and analysis were similar to Matrix Study 3.

The matrices presented to the infants fell into three categories. First, the matrices in Figure 3.27a were designed to investigate whether squares would continue to be selected over lines when the figure–ground brightness ratio of the matrices was reversed, i.e., when the brightness value of the matrix area containing line segments was made appreciably higher than the matrix area containing squares. Matrices 3.27a (i), (ii), (iii), and (iv), then, were merely the 3 × 3 lines–squares matrices of Matrix Study 3, presented again to verify the results of Study 3. Matrices 3.27a (v), (vi), (vii), and (viii) were the straightforward brightness reversal of

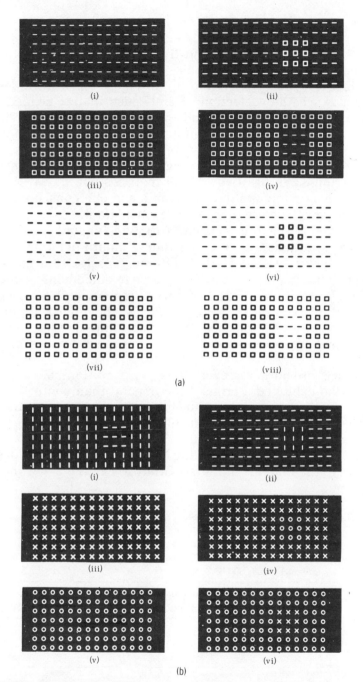

Figure 3.27 (a) Square-in-lines and line-in-squares matrices presented in Matrix Study 4. Matrix elements were 5° high and/or wide near field center. (b) Horizontal–vertical and X–O matrices presented in Matrix Study 4. Matrix elements were 5° high and/or wide near field center.

matrices 3.27a (i), (ii), (iii), and (iv), presented to see if a gross brightness shift would affect choice of squares over lines.

The first two matrices, (i) and (ii), in Figure 3.27b were designed to examine whether detection of embedded matrix elements was possible when the embedded and embedding elements were identical in shape, brightness, and contour density. Orientation of embedded and background elements were varied to study discrimination of horizontal from vertical line segments. In addition to matrices 3.27b (i) and 3.27b (ii), two control matrices not shown, one consisting of only horizontal line segments and one consisting of only vertical segments, were presented to each infant.

Finally, the lower four matrices, (iii), (iv), (v), and (vi), in Figure 3.27b were designed to see whether 2-month-old infants could detect embedded elements that differed grossly from embedding elements in shape, but that were equated to embedding elements in size, brightness, and contour density. The Xs and Os employed differed in many basic shape properties, such as linearity, angularity, and closedness, but had the same contour area, length of contour, and brightness, and a size difference very imperceptible to the adult.

Table 3.6 provides for each stimulus condition the number of infants who exhibited a larger experimental than control HIT–MISS ratio $(E > C)$, an equal experimental and control HIT–MISS ratio $(E = C)$, and a smaller experimental than control HIT–MISS ratio $(E < C)$. Again, as in Matrix Study 3 the results of the first fixation analysis were very clear-cut. In the first place the matrices designed to replicate the findings of Matrix Study 3, i.e., the 3×3 matrix of

TABLE 3.6   **NUMBER OF INFANTS WHOSE EXPERIMENTAL** HIT–MISS
**RATIO EXCEEDED $(E > C)$, EQUALED $(E = C)$, OR
WAS LESS THAN $(E < C)$ THEIR CONTROL** HIT–MISS
**RATIO, FOR EACH TYPE OF MATRIX PRESENTED
IN MATRIX STUDY 4**

	Bright elements dark background		Dark elements bright background		Bright elements dark background			
	— in □	□ in —	— in □	□ in —	| in —	— in |	○ in ×	× in ○
$E > C$	9	23	7	24	9	5	19	10
$E = C$	5	5	8	6	12	6	4	11
$E < C$	20	7	20	5	14	24	12	13

bright horizontal lines embedded in bright squares against a dark background and the 3 × 3 matrix of bright squares embedded in bright lines against a dark background, did so exactly. Infants consistently directed first fixation toward the side with most squares.

When the brightness of figure and ground was reversed, infants in Matrix Study 4 continued to direct first fixation toward the side of the matrix containing squares rather than lines, and to the same extent as in the unreversed condition. This finding strongly suggests that either the contour density, the size, or the shape of the squares, rather than the absolute brightness of the figure, determined direction of first fixation in this study and in Matrix Study 3.

Matrix Study 4 also provided some suggestion that first fixation in a matrix may be influenced by a factor other than brightness, contour density, or shape. In Table 3.6 it may be noted that infants did *not* selectively fixate toward or away from a 3 × 3 matrix of vertical lines embedded in a background of horizontal lines. However, when a 3 × 3 matrix of horizontal lines was embedded in a background matrix of vertical line segments, only 5 infants exhibited higher experimental than control HIT–MISS ratios; an additional 6 infants showed no bias; but 24 infants showed a bias in first fixation toward the side of the matrix containing only vertical lines. These findings suggest that vertical line segments attracted first fixation more strongly than horizontal line segments, but only if a sufficiently high ratio (and perhaps absolute number) of vertical to horizontal segments were present on one side of the visual field versus the other. These data may also partially explain the attractive power of embedded squares (which contain vertical segments) over horizontal line segments.

Finally, it should be noted in Table 3.6 that there was no difference between experimental and control trials for matrices in which Xs were embedded in Os, or the reverse. This finding strongly suggests that gross shape differences do not stand out for the infant when brightness and contour density are equated. It further suggests that the difference in contour density probably played a role in infants' choice of squares over lines. However, more controls are necessary before firm conclusions can be drawn regarding the exact source of effects in the matrix studies.

In an ongoing study six preschool children (3–4 years) have been presented with the matrices of Matrix Study 3, and the horizontal–vertical and X and O matrices of Matrix Study 4, along with their control matrices. Preliminary analysis of data from these first six subjects clearly indicates first fixation of *all* discrepant embeddings, but in interaction with contour density when it is different from one semifield to the other. That is, there was more of a tendency for first fixation to be directed toward the discrepant embedded elements when they were of higher than of lower contour density with respect to the background elements.

V.   EARLY PERCEPTUAL DEVELOPMENT RECONSIDERED

A.   Innate Organization

The bulk of research and literature indicates that the very early perception of two-dimensional visual stimuli must be regarded as the perception of parts rather than wholes. This appears to be true for at least three reasons. First, before 2 months of age visual attention appears to be captured by a single or limited number of features of a figure or pattern. Second, before approximately 1 to 2 months of age there is little evidence that the arrangement or pattern of figural elements plays any role in visual selection or memory. Third, before 1 to 2 months, there is little evidence that the line of sight is attracted by anything more than the greatest number or size of visible contour elements per unit area, regardless of type or arrangement of elements. Although one might argue that contour density, number, or size are, in effect, global properties of the visual stimulus, nevertheless the system cannot distinguish between spatial distributions of contour, roughly equated for density of contour. Even if it turns out that certain types of contour are more preferred than others, e.g., circular rather than linear (cf. Chapter 4 by Fantz *et al.* in this volume), it does not appear at this point that random arrangements of segments of this contour need be any more preferred than regular arrangements. Finally, there is little indication that basic principles of perceptual grouping, such as grouping on the basis of proximity, similarity, or good continuation, or the formation of contours or figure–ground relationships on the basis of these properties, are strong enough in the two-dimensional case to overcome the tendency to select on the basis of contour density.

Even beyond 2 months visual perception often appears to be part as opposed to whole. As we have seen, attention by the 1-month-old is often directed toward a single external feature, and by the

2-month-old toward internal features. Faces appear to be learned initially on the basis of limited cues that gradually become elaborated. Even when many features of a stimulus are learned, their configuration or "gestalt" appears not to be immediately appreciated, as distinct from the parts (Bower, 1966). It appears that for arbitrary configurations, features and their arrangement appear to be learned piecemeal and slowly.

B.   Focal and Peripheral Processing

Partial information has been gathered regarding the two senses (sensory–anatomical versus attentional) of focal versus peripheral processing, but this information remains fragmentary. In the first place, it appears clear that the infant, even the newborn, looking at a patternless field, is sensitive to stimulation introduced far from the fovea. There is also some indication that this sensitivity increases with age. But it is also clear that sensitivity to peripheral targets decreases with increasing target distance from the fovea, and with the presence of a fixated target in the field. These results are perhaps as they should be, given both the anatomy of the visual system, and the nature of focal attention.

It also appears clear that the peripheral retina is heavily involved in initial visual selection by the very young infant. Virtually all visual selection studies theoretically demand initial selection by the peripheral retina, and our own matrix studies indicate that first eye movements are based on peripheral sensitivity. Before 2 months of age, however, it appears that most selection is based on detection of local and largest area of maximum contour density. If this is so, then we have only demonstrated that the peripheral retina detects amount of contour. There are some indications that selection may be for specific shape, e.g., orientation, circularity (Chapter 4 by Fantz *et al.* in this volume; Kessen, Salapatek, & Haith, 1972; Section IV-B-5 in this chapter). However, these studies merit further substantiation. Even if true they may indicate selection for only fragments rather than for figures or patterns.

Spontaneous selection, if present, provides proof of discrimination. But, if absent, it does not indicate that detection and discrimination did *not* occur. In our one study on the "motivated" perception of shape by the peripheral retina (Section IV-B-1) no evidence of discrimination of shape by either peripheral or central vision was obtained. No comparable data on peripheral detection of shape by the infant beyond 2 months are yet available.

Almost paradoxically, studies of shape discrimination by the young infant have yielded more solid data regarding the capacities of the peripheral retina than of the fovea or macula. We do not know, except by inference, whether the fovea is even perceptually functional by 2 months of age. In the first place, the macula is tiny compared to the peripheral retina, and with the error inherent in current eye fixation measures it is possible to assign a target in the visual field with certainty to the periphery, but not to the macula. Even in the eye movement plots reported throughout this chapter where a target has seemingly been foveally fixated, fixation has consisted of a loose scan with a variance greater than the extent of the macula. Second, the one piece of information that could definitely indicate macular processing, namely acuity threshold, is equivocal. Acuity threshold for a stationary target is no better on the average than 20/150 even by the fourth month[28]; and in adults at least, such a high threshold could be readily accomplished further than 15° from the fovea (Alpern, 1962). Acuity threshold for a stationary target at 2 months of age is approximately 20/500, and could be readily accomplished even further from the fovea by adults. About the only data we have that suggest macular functioning at 2 months are those from studies on color vision (e.g., Chase, 1937; Fagan, 1974; see also Chapter 1 by Maurer, in this volume, regarding electroretinograms and visually evoked potentials under scotopic and photopic conditions) indicating photopic functioning before or by 2 months. However, even these results could have been effected by extrafoveal cones. The best working assumption, however, given that there are accurate tendencies to localize peripheral targets, and given that targets localized appear to be generally maintained in central vision, and given that the effective visual field appears to decrease if a target is in central vision, seems to be that the macula is functional and more acute than the periphery in pattern vision during early infancy. The true threshold of infant macular acuity may currently be set too high, since most determinations of this threshold have been based on visual preference data and the infant simply may not strongly prefer weak but visible targets.

Finally, some evidence has now been gathered regarding the

---

[28] These Snellen equivalents of infant visual acuity and the other infant values here reported are based on an average tabulation across all published studies of infant visual acuity up to 1970, along with unpublished data provided by D. Teller. This summary was tabulated by D. Teller (personal communication), and verified by me.

second, "attentional," sense of focal vision during early infancy. Studies on peripheral localization (Aslin & Salapatek, discussed in Section IV-A; Harris & Macfarlane, 1974; Tronick, 1972) clearly indicate that there is greater sensitivity to peripheral targets under conditions with no central target in the visual field. There is some question as to the developmental course of expansion of the effective visual field, but it appears that some expansion does occur during the early months. Because of the very strong localizing tendencies indicated in peripheral localization studies, and because of the early lack of inhibiting systems and memory, it may be that the focal and foveal lines of sight are coincident during early infancy.

C. Oculomotor Involvement in Perceptual Learning

In the introduction we reviewed various theories of early perceptual development with respect to the role they assigned to oculomotor activity in the perception of figure or pattern. It is now possible to consider these theories in the light of the data presented regarding the accuracy of saccadic localization by the human infant. To this writer's mind, the strongest sensorimotor theories are those of Hebb and Festinger. Both theories appear to demand (*1*) that feedback from either eye movements (Hebb) or the efferent commands for eye movements (Festinger) are stored as part of the definition of the shape being learned, and (*2*) that oculomotor feedback from efferent saccadic commands remains constant across perceptual learning or adaptation. Although the latter assumption is rarely stated explicitly, its removal tends to wreak havoc with these theories, considered developmentally, if all components of the eye do not mature in synchrony (see Sections III-C and III-A).

The Aslin and Salapatek data indicate that infant saccades executed to a peripheral target and, therefore, feedback from saccades, are quite different in form from those of the adult. This consideration has interesting implications if viewed within the framework of a strict motor theory, such as that of Hebb or Festinger. The most striking implication is that stimuli well learned during early infancy or childhood, before final growth and calibration of the saccadic and other systems, and never viewed again until final growth and calibration, should appear distorted and disproportionate upon later viewing. This should be true since they should arouse stored local signs inappropriate for motor tendencies to eye movement. There is no question that adults viewing familiar objects through magnifying, minifying, displacing, inverting, or distorting lenses, experience these events as distorted (e.g., Harris, 1965; Rock, 1966).

How does one test to see if such distortion occurs developmentally? To my knowledge, outside of a few clinical claims,[29] none of us has conscious visual imagery from infancy, nor even recognition of objects familiar during infancy but unviewed since that time. Conscious visual imagery for childhood events generally dates back to approximately 3 years. If one forms an image of such early childhood events or scenes, the imagery appears essentially normal in shape (at least to me). On revisiting childhood locales never seen since childhood, I personally have experienced, and others have reported to me, a distortion of sorts. Shape and orientation seem normal, but magnitude appears greatly changed. Fences, houses, rooms, streets appear to have shrunk considerably. One might interpret this shrinking as an indication that the same saccadic programming for distance actually rotates the eye, or at least commands the eye to rotate, considerably further during adulthood than during infancy. However, the fact that magnitude, but not shape or orientation, is distorted suggests a much simpler explanation. What has changed over age is probably the visual point of view of the observer (it was lower in the visual field at a younger age), and the judgment of the size of objects with respect to himself (they are smaller with respect to oneself as one grows larger).

The foregoing considerations, at least for late infancy, suggest that sensory (including optical) and motor components of the visual system may remain interactively constant across age as far as the programming of saccadic eye movements is concerned. During early infancy, however, there is no way to evaluate this issue, since conscious imagery and local sign are not recalled. However, it does appear that even during earliest infancy the saccadic system appears to judge distance and direction in an appropriate fashion *prior* to localization of a peripheral target, since the direction and particularly the magnitude of the *first* eye movement appear to be appropriately and linearly related to target direction and distance, respectively (Aslin & Salapatek, discussed in Section IV-A in this

---

[29] Luria (1968) reports a patient who apparently had clear visual imagery during the first year of life. The patient did not report gross shape distortion in this visual imagery.

chapter). Thus, there may be a constant system across all ages which, in conjunction with other systems, could tag the spatial distribution of features with respect to one another.

In order to examine the necessity of the saccadic eye movement centers for the appreciation of spatial distribution, it may be useful to consider for a moment the consequences of removing all centers having to do with programming of eye, head, and body movement with respect to a stimulus distributed over a fairly broad area, say 30° of the retina. Presumably, retinal, lateral geniculate, and cortical units, or even collicular units, associated with the location of contour features would respond. Moreover, units responding should preserve the spatial arrangement of features since (1) these units are topologically organized even at the level of the cortex in a fashion reflecting spatial arrangement of retinal cells, and (2) on logical grounds spatial information must be preserved since it is this system that would have provided the eye movement centers with information on the basis of which to program a saccade. Theoretically, then, the system *sans* movement is capable of perceiving spatial arrangement.

What would be lost, however, if there were no eye movement centers, would be the "meaning" or definition of spatial arrangement. *There would be no action implications of spatial arrangement.* The stimulus learned would be discriminably different from other patterns learned with different spatial arrangements, or from the same pattern learned but in a different orientation. But there would be no essential meaning beyond that contained in saying that red is different from blue, or white from black. Bower (1974) has argued that concepts of space or distance are meaningless unless ultimately defined in terms of some motor act, and we agree. For example, the concept of distance is not separable from the cues for distance (which may allow discrimination of objects at different distances) unless it may be shown that the organism will program different spatially appropriate action sequences (e.g., calibrated eye movements, defensive reactions, calibrated reaching) for stimuli differing in their cues for depth. We see no reason why this analysis does not apply equally well to *eye movements* in *two-* or three-dimensional space, since we see no essential difference between two- and three-dimensional space (see Section VI) or between eye versus hand or other motor systems. Finally, we believe this is the position held most explicitly by Hochberg (1968), if some extensions are made to his theory. For Hochberg, actual eye movements are apparently not necessary *for the experienced observer* for the

perceptual learning of two-dimensional figures. However, perceptual learning of such figures (1) is typically accompanied by eye
movements for acuity and attentional reasons, and (2) whether
accompanied by eye movements or not, results ultimately in
sensorimotor expectancies: If I move my eyes in such and such a
direction, I shall see such and such. For an experienced observer
who knows space (local sign) well, and for whom the programming
of eye movements to targets in space has been well exercised,
appropriate sensorimotor expectancies could indeed be built up
through exposure to a stimulus if no eye movements occur,
providing identity of the stimulus is maintained (see Section III-C).
However, for a naive, "mindless" infant, it would seem that actual
eye movements and their resultant sensory feedback from the
stimulus would be necessary for the motor definition of a spatially
distributed stimulus, as distinct from simply a discriminable stimulus. In short, the earliest definition or meaning of distance
or space may be that different sensorimotor eye movement expectancies are built up for figures with differing spatial arrangements
of features. This is consistent with the view of the infant as a
sensorimotor rather than a conceptual organism (see Section III-D).

It is unclear at this point whether a strong or some weaker
sensorimotor (oculomotor) position of early perceptual learning is
correct. The data indicating little appreciation of spatial arrangement before a couple of months of age suggest that a strong
position is still possible. Unfortunately, because of the difficulties in
conducting conditioning and habituation studies with infants, we
cannot be sure we have motivated the infant to tell us all he
perceives. However, the burden appears to have shifted toward
demonstrations that amotoric, wholistic perception of pattern does
exist at birth, rather than toward demonstrations that most of
perception is learned piecemeal and laboriously.

D. Mind Interacts with Sensation

Throughout this chapter we have stressed that the newborn and
very young infant is not an adult in his approach to perceptual
learning. By most accounts the very young infant possesses little
stored information regarding specific pattern and form; he does not
possess stored sensorimotor knowledge of spatial direction and
distance. He certainly does not evidence conceptual knowledge of

space and pattern in the sense that he is capable of logically and consciously understanding the implications of space in the absence of action, nor apparently of inhibiting actions in space on the basis of thought or instructions (although this remains to be explored). It is unlikely that he would be capable of maintaining object identity in order to learn an object whose features were serially presented, as in the Hochberg (1968) or Farley (1974) studies, or of *consciously* understanding the sensorimotor implications of a particular action, e.g., an eye movement, given presentation of a feature of a well-learned stimulus. It is unclear whether the infant is capable of presetting peripheral attention to allow the detection of a particular feature or figure. He certainly does not possess conscious concepts of "up–down," "right–left," except on a sensorimotor level, and, therefore, "local sign" defined as a "perceived" direction must differ from the definition of local sign in the child or adult. It would appear, then, that in early infancy, perceptual learning consists largely of identifying pattern features and their arrangement through oculomotor scanning involving foveal inspection of critical features. This activity probably provides the rudimentary meaning of extension of features in space, i.e., figure or pattern, as well as clarifying such features by placing them on the fovea.

VI. TWO VERSUS THREE DIMENSIONS, FIGURE VERSUS OBJECT, AND STATIC VERSUS DYNAMIC CUES: THE LIMITATIONS OF THIS CHAPTER

In 1951 J. J. Gibson criticized the use of two-dimensional displays as a means of gaining knowledge regarding the perception of objects in the real world. Two-dimensional "outline," "pictorial," "plan," "perspective," "nonsense," or "projected" forms were characterized as poor examples of reality since they lacked many dynamic, three-dimensional, immediate cues typically associated with real events. We must agree with Gibson that "representations" of real objects are on a level removed from the real objects. However, if "representations" of real objects are not involved, then it appears to us that two-dimensional stimuli on a surface some distance from the eyes are essentially indistinguishable from so-called real, three-dimensional events. Consider a circle projected on a screen 25 cm from the infant's eyes. To the infant it is a real pattern on a surface in the fronto–parallel plane at a three-dimensional distance of 25 cm. To our minds this pattern on a surface is no different from the pattern a primitive human might have encountered on the surface of a flat rock, the side of a flat fish, or on a flat leaf 25 cm away. The pattern on the surface of a real flat object does not define an object, but it is natural, and apparently, we have evolved to detect such patterns (Trevarthen, 1968). The two-dimensional figures and patterns, then, that we have considered in this chapter, are not objects, but they are natural, and they do have three-dimensional definition since they are on a surface at a discriminable distance from the subject, and we have apparently evolved to detect them (as distinct from having evolved to detect "representations" of objects).

However, there is a sense in which J. J. Gibson is correct. The outlines of real, three-dimensional objects are distinct from the outlines of two-dimensional patterning on the surface of three-dimensional objects. Distance cues for the outlines are different for the two events, different visual centers may be involved in the detection of the two events, and there is some evidence that the two events have different perceptual properties in early infancy. For example, Bower's experiments during early infancy are consistent with the generalization that size and shape constancy, existence constancy, and good continuation hold only for three-dimensional objects, and that movement is a prerequisite to the early perception of common fate (Bower, 1974). We can only reiterate that we have studied the perception of static, two-dimensional, but *real* or *natural* shapes and patterns, and have compared infant perception of such patterns to similar adult perception, and to the predictions made by well-known theories for such patterns.

ACKNOWLEDGMENTS

The author is indebted to Richard Aslin, Emily Bushnell, Bonita Grussing, Deborah Lord, Elizabeth Pulos, and John Simonson who assisted in the preparation of either data or other material for this chapter. Martin Banks and Richard Aslin generously read an early draft of this manuscript and removed errors. For any remaining errors I assume full responsibility.

REFERENCES

Ahrens, R. Beitrage zur Entwicklung des Physiognomie und Mimikerkennes. *Zeitchrift fur Experimentalle und Angewandte Psychologie*, 1954, *2*, 412–454; 599–633.

Alpern, M. Movements of the eyes. In H. Davson (Ed.), *The eye.* Vol. 3. *Muscular mechanisms.* New York: Academic Press, 1962. Pp. 1–187.

Alpern, M. Effector mechanisms in vision. In J. W. Kling & L. A. Riggs (Eds.), *Woodworth & Schlosberg's experimental psychology.* (3rd ed.) New York: Holt, 1971. Pp. 369–394.

Ames, E. & Silfen, C. Methodological issues in the study of age differences in infant's attention to stimuli varying in movement and complexity. Paper presented at meetings of the Society for Research in Child Development, Minneapolis, Minnesota, March, 1965.

Andrews, D. P. Perception of contour orientation in the central fovea. Part I: Short lines. *Vision Research,* 1967, *7,* 975–997. (a)

Andrews, D. P. Perception of contour orientation in the central fovea. Part II: Spatial integration. *Vision Research,* 1967, *7,* 999–1013. (b)

Aserinsky, E., & Kleitman, N. A motility cycle in sleeping infants as manifested by ocular and gross bodily activity. *Journal of Applied Physiology,* 1955, *8,* 11–18.

Aslin, R. N., & Banks, M. S. A critical period for the development of human binocular vision. Paper presented at biennial meetings of the Society for Research in Child Development, Denver, Colorado, April 10–13, 1975.

Aslin, R. N., & Salapatek, P. Saccadic localization of peripheral targets by the very young human infant. *Perception and Psychophysics,* 1975, *17,* 293–302.

Atkinson, J., Braddick, O., & Braddick, F. Acuity and contrast sensitivity of infant vision. *Nature,* 1974, *247,* 403–404.

Atkinson, R. C., & Shiffrin, R. M. Human memory: A proposed system and its control processes. In G. H. Bower & J. T. Spence (Eds.), *The psychology of learning and motivation.* Vol. 2. New York: Academic Press, 1968.

Aulhorn, E., & Harms, H. Visual perimetry. In D. Jameson & L. M. Hurvich (Eds.), *Handbook of sensory physiology. vii/4. Visual psychophysics.* New York: Springer-Verlag, 1972.

Bach-Y-Rita, P., Collins, C. C., & Hyde, J. E. (Eds.), *The control of eye movements.* New York: Academic Press, 1971.

Barlow, H. B., Narasimhan, R., & Rosenfeld, A. Visual pattern analysis in machines and animals. *Science,* 1972, *177,* 567–575.

Barlow, H. B., & Pettigrew, J. D. Lack of specificity of neurones in the visual cortex of young kittens. *Journal of Physiology (London),* 1971, *219,* 98P–100P.

Bartz, A. E. Eye movement latency, duration, and response time as a function of angular displacement. *Journal of Experimental Psychology,* 1962, *64,* 318–324.

Bartz, A. E. Fixation errors in eye movements to peripheral stimuli. *Journal of Experimental Psychology,* 1967, *75,* 444–446.

Becker, W., & Fuchs, A. F. Further properties of the human saccadic system: Eye movements and correction saccades with and without visual fixation points. *Vision Research,* 1969, *9,* 1247–1258.

Bergman, T., Haith, M. M., & Mann, L. Development of eye contact and facial scanning in infants. Paper presented at meetings of Society for Research in Child Development, Minneapolis, Minnesota, March, 1971.

Blakemore, C., & Campbell, F. W. On the existence of neurones in the human visual system selectively sensitive to the orientation and size of retinal images. *Journal of Physiology (London),* 1969, *203,* 237–260.

Blakemore, C., & Cooper, G. F. Development of the brain depends on the visual environment. *Nature,* 1970, *228,* 447–478.

Blakemore, C., Nachmias, J., & Sutton, P. The perceived spatial frequency shift: Evidence for frequency selective neurones in the human brain. *Journal of Physiology (London)*, 1970, *210*, 727–750.

Bodis-Wollner, I. Visual acuity and contrast sensitivity in patients with cerebral lesions. *Science*, 1972, *178*, 769–771.

Bond, E. Perception of form by the human infant. *Psychological Bulletin*, 1972, *77*, 225–245.

Bower, T. G. R. The determinants of perceptual unity in infancy. *Psychonomic Science*, 1965, *3*, 323–324.

Bower, T. G. R. Heterogeneous summation in human infants. *Animal Behavior*, 1966, *14*, 395–398.

Bower, T. G. R. The development of object-permanence: Some studies of existence constancy. *Perception and Psychophysics*, 1967, *2*, 411–418. (a)

Bower, T. G. R. Phenomenal identity and form perception in an infant. *Perception and Psychophysics*, 1967, *2*, 74–76. (b)

Bower, T. G. R. *Development in infancy.* San Francisco: Freeman, 1974.

Brindley, G. S., & Merton, P. A. The absence of position sense in the human eye. *Journal of Physiology (London)*, 1960, *153*, 127–130.

Broadbent, D. E. *Perception and communication.* London: Pergamon Press, 1958.

Broadbent, D. E. Stimulus set and response set: Two kinds of selective attention. In D. I. Mostofsky (Ed.), *Attention: Contemporary theory and analysis.* New York: Appleton, 1970. Pp. 51–60.

Broadbent, D. E. *Decision and stress.* New York: Academic Press, 1971.

Bronson, G. W. The postnatal growth of visual capacity. *Child Development*, 1974, *45*, 873–890.

Brooks, B., & Jung, R. Neuronai physiology of the visual cortex. In R. Jung (Ed.), *Handbook of sensory physiology.* Vol. VII/3. Part B: *Central processing of visual information: Visual centers in the brain.* New York: Springer-Verlag, 1973. Pp. 325–440.

Brown, J. L. Visual sensitivity. *Annual Review of Psychology*, 1973, *24*, 151–186.

Campbell, F. W., Cleland, B. G., Cooper, G. F., & Enroth-Cugell, C. The angular selectivity of visual cortical cells to moving gratings. *Journal of Physiology (London)*, 1968, *198*, 237–250.

Campbell, F. W., & Kulikowski, J. J. The visual evoked potential as a function of contrast of a grating pattern. *Journal of Physiology (London)*, 1972, *222*, 345–356.

Campbell, F. W., & Robson, J. G. Application of Fourier analysis to the visibility of gratings. *Journal of Physiology (London)*, 1968, *197*, 551–566.

Chase, W. P. Color vision in infants. *Journal of Experimental Psychology*, 1937, *20*, 203–222.

Collier, R. M. An experimental study of form perception in indirect vision. *Journal of Comparative Psychology*, 1931, *11*, 281–289.

Conel, J. L. *The postnatal development of the human cerebral cortex.* Vol. 1. *The cortex of the newborn.* Cambridge, Massachusetts: Harvard Univ. Press, 1939.

Conel, J. L. *The postnatal development of the human cerebral cortex.* Vol. 2. *The cortex of the one-month infant.* Cambridge, Massachusetts: Harvard Univ. Press, 1941.

Conel, J. L. *The postnatal development of the human cerebral cortex.* Vol. 3. *The cortex of the three-month infant.* Cambridge, Massachusetts: Harvard Univ. Press, 1947.

Cooper, G. F., & Robson, J. G. The yellow colour of the lens of man and other primates. *Journal of Physiology (London)*, 1969, *203*, 411–417.

Cornsweet, T. N. *Visual perception.* New York: Academic Press, 1970.

Cosgrove, M. P., Schmidt, M. J., Fulgham, D. D., & Brown, D. R. Stabilized images: Dependent variable specificity of pattern-specific effects with prolonged viewing. *Perception and Psychophysics*, 1972, *11*, 398–402.

Crannell, C. W., & Christensen, J. M. Expansion of the visual form field by perimeter training. *USAF WADC Technical Report*, 1955, 55–368.

Crawford, B. H. The Stiles-Crawford effects and their significance in vision. In D. Jameson & L. Hurvich (Eds.), *Handbook of sensory physiology.* Vol. 7/4. *Visual psychophysics.* New York: Springer-Verlag, 1972. Pp. 470–483.

Cunningham, M. *Intelligence: Its organization and development.* New York: Academic Press, 1972.

Davson, H. *The physiology of the eye.* (3rd ed.) New York: Academic Press, 1972.

Day, R. H. The physiological basis of form perception in the peripheral retina. *Psychological Review*, 1957, *64*, 38–48.

Dayton, G. O., Jr., & Jones, M. H. Analysis of characteristics of fixation reflex in infants by use of direct current electrooculography. *Neurology*, 1964, *14*, 1152–1156.

Dayton, G. O., Jr., Jones, M. H., Aiu, P., Rawson, R. A., Steele, B., & Rose, M. Developmental study of coordinated eye movements in the human infant. I. Visual acuity in the newborn human: A study based on induced optokinetic nystagmus recorded by electro-oculography. *Archives of Ophthalmology*, 1964, *71*, 865–870. (a)

Dayton, G. O., Jr., Jones, M. H., Steele, B., & Rose, M. Developmental study of coordinated eye movements in the human infant. II. An electro-oculographic study of the fixation reflex in the newborn. *Archives of Ophthalmology*, 1964, *71*, 871–875. (b)

Deutsch, J. A. *The structural basis of behavior.* Chicago: Chicago Univ. Press, 1960.

Dews, P. B., & Wiesel, T. N. Consequences of monocular deprivation on visual behavior in kittens. *Journal of Physiology (London)*, 1970, *206*, 437–455.

Diamond, I. T., & Hall, W. C. Evolution of neocortex. *Science*, 1969, *164*, 251–262.

Dodwell, P. C. A coupled system for coding and learning in shape discrimination. *Psychological Review*, 1964, *71*, 148–159.

Dodwell, P. C. *Visual pattern recognition.* New York: Holt, 1970.

Donnee, L. H. Infants' developmental scanning patterns to face and nonface stimuli under various auditory conditions. Paper delivered at meetings of Society for Research in Child Development, Philadelphia, Pennsylvania, March, 1973.

Doty, R. W. Ablation of visual areas in the central nervous system. In R. Jung (Ed.), *Handbook of Sensory Physiology.* Vol. VII/3. *Central processing of visual information.* Part B. *Visual centers in the brain.* New York: Springer-Verlag, 1973. Pp. 483–541.

Dreyfus-Brisac, C. Sleep ontogenesis in early human prematurity from 24 to 27 weeks of conceptional age. *Developmental Psychobiology*, 1968, *1*, 162–169.

Dreyfus-Brisac, C., & Monod, N. Sleeping behavior in abnormal newborns. *Neuropädiatrie*, 1970, *1*, 354–366.

Dreyfus-Brisac, C., Monod, N., Parmelee, A. H., Prechtl, H. F. R., & Schulte, F. J. For what reason should the pediatrician follow the rapidly expanding literature on sleep? *Neuropädiatrie*, 1970, *1*, 349–372.

Easterbrook, J. A. The effect of emotion on cue utilization and the organization of behavior. *Psychological Review*, 1959, *66*, 183–201.

Evans, C. R. Further studies of pattern perception and a stabilized retinal image: The use of prolonged after-images to achieve perfect stabilization. *British Journal of Psychology*, 1967, *58*, 315–327.

Evarts, E. V. Motor cortex reflexes associated with learned movement. *Science*, 1973, *179*, 501–503.

Evarts, E. V., Bizzi, E., Burke, R. E., DeLong, M., & Thach, W. T., Jr. Central control of movement. *Neurosciences Research Program Bulletin*, 1971, No. 9.

Fagan, J. F. Infant color perception. *Science*, 1974, *183*, 973–975.

Fantz, R. L. Pattern vision in young infants. *Psychological Record*, 1958, *8*, 43–47.

Fantz, R. L. The origin of form perception. *Scientific American*, 1961, *204*, 66–72.

Fantz, R. L. Pattern vision in newborn infants. *Science*, 1963, *140*, 296–297.

Farley, A. M. VIPS: A visual imagery and perception system. The results of a protocol analysis. Unpublished doctoral dissertation, Carnegie Mellon Univ., 1974.

Ferree, C. E., & Rand, G. The effect of relation to background on the size and shape of the form field for stimuli of different sizes. *American Journal of Ophthamology*, 1931, *14*, 1018–1029.

Ferree, C. E., & Rand, G. Two important factors in the size and shape of the form field and some of their relations to practical perimetry. *Journal of General Psychology*, 1932, *6*, 414–428.

Ferree, C. E., Rand, G., & Hardy, C. Refraction for the peripheral field of vision. *Archives of Ophthalmology*, 1931, *5*, 717–731.

Ferree, C. E., Rand, G., & Monroe, M. M. A study of the factors which cause individual differences in the size of the form field. *American Journal of Psychology*, 1930, *42*, 63–71.

Festinger, L. Eye movements and perception. In P. Bach-Y-Rita, C. C. Collins, & J. E. Hyde (Eds.), *The control of eye movements*. New York: Academic Press, 1971. Pp. 259–273.

Festinger, L., Burnham, C. A., Ono, H., & Bamber, D. Efference and the conscious experience of perception. *Journal of Experimental Psychology Monograph*, 1967, *74* (4, Pt. 2).

Festinger, L., & Canon, L. K. Information about spatial location based on knowledge about efference. *Psychological Review*, 1965, *72*, 373–384.

Festinger, L., & Easton, A. M. Inferences about the efferent system based on a perceptual illusion produced by eye movements. *Psychological Review*, 1974, *81*, 44–58.

Fiorentini, A., Ghez, C., & Maffei, L. Physiological correlates of adaptation to a rotated visual field. *Brain Research*, 1972, *42*, 544–545. (a)

Fiorentini, A., Ghez, C., & Maffei, L. Physiological correlates of adaptation to a rotated visual field. *Journal of Physiology (London)*, 1972, *227*, 313–322. (b)

Freeman, R. D., Mitchell, D. E., & Millodot, M. A. Neural effect of partial visual deprivation in humans. *Science*, 1972, *175*, 1384–1386.

Freeman, R. D., & Thibos, L. N. Electrophysiological evidence that abnormal early visual experience can modify the human brain. *Science*, 1973, *180*, 876–878.

Geissler, L. R. Form perception in indirect vision. *Psychological Bulletin*, 1926, *23*, 135–136.

Gibson, E. J. *Principles of perceptual learning and development.* New York: Appleton, 1969.

Gibson, J. J. *The perception of the visual world.* Boston: Houghton Mifflin, 1950.

Gibson, J. J. What is form? *Psychological Review,* 1951, *58,* 403–412.

Gibson, J. J. *The senses considered as perceptual systems.* Boston: Houghton Mifflin, 1966.

Gibson, J. J., & Gibson, E. J. Perceptual learning: Differentiation or enrichment? *Psychological Review,* 1955, *62,* 32–41.

Gordon, B. The superior colliculus of the brain. *Scientific American,* 1972, *227,* 72–83.

Graefe, O. Qualitative Untersuchungen über Kontur und Fläche in der optischen Figurwahrnehmung. *Psychologische Forschung,* 1964, *27,* 260–306.

Graham, N. Spatial frequency channels in the human visual system: Effects of luminance and pattern drift rate. *Vision Research,* 1972, *12,* 53–68.

Graham, N., & Nachmias, J. Detection of grating patterns containing two spatial frequencies: A comparison of single-channel and multiple-channel models. *Vision Research,* 1971, *11,* 251–259.

Gregory, R. L., & Wallace, J. G. Recovery from early blindness: A case study. *Experimental Psychology and Sociology Monographs,* 1963, No. 2, Cambridge.

Gresty, M. A. Coordination of head and eye movements to fixate continuous and intermittent targets. *Vision Research,* 1974, *14,* 395–403.

Grindley, G. C. Psychological factors in peripheral vision. *Medical Research Council Special Report Series, No. 163.* London: His Majesty's Stationery Office, 1931.

Guillery, R. W. Visual pathways in albinos. *Scientific American,* 1974, *230,* 44–54.

Guillery, R. W., & Kaas, J. H. A study of normal and congenitally abnormal retinogeniculate projections in cats. *Journal of Comparative Neurology,* 1971, *143,* 73–100.

Guzman, A. Decomposition of a visual scene into three-dimensional bodies. *Proceedings of the Fall Joint Computer Conference,* 1968, 291–304.

Gyr, J. W. Is a theory of direct visual perception adequate? *Psychological Bulletin,* 1972, 77, 246–261.

Gyr, J. W., Brown, J. S., Willey, R., & Zivian, A. Computer simulation and psychological theories of perception. *Psychological Bulletin,* 1966, *65,* 174–192.

Haber, R. N. The nature of the effect of set on perception. *Psychological Review,* 1966, *73,* 335–350.

Haber, R. N., & Hershenson, M. The effects of repeated brief exposures on the growth of a percept. *Journal of Experimental Psychology,* 1965, *69,* 40–46.

Haber, R. N., & Hershenson, M. *The psychology of visual perception.* New York: Holt, 1973.

Haith, M. M. Infrared television recording and measurement of ocular behavior in the human infant. *American Psychologist,* 1969, *24,* 279–283.

Haith, M. M. Visual competence in early infancy. In R. Held, H. Leibowitz, & H. L. Teuber (Eds.), *Handbook of sensory physiology.* Vol. VIII. New York: Springer-Verlag, in press.

Haith, M. M., Morrison, F. J., Sheingold, K., & Mindes, P. Short-term memory for visual information in children and adults. *Journal of Experimental Child Psychology,* 1970, *9,* 454–469.

Hamasaki, D., Ong, J., & Marg, E. The amplitude of accommodation in presbyopia. *American Journal of Optometry,* 1956, *33,* 3–14.

Harris, C. S. Perceptual adaptation to inverted, reversed, and displaced vision. *Psychological Review*, 1965, *72*, 419–444.

Harris, P., & Macfarlane, A. The growth of the effective visual field from birth to seven weeks. *Journal of Experimental Child Psychology*, 1974, *18*, 340–348.

Haynes, H., White, B. L., & Held, R. Visual accommodation in human infants. *Science*, 1965, *148*, 528–530.

Hebb, D. O. The innate organization of visual activity: I. Perception of figures by rats reared in total darkness. *Pedagogical Seminary and Journal of Genetic Psychology*, 1937, *51*, 101–126.

Hebb, D. O. *The organization of behavior*. New York: Wiley, 1949.

Hebb, D. O. The semiautonomous process: Its nature and nurture. *American Psychologist*, 1963, *18*, 16–27.

Hebb, D. O. Concerning imagery. *Psychological Review*, 1968, *75*, 466–477.

Hebb, D. O. *Textbook of psychology*. (3rd ed.) Philadelphia: Saunders, 1972.

Heckenmueller, E. G. Stabilization of the retinal image: A review of method, effects, and theory. *Psychological Bulletin*, 1965, *63*, 157–169.

Held, R. Exposure-history as a factor in maintaining stability of perception and coordination. *Journal of Nervous and Mental Disease*, 1961, *132*, 26–32.

Held, R. Plasticity in sensory-motor systems. *Scientific American*, 1965, November, 84–94.

Held, R. Dissociation of visual functions by deprivation and rearrangement. *Psychologische Forschung*, 1968, *31*, 338–348.

Held, R. Two modes of processing spatially distributed visual stimulation. In F. O. Schmitt (Ed.), *The neurosciences: Second study program*. New York: Rockefeller Univ. Press, 1969.

Held, R., & Freedman, S. J. Plasticity in human sensorimotor control. *Science*, 1963, *142*, 455–462.

Helson, H. The fundamental propositions of gestalt psychology. *Psychological Review*, 1933, *40*, 13–32.

Hershenson, M. Visual discrimination in the human newborn. *Journal of Comparative and Physiological Psychology*, 1964, *58*, 270–276.

Hershenson, M. Development of the perception of form. *Psychological Bulletin*, 1967, *67*, 326–336.

Hershenson, M. The development of visual perceptual systems. In H. Moltz (Ed.), *The ontogeny of vertebrate behavior*. New York: Academic Press, 1970. Pp. 30–56.

Hess, E. H. Ethology and developmental psychology. In P. Mussen (Ed.), *Carmichael's manual of child psychology*. Vol. 1. New York: Wiley, 1970. Pp. 1–38.

Hirsch, H. V. B. Visual perception in cats after environmental surgery. *Experimental Brain Research*, 1972, *15*, 405–423.

Hirsch, H. V. B., & Spinelli, D. N. Visual experience modifies distribution of horizontally and vertically oriented receptive fields in cats. *Science*, 1970, *168*, 869–871.

Hochberg, J. In the mind's eye. In R. N. Haber (Ed.), *Contemporary theory and research in visual perception*. New York: Holt, 1968. Pp. 309–331.

Hochberg, J. Attention, organization and consciousness. In D. Mostofsky (Ed.), *Attention: Contemporary theory and analysis*. New York: Appleton, 1970. Pp. 99–124.

Hochberg, J. Perception: I. Color and shape. In J. A. Kling & L. A. Riggs (Eds.),

Woodworth and Schlosberg's experimental psychology. (3rd ed.) New York: Holt, 1971. Pp. 395–474. (a)

Hochberg, J. Perception: II. Space and movement. In J. A. Kling & L. A. Riggs (Eds.), *Woodworth and Schlosberg's experimental psychology.* (3rd ed.) New York: Holt, 1971. Pp. 475–550. (b)

Hosoya, Y. Über die Altersverschiedenheit der Ultraviolettabsorption der menschlichen Augenmedien. *Tohoku Journal of Experimental Medicine, 1929, 13,* 510–523.

Hubel, D. H., & Wiesel, T. N. Receptive fields of single neurones in the cat's striate cortex. *Journal of Physiology (London), 1959, 148,* 574–591.

Hubel, D. H., & Wiesel, T. N. Receptive fields, binocular interaction and functional architecture in the cat's visual cortex. *Journal of Physiology (London), 1962, 160,* 106–154.

Hubel, D. H., & Wiesel, T. N. Receptive fields of cells in striate cortex of very young visually inexperienced kittens. *Journal of Neurophysiology, 1963, 26,* 994–1002.

Hubel, D. H., & Wiesel, T. N. Binocular interaction in striate cortex of kittens reared with artificial squint. *Journal of Neurophysiology, 1965, 28,* 1041–1059.

Hubel, D. H., & Wiesel, T. N. Receptive fields and functional architecture of monkey striate cortex. *Journal of Physiology (London), 1968, 195,* 215–243.

Hubel, D. H., & Wiesel, T. N. The period of susceptibility to the physiological effects of unilateral eye closure in kittens. *Journal of Physiology (London), 1970, 206,* 419–436.

Hubel, D. H., & Wiesel, T. N. Aberrant visual projections in the Siamese cat. *Journal of Physiology (London), 1971, 218,* 33–62.

Humphrey, N. K. What the frog's eye tells the monkey's brain. *Brain, Behavior and Evolution, 1970, 3,* 324–337.

Humphrey, N. Seeing and nothingness. *New Scientist,* 1972, 30 March, 682–684.

Humphrey, N. K., & Weiskrantz, L. Vision in monkeys after removal of the striate cortex. *Nature, 1967, 215,* 595–597.

Jeffrey, W. The orienting reflex and attention in cognitive development. *Psychological Review, 1968, 75,* 323–334.

Keibel, F. Development of the sense organs. In F. Keibel & F. Mall (Eds.), *Human embryology.* Philadelphia: Lippincott, 1912. Pp. 180–290.

Kessen, W., Haith, M., & Salapatek, P. Human infancy: A bibliography and guide. In P. Mussen (Ed.), *Carmichael's manual of child psychology.* Vol. 1. New York: Wiley, 1970. Pp. 287–446.

Kessen, W., Salapatek, P., & Haith, M. The visual response of the human newborn to linear contour. *Journal of Experimental Child Psychology, 1972, 13,* 9–20.

Kestenbaum, A. *Applied anatomy of the eye.* New York: Grune & Stratton, 1963.

King, S. J. A system for separating objects from the background in automatic picture processing. Unpublished doctoral dissertation, Cornell Univ., 1971.

Kleitman, N., & Blier, Z. A. Color and form discrimination in the periphery of the retina. *American Journal of Physiology, 1928, 85,* 178–190.

Klopfer, P. H. *Behavioral aspects of ecology.* Englewood Cliffs, New Jersey: Prentice-Hall, 1962.

Knighton, W. S. Development of the normal eye in infancy and childhood. *Sight-Saving Review, 1939, 9,* 3–10.

Koehler, W. *Die physischen Gestalten in Ruhe und im stationaeren Zustand.* Erlangen: Philosophische Akademie, 1924.

Koehler, W. *Gestalt psychology.* New York: Mentor, 1959 (1947).

Koffka, K. *Principles of Gestalt psychology.* New York: Harcourt, 1935.

Komoda, M. K., Festinger, L., Phillips, L. J., Duckman, R. H., & Young, R. A. Some observations concerning saccadic eye movements. *Vision Research,* 1973, *13,* 1009–1020.

Kris, E. Bi-dimensional, binocular eye-position and motion electrooculogram measurement in infants and children with nystagmus and strabismus. *Digest of the Seventh International Conference of Medical and Biological Engineering,* 1967, 248.

Lamont, A., & Millodot, M. Dioptrics of the periphery of the eye. *Science,* 1973, *182,* 86.

Larroche, J. Development of the nervous system in early life. Part II: The development of the central nervous system during intrauterine life. In F. Falkner (Ed.), *Human development.* Philadelphia: Saunders, 1966. Pp. 257–276.

Le Grand, Y. *Form and space vision.* (Translated by M. Millodot and G. G. Heath). Bloomington, Indiana: Indiana Univ. Press, *Revised Edition,* 1967.

Leibowitz, H. W., & Harvey, L. O., Jr. Perception. *Annual Review of Psychology,* 1973, *24,* 207–240.

Leibowitz, H. W., Johnson, C. A., & Isabelle, E. Peripheral motion detection and refractive error. *Science,* 1972, *177,* 1207.

Leushina, L. I. On estimation of position of photostimulus and eye movements. *Biofizika,* 1965, *10,* 130–136.

Levy, J., Trevarthen, C., & Sperry, R. W. Perception of bilateral chimeric figures following hemispheric deconnexion. *Brain,* 1972, *95,* 61–78.

Ling, B. C. A genetic study of sustained visual fixation and associated behavior in the human infant from birth to six months. *Pedagogical Seminary and Journal of Genetic Psychology,* 1942, *61,* 227–277.

Liss, P. H., & Haith, M. M. The speed of visual processing in children and adults: Effects of backward and forward masking. *Perception and Psychophysics,* 1970, *8,* 396–398.

Locher, P. J., & Nodine, C. F. The role of scanpaths in the recognition of random shapes. *Perception and Psychophysics,* 1974, *15,* 308–314.

Lorenz, K. *Evolution and modification of behavior.* Chicago: Univ. of Chicago Press, 1965.

Ludlam, W. M., & Twarowski, C. J. Ocular-dioptric-component changes in the growing rabbit. *Journal of the Optical Society of America,* 1973, *63,* 95–98.

Luria, A. R. *The mind of a mnemonist.* New York: Basic Books, 1968.

Mach, E. *The analysis of sensations.* New York: Dover Publications, 1959. (Original edition, 1885.)

Mack, A., & Herman, E. A new illusion: The underestimation of distance during pursuit eye movements. *Perception and Psychophysics,* 1972, *12,* 471–473.

MacKay, D. M., & Jeffreys, D. A. Visually evoked potentials and visual perception in man. In R. Jung (Ed.), *Handbook of sensory physiology.* Vol. VII/3. *Part B: Visual centers in the brain.* New York: Springer-Verlag, 1973. Pp. 647–678.

Mackworth, N. H. Visual noise causes tunnel vision. *Psychonomic Science,* 1965, *3,* 67–68.

Maffei, L., & Fiorentini, A. Processes of synthesis in visual perception. *Nature,* 1972, *240,* 479–481.

Mann, I. C. *The development of the human eye.* London: British Medical Association, 1964.

Marg, E. Recording from single cells in the human visual cortex. In R. Jung (Ed.), *Visual centers in the brain. Handbook of sensory physiology*, Vol. VII/3. New York: Springer-Verlag, 1973. Pp. 441–449.

Marg, E., & Adams, J. E. Evidence for a neurological zoom system in vision from angular changes in some receptive fields of single neurons with changes in fixation distance in the human visual cortex. *Experientia*, 1970, *26*, 270–271.

Marg, E., Adams, J. E., & Rutkin, B. Receptive fields of cells in the human visual cortex. *Experientia*, 1968, *24*, 348–350.

Markoff, J. I., & Sturr, J. F. Spatial and luminance determinants of the increment threshold under monoptic and dichoptic viewing. *Journal of the Optical Society of America*, 1971, *61*, 1530–1537.

Matin, L. Eye movements and perceived visual direction. In D. Jameson & L. M. Hurvich (Eds.), *Handbook of sensory physiology*. Vol. VII/4. *Visual psychophysics*. New York: Springer-Verlag, 1972. Pp. 331–380.

Maurer, D., & Salapatek, P. Developmental changes in the scanning of faces by infants. Paper presented at biennial meetings of the Society for Research in Child Development, Denver, Colorado, April 10–13, 1975.

Mayzner, M. S., & Tresselt, M. E. Sequential blanking: A function of geometric analyzers in the human visual system. *Psychonomic Science*, 1969, *17*, 77–78.

McCollough, C. Color adaptation of edge detectors in the human visual system. *Science*, 1965, *149*, 1115–1116.

McIlwain, J. T. Central vision: Visual cortex and superior colliculus. *Annual Review of Physiology*, 1972, *34*, 291–314.

McLaughlin, S. C. Parametric adjustment in saccadic eye movements. *Perception and Psychophysics*, 1967, *2*, 359–362.

Michotte, A., Thines, G., & Crabbe, G. Les complements amodaux des structures perceptives. *Studia Psychologica*. Louvain: Publications Universitaires de Louvain, 1964.

Minsky, M., & Pappert, S. *Perceptrons: An introduction to computational geometry*. Cambridge, Massachusetts: MIT Press, 1969.

Mitchell, D. E., Freeman, R. D., Millodot, M., & Haegerstrom, G. Meridional amblyopia: Evidence for modification of the human visual system by early visual experience. *Vision Research*, 1973, *13*, 535–558.

Mize, R. R., & Murphy, E. H. Selective visual experience fails to modify receptive field properties of rabbit striate cortex neurons. *Science*, 1973, *180*, 320–323.

Mooney, C. M. Closure as affected by viewing time and multiple visual fixation. *Canadian Journal of Psychology*, 1957, *11*, 21–28.

Mooney, C. M. Recognition of novel visual configurations with and without eye movements. *Journal of Experimental Psychology*, 1958, *56*, 133–138.

Mooney, C. M. Recognition of symmetrical and non-symmetrical ink blots with and without eye movements. *Canadian Journal of Psychology*, 1959, *13*, 11–19.

Moray, N. *Attention: Selective processes in vision and hearing*. New York: Academic Press, 1970.

Mostofsky, D. I. (Ed.), *Attention: Contemporary theory and analysis*. New York: Appleton, 1970.

Mundy-Castle, A., & Anglin, J. M. Looking strategies in infants. Paper presented at Society for Research in Child Development Conference Santa Barbara, 1969.

Munn, N. L., & Geil, G. A. A note on peripheral form discrimination. *Journal of General Psychology*, 1931, *5*, 78–88.

Neisser, U. *Cognitive psychology*. New York: Appleton, 1967.

Nelson, K., & Kessen, W. Visual scanning by human newborns: Responses to complete triangle, to sides only, and to corners only. Paper presented at meetings of the American Psychological Association, 1969.

Norman, D. A. *Models of human memory.* New York: Academic Press, 1970.

Noton, D., & Stark, L. Scanpaths in eye movements during pattern perception. *Science,* 1971, *171,* 308–311.

O'Brien, B. Vision and resolution in the central retina. *Journal of the Optical Society of America,* 1951, *41,* 882–894.

Pantle, A., & Sekuler, R. Size detecting mechanisms in human vision. *Science,* 1968, *162,* 1146–1148.

Parmelee, A. H., Wenner, W. H., Akiyama, Y., Stern, E., & Fleischer, J. EEG and brain maturation. In A. Minkowsky (Ed.), *Regional development of the brain in early life.* Oxford: Blackwell, 1967. Pp. 459–476.

Pettigrew, J. D., & Freeman, R. D. Visual experience without lines: Effect on developing cortical neurons. *Science,* 1973, *182,* 599–601.

Piaget, J. *The origins of intelligence in children:* New York: W. W. Norton and Company, Inc., 1952.

Piaget, J. *Play, dreams, and imitation in childhood.* New York: W. W. Norton, 1962.

Piaget, J. *The mechanisms of perception.* New York: Basic Books, 1969.

Piaget, J., & Vinh-Bang. Comparaison des mouvements oculaires et des centrations du regard chez l'enfant et chez l'adulte. *Archives de Psychologie,* Genève, 1961, *38,* 167–200.

Pick, H. L., Jr. Perception in Soviet psychology. *Psychological Bulletin,* 1964, *62,* 21–35.

Pick, H. L., Jr., & Hay, J. C. Adaptation to prismatic distortion. *Psychonomic Science,* 1964, *1,* 199–200.

Pirenne, M. *Vision and the eye* (2nd ed.). London: Associated Book Publishers, 1967.

Pola, J. The relation of the perception of visual direction to eye position during and following a voluntary saccade. Unpublished doctoral dissertation, Columbia University, 1974.

Pollen, D. A., Lee, J. R., & Taylor, J. H. How does the striate cortex begin the reconstruction of the visual world? *Science,* 1971, *173,* 74–77.

Polyak, S. *The vertebrate visual system.* Chicago: Univ. of Chicago Press, 1957.

Posner, M. I. Abstraction and the process of recognition. In G. H. Bower & J. T. Spence (Eds.), *The psychology of learning and motivation.* New York: Academic Press, 1969. Pp. 44–100.

Prechtl, H. F. R. Brain and behavioral mechanisms in the human newborn infant. In R. J. Robinson (Ed.), *Brain and early behavior.* New York: Academic Press, 1969. Pp. 115–138.

Prechtl, H. F. R. & Lenard, H. G. A study of eye movements in sleeping newborn infants. *Brain Research,* 1967, *5,* 477–493.

Pritchard, R. M., Heron, W., & Hebb, D. O. Visual perception approached by the method of stabilized images. *Canadian Journal of Psychology,* 1960, *14,* 67–77.

Rashbass, C. The relationship between saccadic and smooth tracking eye movements. *Journal of Physiology (London),* 1961, *159,* 326–338.

Reading, V. M., & Weale, R. A. Macular pigment and chromatic aberration. *Journal of the Optical Society of America,* 1974, *64,* 231–234.

Riggs, L. A. Progress in the recording of human retinal and occipital potentials. *Journal of the Optical Society of America,* 1969, *59,* 1558–1566.

Riggs, L. A., & Wooten, B. R. Electrical measures and psychophysical data on human vision. In D. Jameson & L. M. Hurvich (Eds.), *Handbook of sensory physiology.* Vol. VII/4. *Visual psychophysics.* New York: Springer-Verlag, 1972. Pp. 690–731.

Riggs, L. A. Curvature as a feature of pattern vision. *Science,* 1973, *181,* 1070–1072.

Riggs, L. A. Curvature detectors in human vision. *Science,* 1974, *184,* 1200–1201.

Roberts, L. G. Pattern recognition with an adaptive network. *IRE Convention Record,* 1960, *8,* part 2, 66–70.

Robinson, D. A. Eye movement control in primates. *Science,* 1968, *161,* 1219–1224.

Rock, I. *The nature of perceptual adaptation.* New York: Basic Books, 1966.

Roffwarg, H. P., Muzio, J. N., & Dement, W. C. Ontogenetic development of the human sleep-dream cycle. *Science,* 1966, *152,* 604–619.

Rubin, E. Figure and ground. (Abridged by M. Wertheimer.) In D. C. Beardslee & M. Wertheimer (Eds.), *Readings in perception.* New York: Van Nostrand, 1958. Pp. 194–203.

Ruddock, K. H. Light transmission through the ocular media and macular pigment and its significance for psychological investigation. In D. Jameson & L. M. Hurvich (Eds.), *Handbook of sensory physiology.* Vol. VII/4. *Visual psychophysics.* New York: Springer-Verlag, 1972. Pp. 455–469.

Sachs, M. B., Nachmias, J., & Robson, J. G. Spatial frequency channels in human vision. *Journal of the Optical Society of America,* 1971, *61,* 1176–1186.

Salaman, M. Some experiments on peripheral vision. *Medical Research Council Special Report Series No. 136. (London):* His Majesty's Stationery Office, 1929.

Salapatek, P. Visual scanning of geometric figures by the human newborn. *Journal of Comparative and Physiological Psychology,* 1968, *66,* 247–258.

Salapatek, P. The visual investigation of geometric pattern by the one and two month old infant. Paper presented at the meetings of the American Association for the Advancement of Science, Boston, Massachusetts, December, 1969.

Salapatek, P. Visual investigation of geometric pattern by the human infant. Paper presented at meetings of the Society for Research in Child Development, Philadelphia, March 27–30, 1973.

Salapatek, P., Haith, M., Maurer, D., & Kessen, W. Error in the corneal reflection technique: A note on Slater and Findlay. *Journal of Experimental Child Psychology,* 1972, *14,* 493–497.

Salapatek, P., & Kessen, W. Visual scanning of triangles by the human newborn. *Journal of Experimental Child Psychology,* 1966, *3,* 155–167.

Salapatek, P., & Kessen, W. Prolonged investigation of a plane geometric triangle by the human newborn. *Journal of Experimental Child Psychology,* 1973, *15,* 22–29.

Sanders, A. *The selective process in the functional visual field.* Institute for Perception, RVO-TNO, Soesterberg, The Netherlands, 1963.

Saslow, M. G. Latency for saccadic eye movement. *Journal of the Optical Society of America,* 1967, *57,* 1030–1033.

Schneider, G. E. Two visual systems. *Science,* 1969, *163,* 895–902.

Schulman, C. A. Eye movements in infants using DC recording. *Neuropädiatrie,* 1973, *4,* 76–87.

Sekuler, R. Spatial vision. *Annual Review of Psychology,* 1974, *25,* 195–232.

Skavenski, A. A., Haddad, G., & Steinman, R. M. The extraretinal signal for the visual perception of direction. *Perception and Psychophysics,* 1972, *11,* 287–290.

Slater, A. M., & Findlay, J. M. The measurement of fixation position in the newborn baby. *Journal of Experimental Child Psychology,* 1972, *14,* 349–364.

Spears, W., 7 Hohle, R. Sensory and perceptual processes in infants. In Y. Brackbill (Ed.), *Infancy and early childhood*. New York: Free Press, 1967. Pp. 49–121.

Sperling, G. The information available in brief visual presentations. *Psychological Monographs*, 1960, *74* (11, Whole No. 498).

Sperling, G. A model for visual memory tasks. *Human Factors*, 1963, *5*, 19–31.

Sperling, G. Successive approximation to a model for short term memory. *Acta Psychologica*, 1967, *27*, 285–292.

Spitz, R. A., & Wolf, K. M. The smiling response: A contribution to the ontogenesis of social relations. *Genetic Psychology Monographs*, 1946, *34*, 57–125.

Sprague, J. M. Interaction of cortex and superior colliculus in mediation of visually guided behavior in the cat. *Science*, 1966, *153*, 1544–1547.

Sprague, J. M., Berlucchi, G., & Rizzolatti, G. The role of the superior colliculus and pretectum in vision and visually guided behavior. In R. Jung (Ed.), *Handbook of sensory physiology*. Vol. VII/3. *Central processing of visual information*. Part B. *Visual centers in the brain*. New York: Springer-Verlag, 1973. Pp. 27–101.

Stechler, G., & Latz, E. Some observations on attention and arousal in the human infant. *Journal of the American Academy of Child Psychiatry*, 1966, *5*, 517–525.

Stern, E., Parmelee, A. H., Akiyama, Y., Schultz, M. A., & Wenner, W. H. Sleep cycle characteristics in infants. *Pediatrics*, 1969, *43*, 65–70.

Stiles, W. S., & Burch, J. M. N. P. L. color matching investigation: Final report (1958). *Optica Acta*, 1959, 1–26.

Stiles, W. S., & Crawford, B. H. The luminous efficiency of rays entering the eye pupil at different points. *Proceedings of the Royal Society (London)*. Series B, 1933, *112*, 428–450.

Streiff, E. B. (Ed.). Cerebral control of eye movements and motion perception. *Bibliotheca Ophthalmologica*, 1972, *82*, 1–403.

Stromeyer, C. F., III. Curvature detectors in human vision? *Science*, 1974, *184*, 1199–1200.

Sutherland, N. S. Object recognition. In E. C. Carterette & M. P. Friedman (Eds.) *Handbook of perception*. Vol. III. New York: Academic Press, 1973.

Taylor, D. M. Is congenital esotropia functionally curable? *Journal of Pediatric Ophthalmology*, 1974, *11*, 3–35.

Thomas, H. Unfolding the baby's mind: The infant's selection of visual stimuli. *Psychological Review*, 1973, *80*, 468–488.

Tinbergen, N. Social releasers and the experimental method required for their study. *Wilson Bulletin*, 1948, *60*, 6–51.

Tinbergen, N., & Perdeck, A. C. On the stimulus situation releasing the begging response in the newly hatched Herring Gull chick (Larus argentatus argentatus Pont.). *Behavior*, 1951, *3*, 1–39.

Todd, T., Beecher, H., Williams, G., & Todd, A. The weight and growth of the human eyeball. *Human Biology*, 1940, *12*, 1–20.

Treisman, A. M. Strategies and models of selective attention. *Psychological Review*, 1969, *76*, 282–299.

Trevarthen, C. B. Two mechanisms of vision in primates. *Psychologische Forschung*, 1968, *31*, 299–337.

Trevarthen, C. Analysis of cerebral activities that generate and regulate consciousness in commissurotomy patients. In S. J. Dimond & J. G. Beaumont (Eds.), *Hemisphere function in the human brain*. London: Paul Elek (Scientific Books), in press.

Trevarthen, C., & Sperry, R. W. Perceptual unity of the ambient visual field in human commissurotomy patients. *Brain*, 1973, *96*, 547–570.

Tronick, E. Stimulus control and the growth of the infant's effective visual field. *Perception and Psychophysics*, 1972, *11*, 373–375.

Tronick, E., & Clanton, C. Infant looking patterns. *Vision Research*, 1971, *11*, 1479–1486.

Uhr, L. "Pattern recognition" computers as models for form perception. *Psychological Bulletin*, 1963, *60*, 40–73.

Uhr, L. & Vossler, C. A pattern recognition program that generates, evaluates, and adjusts its own operators. *Proceedings of the Western Joint Computer Conference*, 1961, *19*, 555–569.

Uttley, A. M. Conditional probability computing in a nervous system. *The mechanisation of thought processes*. Vol. 1. London: Her Majesty's Stationery Office, 1958. Pp. 119–147.

von Noorden, G. K. Classification, diagnosis and natural history of amblyopia. *Israel Journal of Medical Sciences*, 1972, *8*, 1465–1468.

von Noorden, G. K., Dowling, J. E., & Ferguson, D. C. Experimental amblyopia in monkeys. I. Behavioral studies of stimulus deprivation amblyopia. *Archives of Ophthalmology*, 1970, *84*, 206–214.

von Senden, M. *Space and sight*. New York: Methuen, 1960. (Translated by P. Heath.)

Walls, G. L. *The vertebrate eye*. Bloomfield Hills, Michigan: The Cranbrook Press, 1942.

Weale, R. A. Presbyopia. *British Journal of Ophthalmology*, 1962, *46*, 660–668.

Weber, R. B., 7 Daroff, R. B. The metrics of horizontal saccadic eye movements in normal humans. *Vision Research*, 1971, *11*, 921–928.

Weisstein, N. What the frog's eye tells the human brain: Single cell analyzers in the human visual system. *Psychological Bulletin*, 1969, *72*, 157–176.

Wertheimer, M. Untersuchungen zur Lehre von der Gestalt, II. *Psychologische Forschung*, 1923, *4*, 301–350.

Westheimer, G. Eye movement responses to a horizontally moving visual stimulus. *A.M.A. Archives—Ophthalmology*, 1954, *52*, 932–943.

Wheeless, L. L., Jr., Boynton, R. M., & Cohen, G. H. Eye movement responses to step and pulse-step stimuli. *Journal of the Optical Society of America*, 1966, *56*, 956–960.

White, B. L. *Human infants*. Englewood Cliffs, New Jersey: Prentice-Hall, 1971.

White, C. T., Eason, R. G., & Bartlett, N. R. Latency and duration of eye movements in the horizontal plane. *Journal of the Optical Society of America*, 1962, *52*, 210–213.

Whiteside, J. A. Eye movements of children, adults, and elderly persons during inspection of dot patterns. *Journal of Experimental Child Psychology*, 1974, *18*, 313–332.

Whitmer, C. A. Peripheral form discrimination under dark adaptation. *Journal of General Psychology*, 1933, *9*, 405–419.

Whitteridge, D. Projection of optic pathways to the visual cortex. In R. Jung (Ed.), *Handbook of sensory physiology*. Vol. VII/7. Part B: *Central processing of visual information. Visual centers in the brain*. New York: Springer-Verlag, 1973. Pp. 247–268.

Wickelgren, L. W. Convergence in the human newborn. *Journal of Experimental Child Psychology*, 1967, *5*, 74–85.

Wiesel, T. N., & Hubel, D. H. Comparison of the effects of unilateral and bilateral eye closure on cortical unit responses in kittens. *Journal of Neurophysiology,* 1965, *28,* 1029–1040. (a)

Wiesel, T. N., & Hubel, D. H. Extent of recovery from the effects of visual deprivation in kittens. *Journal of Neurophysiology,* 1965, *28,* 1060–1072. (b)

Wilmer, H. A., & Scammon, R. E. Growth of the components of the human eyeball. I. Diagrams, calculations, computation and reference tables. *Archives of Ophthalmology,* 1950, *43,* 599–619.

Yakovlev, P. I., & Le Cours, A. The myelogenetic cycles of regional maturation of the brain. In A. Minkowski (Ed.), *Regional development of the brain in early life.* Philadelphia: F. A. Davis Co., 1967.

Yamada, E., & Ishikawa, T. Some observations on the submicroscopic morphogenesis of the human retina. In J. W. Rohen (Ed.), *The structure of the eye.* II. Stuttgart: Schattauer-Verlag, 1965. Pp. 5–16.

Zaporozhets, A. V. The development of perception in the preschool child. In P. H. Mussen (Ed.), European research in cognitive development. *Monographs of the Society for Research in Child Development,* 1965, *30.* Pp. 82–101.

Zaporozhets, A. V., & Zinchenko, V. P. Development of perceptual activity and formation of a sensory image in the child. In A. Leontyev, A. Luriya, & A. Smirnov (Eds.), *Psychological research in the U.S.S.R.* Vol. 1. Moscow: Progress Publishers, 1966. Pp. 393–421.

Zinchenko, V. P. Vospriyatie kad deistvie. (Perception as activity.) *Voprosy Psikhologii,* 1967, *13,* 17–24.

Zuckerman, C. B., & Rock, I. A reappraisal of the roles of past experience and innate organizing processes in visual perception. *Psychological Bulletin,* 1957, *54,* 269–296.

Zusne, L. *Visual perception of form.* New York: Academic Press, 1970.

Zusne, L., & Michels, K. M. Nonrepresentational shapes and eye movements. *Perceptual and Motor Skills,* 1964, *18,* 11–20.

chapter 4:   Early Visual Selectivity

As a Function of Pattern Variables,
Previous Exposure, Age from Birth and Conception,
and Expected Cognitive Deficit

ROBERT L. FANTZ
Case Western Reserve University

JOSEPH F. FAGAN, III
Case Western Reserve University

SIMÓN B. MIRANDA
Case Western Reserve University

I. INTRODUCTION

Much of the information in this book indicates that young infants show high selectivity in attending to their environment. This selectivity establishes the young infant as a sentient being who receives visual and other sensory information from the environment, even if the information received cannot then be used to direct behavior other than attentional responses. The limited response capabilities during the early months of life had in earlier decades led to the assumption of a visual–perceptual void until the infant was able to interact actively with the environment and so "learn to perceive." In place of this view that action precedes perception, recent findings give further basis for the assertion that in humans perception precedes action (Fantz, 1966). One might go further and assume that perception is ready to be used from the beginning and only waits for motor development to catch up. But there is as much evidence against this extreme view as against the opposite one of an initial perceptual void. The development of visually directed behavior requires much improvement of perceptual abilities including oculomotor skills, as well as the acquisition of information from the environment. The early months of life, instead of being a waiting period, are well suited for such a complex perceptual development process, especially for vision. The infant has much time for visual practice and for casually exploring and learning about and from the surroundings. Intake of environmental information is possible by initially poor but rapidly developing pattern fixation and discrimination capacities; it is guided throughout development by intrinsic selectivities among parts or aspects of the environment; it is, after several months, aided by recognition of what has been seen, with novel stimuli then receiving special attention, and with additional developmental contributions of recognition memory through the resulting accumulation of knowledge. We will propose that the selectivities among the myriad features of the environment, whether based on specific and general experiences or intrinsic to a given phase of development, are crucial at all ages both for immediate visual-directed behavior and for facilitating perceptual learning through infancy and beyond.

This tentative and schematic description of early perceptual development points up three functions in the young infant of known importance for later behavior: visual capacity (discrimination), visual selectivity (attention), and visual recognition (memory). The research presented in this chapter studied these three basic functions—their course of development, the relevant stimulus variables, and certain environmental and organismic influences. Selective visual attention was not only one of the functions under study but also provided the response measure (i.e., differential fixation times) for studying all three functions. In the next section, this special role of visual selectivity and other methodological–conceptual points of general relevance will be taken up, along with essential details of the method.

II. METHOD AND CONCEPTS

A. The Response

If subjects repeatedly look longer at one of two paired stimuli, regardless of position, they see the stimuli as different in some way. The pertinent difference can be further specified with careful choice and variation of stimuli. A reliable differential fixation response also indicates a behavioral choice by infants among stimuli that here is called a "visual preference" as an operational term (without implying that the preferred stimulus is "liked"). The direction of this visual selectivity can be as important for perceptual development as the ability to discriminate thereby shown. This point will be illustrated in two applications of the visual preference method.

Visual acuity has been estimated in newborn and older infants (Fantz, 1965a; Fantz, Ordy, & Udelf, 1962; Miranda, 1970a) by presenting pattern details of varying size paired with an unpatterned stimulus. Finding the minimum size of patterning that is selectively fixated over the plain stimulus indicates resolution of pattern details at least that fine. The same visual resolution would be shown in a particular pairing if the differential fixation was consistently for the plain over the patterned stimulus; however this opposite direction of preference would imply that the infant attends more to those parts of the environment that contain less information and give less opportunity for oculomotor practice, perceptual learning, or recognition of objects. The actual finding of selective fixation of patterned over unpatterned areas suggests instead the adaptive use of pattern vision ability in visual explorations.

The direction of visual preference may have more specific implications. For example, whether the infant attends to patterns of higher or lower "complexity" has been related to development of the capacity for processing visual information. While studies in this broad area have varied many stimulus parameters and often obtained divergent results (Section IV), it is the presence and direction of differential response at particular ages that is given importance rather than the demonstration of discrimination among certain patterns. In the research that follows we will consider additional stimulus features such as form, contrast, and depth (Sections III and V) for which the direction of the selective responses may have as much or more significance for perceptual development than the discrimination capacities revealed by the preference. Particular significance will be attributed to changes in direction or strength of selectivity with age, both within a given stimulus variation and among different variations. These developmental changes in selectivity underly some theoretical interpretations presented in Section VII.

The research presented here is restricted to the response measure of differential duration of fixation to paired stimuli, a measure considered of special relevance to adaptive behavior both in infancy and in subsequent development, and, furthermore, a measure of proven research usefulness.

B. The Stimuli

The experimenter's choice of stimuli is especially critical for a method based on a naturally existing differential response. Finding the stimulus targets that will give best evidence of discrimination ability and selectivity relative to a certain category of stimulus variation may require many trials by the experimenter. For example, only after years of research using many stimuli have we found clear evidence of form discrimination by newborn infants (Section III-D). But the problems in choosing stimuli have not interfered with the usefulness of the preference method as illustrated by the large number and wide variety of differential responses shown in the results in this and other chapters.

A more fundamental problem—one that is pervasive in perceptual experiments—is to specify objectively the stimulus difference perceived by the subject and which is the basis of the differential response. The traditional psychophysical approach is to select stimuli along a quantitatively ordered "stimulus dimension" and to find whether responses give a similar ordering of the stimuli. This approach has been largely dropped in research with adults and with animals, at least in form and pattern perception. This is due, first, to the difficulty of analyzing the complexities and interactions of dimensions in even relatively simple pattern discrimination performances (Dodwell, 1971); and second, to the practical difficulty of varying any single dimension without covarying or confounding other dimensions. But in perceptual research with infants, the psychophysical approach is much used, with some logical basis. The perceptual performances of the adult are preceded by a long and intricate developmental process, even though this process is not well understood. Therefore, it is reasonable to hypothesize that the early stages of this process can be adequately explained in terms of a few simple dimensions. But this hypothesis neglects the second difficulty, of isolating single dimensions, that is equally present in infant and adult research. And two examples will show that the first difficulty of the psychophysical approach is also present with infants in spite of their less sophisticated perceptions. Each example at the same time illustrates an alternative approach that can give more information on early perceptual development than the single-dimension approach.

The first example concerns infant preference experiments using a series of checkerboard patterns with increasing number but decreasing size of light and dark elements, a series considered to vary in the "dimension" of "pattern complexity" (Section IV-C). Of the several stimulus variations present in such a series, size and number of elements can be varied independently if unconnected black elements on a white ground are used in place of checkerboards. As we will see, patterns of either larger size or larger number of elements are strongly preferred even by newborns (Section IV-A). But the number and size preferences differ in degree at different ages (Section IV-B) with the result that previous interpretations of developmental changes for a series of patterns inversely varying size and number are challenged (Section IV-C). This technique of bidimensional stimulus variation thus gave more information and different conclusions than the single-dimension technique.

The second example concerns attempts to analyze the stimulus basis for the preference for a bull's-eye over a striped pattern (Section III-A). The psychophysical approach, as it has been applied to infant visual preference studies (Hershenson, Kessen, & Munsinger, 1967), suggests that a way of establishing a dimension is transitivity in the responses to three or more ordered stimuli. Accordingly, an orderly variation of degree of curvature was devised, starting with a bull's-eye and ending with stripes. A pattern of intermediate degree of curvature was found to give an intermediate degree of response, with transitivity among the three patterns. But this unidimensional approach gave no additional information, since other variations, such as concentricity, covaried with curvature. An approach that did give better specification of relevant stimulus variations was comparable to the method of equivalent stimuli (Kluver, 1933; Dodwell, 1971) which employs stimulus pairs that differ in certain features from a trained pair and are presented to the subject to determine what features are necessary for the discrimination. But in our example the initial discrimination, instead of being learned, was the intrinsic preference for bull's-eye over stripes. The use of a number of other stimulus pairs indicated equivalence of response to those varying in curvature but equated in concentricity. In addition, other interacting variables such as regularity of element arrangement were found to influence the response (Sections III-A-2 and III-B-2). Other chapters in this book have shown the value of comparable techniques with infants.

Both the bidimensional design and the equivalent stimulus approach can help to provide more, or better, information than the unidimensional design on stimulus features the infant perceives and selects and to reduce predetermination of results by the experimenter's choice of stimuli. Another approach with similar aims, used in experiments with infants and older subjects, is to use a set of "random" stimuli; but the technique chosen for generating such a stimulus set, usually but not necessarily unidimensional (McCall & Kagan, 1967), somewhat restricts and determines the possible findings. Brunswik (1949) had a similar aim in using a "representative sampling of stimuli" within a given area of perception, emphasizing the goal of stimulus descriptions relevant to the subject's perceptions rather than to the experimenter's perceptions or theories. This goal is more important for infants, whose perceptions differ more from the experimenter's, than do those of adult subjects. This goal might also be more approachable for infants with less developed perceptions, even though not describable by a few simple dimensions.

C. The Subjects

Variations in age are basic for studies of the early development of perception and attention. Many age-related changes in the direction or strength of visual preferences have been found in previous research and in research reported in this chapter. But such changes are only the beginning point for the more difficult tasks of determining the cause and significance of the changes. Is a particular preference change due to specific experiences, to more general effects of the type of rearing environment, or only to maturation accompanied by a necessary minimum of visual experience? The possibilities for experimentally varying experience in human infants are limited, but in our data are illustrated by perceptual enrichment of some institution-reared infants (Section VI-B).

Just as important as knowing the environmental influences is knowing what processes underly the preference change and, hence, what effects there may be on present and future behavior of the subject. Is the change in preference due to improvement of discrimination capacities, to increasing selectivity in attention, or to development of memory? And, at another conceptual level, is the preference change related to peripheral sensory mechanisms, to perceptual abilities, or to higher cognitive processes? Much of the research that will be presented had as one aim the differentiation among these possible processes underlying the change. For this purpose, we compared the course of development in groups of infants expected to differ in perceptual–cognitive abilities.

This experimental technique of using highly selected groups of subjects, rather than a representative sample or one restricted to normal subjects, is illustrated by experiments (Sections VI-D and VI-E) comparing normal infants with Down's Syndrome (mongoloid) infants who have high likelihood of mental retardation in later years. The main purpose was not to assess the early capabilities of a defective population through comparison with a normal population, but rather the opposite purpose of understanding the development of normal infants by comparison with retarded development of defective infants: Are certain age-dependent changes in differential visual responsiveness related to cognition and later intelligent behavior?

Another type of subject variation is relevant to much of the research reported later in this chapter. Age has been discussed in the preceding paragraphs as if it were a simple and unambiguous measure, whereas actually the age of an infant at a given point in time may be measured either from birth or from conception. For infants having the same length of gestation it is immaterial which age is used; but in comparing term and preterm infants the two age measures differ by several weeks or months. Measuring age from birth has the weight of tradition behind it as well as the practical advantage of giving the only unequivocal starting point. It also has a sound rationale from a psychological viewpoint since it marks the beginning of extrauterine experience. But from a biological viewpoint the time of conception is the starting point of development, while the time of birth is somewhat unpredictable and may or may not have effects on particular aspects of development. For tracing somatic development, age from conception is more appropriate; also the early neurological development of the infant is usually closely related to age from conception in both term and preterm infants (Amiel-Tison, 1968).

The question is whether it is more appropriate for studying the early development of perception and attention to use age from birth, with the assumption that a longer or shorter period of prenatal maturation is irrelevant; or to use age from conception, with the assumption that a period of some weeks more or less of postnatal experience is irrelevant. This question is most critical during early infancy when development proceeds at a very rapid rate and several weeks can make a big difference. A partial solution is to restrict the sample to carefully selected full-term infants. But additional information may come with another solution: Instead of making an a priori choice between conception and birth as the starting place, use both scales and determine which best fits the data. This was accomplished in the results described in Section VI-C by comparing a term group with a group of about a month less gestation but consequently having had about a month more postnatal experience. If development of the two groups is the same when plotted by postnatal (PN) age, but the preterm group is ahead when plotted by age from conception (based conventionally on the first day of the last menstrual period, and called postmenstrual or PM age), then early postnatal experience is shown to be important for the development. If, however, development of the two groups is the same when plotted by PM age, this suggests that development was a function of the combined prenatal and postnatal periods and that the PM age scale is more appropriate for the behavior in question. In addition, no effect of the extra weeks of visual experience of the preterm infants is then apparent, but this must be interpreted with caution: Preterm infants at first may not be sufficiently mature to profit from the experiences; even if they are, the experiential opportunities of preterm infants in a hospital are atypical.

D. The Technique

1. General Features

For visual preference testing, the situation must be carefully adjusted for both comfort and stimulation of the subjects—without too much of either if both sleeping and crying are to be prevented. For a technique utilizing natural tendencies for visual explorations, it is not surprising that we have found the state of the infant to be most effectively controlled by the nature of the environment. We have largely avoided unpatterned stimuli not only because of our interest in variations in patterning, but also because it is difficult to obtain much response and maintain alertness with unpatterned stimuli. Additional devices that can aid in maintaining alertness are interesting between-exposure stimulation, a semireclining rather than supine posture, and a pacifier.

With predominantly light stimuli against a darker, homogeneous background, corneal reflections of the stimuli are clearly visible. The location of the right or left reflection over the center of the pupil is a simple, objective, and reliable criterion of fixation of the right or left stimulus. High reliability has frequently been shown between simultaneous observers, even with newborn or premature infants (Section III-D; Miranda, 1970a), or between different readers of photographic records using a similar criterion (Fantz, 1956). Similar results have also been obtained in repeated testing of the same subjects. The response measurement, whether by one or two persons and whether made directly or via camera, is still subject to several possible sources of error—that is, factors that might slightly displace the reflection of the point of fixation from the center of the pupil (cf. Chapter 1 by Maurer, in this volume). But these errors are equal for two stimuli presented equally often to the right and left of a central observation point, and, therefore, cannot give a spurious differential for one of the stimuli, although without these errors the recorded preferences might be a bit larger.

2.   PORTABLE TESTING EQUIPMENT

The trip by a mother and infant to the laboratory at a prearranged time results in many incomplete tests. And when weekly tests are needed or the subjects are twins or defective infants, cooperation of the mothers is sorely taxed. One solution that we have used for many years is to take to the home an apparatus that is light, compact, and quickly assembled (Fantz & Nevis, 1967b). The infant is secured in a special canvas baby seat held semiupright on the lap of a seated assistant. A stimulus chamber is pushed above and in front of the subject, covering the field of view and allowing presentation of two stimulus plaques about a foot away and a foot apart. The chamber is lined with blue felt to give a light-diffusing, homogeneous, contrasting background. The observer looks through a tiny hole between the stimuli and records looking time by a two-way lever switch. A second observer can see the eyes of the subject through a hole in the chamber ceiling by means of a small front-surface mirror above the main observation hole and can make simultaneous response records by a second silent switch, with the noise of the recorder relays masked by a randomly activated relay to prevent contamination between observers.

This portable apparatus was also adapted for use with newborn or premature infants at University Hospitals (Miranda, 1970a). A self-supporting infant seat permits adjustments for size of head and body and maintains positioning of the head toward the stimuli, with minimal tendency to favor the right or left side. A nurse watches the infant through a hole in the side of the chamber, provides needed care, and interrupts testing when the subject is not in a quiet–alert state. Illumination of the chamber and stimuli can be dimmed for photophobic subjects. Additional dim illumination directed on the subject's eyes from either side is usually necessary to make visible the irises of the newborn.

3. MOBILE LABORATORY

A second solution for testing infants beyond the neonatal period has been to equip a specially designed school bus with a power generator and testing equipment (Fantz & Sockel, in preparation; Fantz & Fagan, 1975) for use close to the subject's home. This permits the use of fixed and more elaborate apparatus, and is even more convenient for the mother than testing inside the home. Infants usually cooperate well in testing sessions taking up to 15 to 20 min and including as many as 100 stimulus exposures. This efficiency in obtaining a large amount of data from alert infants is in part attributable to the stimulus situation: high pattern contrast, high homogeneity of the background that fully cover the subject's field of view, and short intervals between exposures, filled with centering and attention-getting stimulation.

Figure 4.1 shows the inside of the chamber and the right one of two stimulus patterns projected on Polacoat rear-surface projection plastic lining the chamber. A center stimulus comes from a rotating color-patterned disk in a kaleidoscopic projector. Control panels on the experimenter's side operate the equipment for programming the number and duration of exposures, the slide changes, and the onset of the kaleidoscopic stimulus following each exposure. The onset of each exposure of a pair of stimuli is initiated manually, when the subject is alert and fixating the kaleidoscopic stimulus above the center observation hole. The subject is secured in a holder that is adjustable for length of torso, for width and depth of head, and for height and tilt of seat, so that at 16 inches the eyes and head of the subject are directed toward the center stimulus. Diffused side lighting illuminates the subject's eyes for better observation of the pupils to indicate direction of gaze. Corneal reflections of the stimuli are easily visible, even though the projector lights are dimmed to a level tolerable to the infants, and which has been found to be about optimal for acuity testing using three different light levels (Fantz, in preparation, b).

III. FORM VARIATIONS

The presentation of research in this part and in Sections IV and V is largely organized in terms of types of variations among stimuli. Form is a stimulus area with several claims to foremost consideration. Adaptively, the discrimination of form is essential for the later

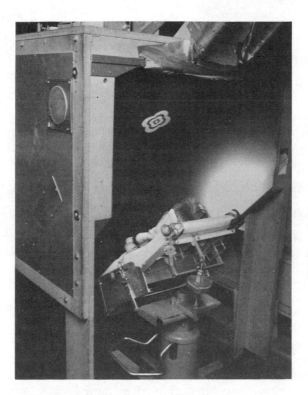

Figure 4.1   Photograph of the mobile laboratory testing apparatus (Section II-D-3), showing the subject in adjustable seat in position for looking at two projected stimulus targets, of which the right is visible here. Between them (not visible) is a small observation hole, and above this a projected kaleidoscopic color pattern comes on between stimulus exposures.

use of vision. Phylogenetically, form perception has advanced remarkably in the evolution of the vertebrate visual system. Historically, it has been the main battlefield for nativists and empiricists on the origin of knowledge of the environment, and, consequently, the main focus of research on newborn or visually deprived animals that preceded the development of techniques appropriate to human infants. Theoretically, form perception is a challenging aspect of vision in any organism of any age, one that has dominated perceptual theories. Empirically, form preference results comprise a large and crucial part of the data of this chapter. Those form results involving variations in populations will be considered mainly in Section VI. In the present section, a rough division is made between form of contour variations in Section III-A and other form variations in Section III-B.

A. Curved versus Straight Contour

Marked visual preferences and developmental changes have previously been obtained using patterns that differed in form of contour and in other respects (Fantz, 1958; Fantz & Nevis, 1967a; Spears, 1964). Specifically, bull's-eye versus striped patterns have also differed in concentricity, perhaps in regularity, and sometimes in number of angles and elements. Therefore, an experiment (Fantz, in preparation, a) was designed in part to differentiate among the influences of these or other possible stimulus features, and thereby verify the ability to discriminate differences in form.

1. SUBJECTS AND PROCEDURE

For this experiment and some others described in this chapter, the subjects were twins. Twins were used in part for purposes not reported here, but also because they provided an economical means for replicating findings, or for controlling incidental variations, and a good population for studying effects of length of gestation. Subjects were all normal and healthy and had known PM ages, based on unambiguous menstrual information and checked by birth measurements. The 46 pairs of twins ranged from 32 to 43 weeks PM age at birth, divided for analysis into a preterm group of 22 pairs under 38 weeks (mean 36.2) and a term group of 24 pairs (mean 39.9). Postnatal ages at testing ranged from 5 to 19 weeks. Each pair was given four different testing sessions, usually on successive weeks, with order balanced among pairs. One of the sessions consisted of acuity tests (see Section III-A-5), while the other three were pertinent to curved versus straight and other form variations. The stimulus patterns are shown in Figure 4.2—including, on the right side, separate stimulus pairings and, on the left, sets of stimuli that were combined in various pairings. The usual procedure was successive exposure of a stimulus pair in each right–left arrangement. Results from the three sessions, varying the sequence of presentation of the stimulus pairs and the exposure time (10 sec versus 5 sec), did not differ and so were averaged together. The testing was done in the mobile laboratory with projected stimuli (Section II-D-3).

2. RESULTS ON STIMULUS VARIATIONS

The overall results for three tests of 42 term infants ranging from 9 to 19 weeks are presented first to allow concentration on effects of different stimulus variations during the age range when differentials were most often shown. The percentage of fixation time is given in Figure 4.2 for the pattern indicated by the arrow. For example, the infants spent 66% of response time looking at the bull's-eye rather than the stripes (E1–E2), a difference from the chance value of 50% that was highly significant, as indicated by underlinings, according to a two-tailed *t* test. This pair, similar to some used previously, was transformed in three ways to see whether the preference would hold. It did with reversal of light and dark areas (E3–E4), but not reliably so with the other two. The fact that reduction to half-sized patterns and ¼-inch elements (E5–E6) resulted in such a decrease in preference is surprising, but subsequent results have supported this importance of size. The low preference for E7–E8 is less surprising: Breaking up the patterns into segments disrupts both the shape of contours and the overall configurations. This disruption was less true for the segmented patterns of G1–G2, a pairing that also controlled number of elements and angles, while retaining the bull's-eye over striped preference as in previous results with this pair (Fantz & Nevis, 1967a).

The "A" series of patterns achieved better control of prominence of details as well as number. The elements were designed so that the degree of curvature could be varied continuously from bull's-eye to stripes by increasing the radius of curvature of the arcs. One intermediate pattern was used and was intermediate in attention value. Rotating the three patterns (A1–A2–A3 versus A4–A5–A6) changed the differentials little, indicating at most a minor importance of orientation of lines relative to degree of curvature. Combining results for the two orientations of each pattern, 26 of 42 infants looked longest at the most curved patterns, next longest at the intermediate patterns, and least at the straight patterns (with chance expectancy being 7 of 42). This shows transitivity of response along a quantifiable series—a criterion sometimes given for a stimulus dimension (Section II-B). However, several stimulus features covary along this dimension and the remaining curved–straight variations were designed to distinguish among these as well as to determine the generality of the preference.

A prominent feature of a bull's-eye that is lacking in stripes is concentricity or "centeredness." This was controlled by pairs of

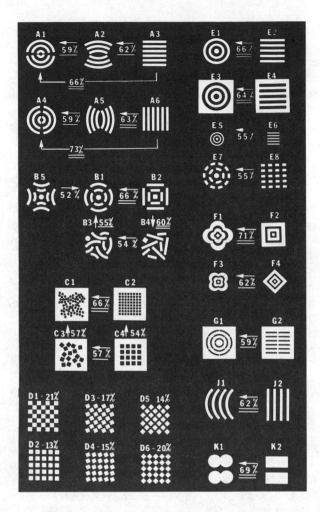

Figure 4.2 Projected stimulus patterns used in the experiment on curved versus straight contour and other form variations (Sections III-A and III-B), along with mean results for 42 term subjects. Percentages shown between two patterns are for the pattern indicated by the arrow in repeated paired exposures. Underlining indicates a difference from 50% significant at .05 level by the two-tailed *t* test; double underlining at .001 level. For D patterns, percentages are of total fixation times for the six patterns presented in all pairings. In most cases the line elements were ½-inch wide. The white square stimuli measured 6 inches; other patterns were to the same scale. Patterns within each pair or set were equated in area of light and dark; all pairs except the "C" set also equated total contour length for the pair or set of patterns.

curvilinear and rectilinear patterns in which the elements of both patterns were arranged around the center (B1–B2, F1–F2, F3–F4), or in which this was true of neither pattern (J1–J2, K1–K2). A reliable curvature preference was shown for each of these five pairs, and was usually as strong or stronger than that shown for bull's-eye versus stripes pairs. The differential for F1–F2 was maintained, but with reduced strength when the patterns were rotated and reduced in size (F3–F4). For both of these pairs and for B1–B2, the member with straight contours bore little resemblance to a pattern of stripes and was less redundant by including lines in two directions. In pairs J1–J2 and K1–K2, on the other hand, the member with curved contours bore little resemblance to a bull's-eye pattern, again without diminishing the curvature preference.

Outstanding in these data is the wide diversity of stimulus pairs that elicited preference for the curved member, including differences among pairs in size, orientation, degree of curvature, concentricity, figure–ground relationship, as well as in the specific nature of the forms. Most of the preferences cannot be accounted for by nonconfigurational features such as number of angles and elements, total contour length, mean contour per detail, and area of light and dark, which were controlled. This gives considerable support for the generalization that a preference for curved over straight contours is shown by infants 2 to 4 months of age. However, certain qualifications are indicated by the described results from two E pairings and, in addition, from the pair B3–B4: No reliable differential was shown between irregular arrangements of pattern elements that had elicited a strong curvature preference with regular arrangements (B1–B2). It would appear from this and from the E7–E8 result that overall curvilinear versus rectilinear configuration is important as well as the form of separate elements.

3. RELATED RESULTS OF OTHERS

Spears (1964) found a visual preference in 4-month infants for a bull's-eye over four other patterns that differed in numerous stimulus dimensions. In a more systematic experiment (Spears, 1966), no reliable preferences were shown among a series of patterns: triangle, square, pentagon, hexagon, and circle. However, his series decreased in angularity while increasing in approximation to curvature—two prepotent stimulus features that may have canceled each other when opposed (Section V-C).

An experiment of Ruff and Birch (1974) did attempt to separate curvature from other features. The purpose was that of analyzing the stimulus variations underlying the bull's-eye over stripes preference, similar to that of the above experiment, but the approach was that of tridimensional variations among an array of patterns. Three-month infants were shown all pairings of 10 patterns that differed in one or more of the dimensions of curvilinearity, concentricity, and number of line directions. Ruff and Birch found visual responses to be influenced most by curvilinearity and concentricity. Of the 10 patterns, a bull's-eye ranked highest in preference, followed by a similar curved–concentric pattern; while the two lowest ranking patterns contained straight elements either all horizontal or half in vertical orientation. These results are in good agreement with ours in showing contour curvature to be an important determinant of infant attention. They also indicate the importance of another form variation—concentricity—that we had attempted to control rather than to vary separately from form of contour.

4. DEVELOPMENTAL RESULTS

Early results from bull's-eye–stripes pairings (Fantz, 1958; Fantz & Nevis, 1967a) were notable not only for the consistency of the bull's-eye preference after 2 months of age but also for the earlier absence of this preference. This developmental change was again shown in the present experiment for most of the curved versus straight pairs. Average postnatal developmental curves are shown for two sets of these pairs: six pairs with clear resemblance to bull's-eye versus stripes (Figure 4.3, top) and seven other pairs with curved versus straight contours in other regular configurations (Figure 4.3, bottom). In each case the term infants increased from close to chance to about 70% of response for curved by 12 weeks. A similar trend in development for the preterm infants was less regular and somewhat delayed, not reaching maximum preference until 16 weeks, a difference corresponding to the 4-week shorter gestation of this group. This suggested that preferences for curvilinear over rectilinear patterns were a function of age from conception rather than age from birth (Section II-C). So, in another analysis of the same data (Figure 4.4), the age groupings were based on postmenstrual age. Here the term and preterm groups are in better agreement on the age of development of the preference in each stimulus grouping.

Results from term and preterm groups together, for both sets of pattern pairings, indicate that the preference for curved over straight contours developed at about 49 weeks PM age, when a significant differential was present for all four curves. For term infants this is similar to the 2-month development in previous findings. The processes underlying this development are of much

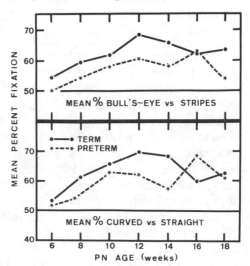

Figure 4.3   Postnatal developmental preference results on form of contour variations, for both term and preterm infants (Section III-A-4). Top curves are based on mean percentages for bull's-eye for stimulus pairs A1–A3; A4–A6; E1–E2; E3–E4; E5–E6; G1–G2. Bottom curves are based on mean percentage for the curved member of pairs A2–A3; A5–A6; B1–B2; F1–F2; F3–F4; J1–J2; K1–K2.

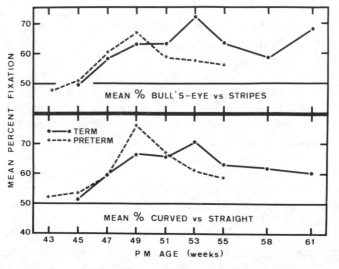

Figure 4.4   Developmental preference results on form of contour variations from the same term and preterm subjects and stimulus pairs as in Figure 4.3, but using age from conception (postmenstrual age) instead of age from birth as the basis for inclusion in a given age grouping.

interest and will come up in several parts of the chapter. A possibility explored but ruled out in the next section is that form preference development is related to the development of visual acuity.

5.   VARIATIONS IN WIDTH OF LINES

One of the four testing sessions given to the subjects in the experiment previously described (Section III-A-1) consisted of three types of visual acuity tests, corresponding roughly to three of the acuity tasks distinguished by Riggs (1965). One was pattern resolution or minimum-separable acuity, using equal dark and light striations that varied in width for different patterns, as have been used in previous acuity tests of young infants (Chapter 1 by Maurer, this volume). The second was pattern detection or minimum-visible acuity, using six separated dark lines on a light field, the lines being curved in some pairings and straight in others, both paired with unpatterned light fields. Overall results for these two types of visual acuity are described later in this chapter (Section VI-C-3) and given in more detail elsewhere (Fantz, in preparation, b). As with older subjects, finer lines were detected against a plain ground (visual angles of 13 min of arc at 1 month, 6 min at 2 months, and 3 min at 3 to 4 months) than were resolved in patterns of striations (25 min at 1, 13 min at 2, and 6 min at 4 months). In addition, curved lines were detected earlier than straight lines of the same width and same total contour length. This dependence of pattern-threshold measurements upon the nature of the pattern has also been found in older subjects (Riggs, 1965) and is another instance of the interaction of stimulus variations in the area of form and pattern perception. The fact that the interaction involved curved versus straight contours suggests that differential-visibility of curved and straight contours might underly the curvature preference. The third part of the acuity experiment provided a test of this possibility.

A third acuity task distinguished by Riggs was pattern recognition, such as discrimination of the form or direction of letters. As an approximation we paired together the curved and linear patterns used in separate parts of the pattern detection test. The visual preference expected after 2 months of age was in essence a substitute for an instructed discriminative response. Circular and linear patterns—equated in area, number of details, and total contour—were paired for five widths of line. Figure 4.5 gives the resulting development curves for four of these widths, using the

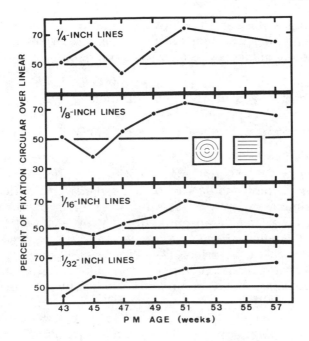

Figure 4.5 Developmental preference results from four circular versus linear pairs differing only in width (subtending 51, 25, 13, and 6 minutes of arc) of curved and straight lines (Section III-A-5). In each case a significant (.01) differential for the circular pattern developed at 51 weeks postmenstrual age for combined term and preterm infants. Form of the patterns on 6-inch squares is illustrated for the ⅛-inch lines.

postmenstrual age scale that gave the best fit for term and preterm groups in other acuity results (Section VI-C-3). In spite of early high variability of response (based on only 2 10-sec exposures for 12 to 18 infants at each point), the general trend for each width of line was upward until 51 weeks, at which age the curvature preference first became significant at the .01 probability level for each of the four curves, even though the preference was then stronger for patterns of wider lines. A significant differential was not shown for the fifth pair of patterns with $\frac{1}{64}$-inch lines. The essential similarity of development for the four widths of lines indicated that this third discrimination task did not measure acuity of any variety. Stating this in another way, the similar development of preference for curved over straight contours over a wide range of line widths indicates that the development of visual acuity cannot explain the development of curvature preference. The explanation must be sought at higher levels of perceptual–cognitive functioning, as has been attempted in the studies discussed in a later section, through the selection of subjects (Section VI).

B. Pattern Arrangement and Configuration

1. INTRODUCTION

The curvature or linearity of contours is one of many types of form variation. Other variations also fit the attentional predilections of the young infant and so can provide visual preference data on form discrimination. While patterns differing in form of contour also often differ in overall configuration, in this section we are focusing on configurational differences that are produced by different arrangements or orientations of the same pattern elements. This restriction gives good control of variables that do not clearly involve form discrimination, and yet could influence visual attention.

The three types of difference in arrangement of elements that have elicited differentials are all illustrated in results from an earlier study (Fantz & Nevis, 1967a), reproduced in Figure 4.6. At least by 3 months, pattern D was looked at reliably less than each of the other three patterns. Patterns A and D differ in circular versus linear configuration, comparable to some differences in the results reported in the preceding paragraphs and thus extend those findings to preference for a circular configuration not produced by contour curvature. Patterns B and D present a difference comparable to the checkerboard versus lattice pairings to be considered later (Section III-B-3); while C and D present a difference in irregular versus regular configuration, comparable to some variations to be considered now.

2. REGULAR VERSUS IRREGULAR ARRANGEMENT

This stimulus variation has in the past been studied from several viewpoints. Since regular patterns contain more redundant information than random ones, this variation has entered into many studies of the preferred complexity or amount of information in a pattern (e.g., Chapter 2 by Karmel and Maisel, in this volume). Since facelike patterns are often somewhat regular and symmetrical, this variation is pertinent to investigations of attention and recognition of faces. But discrimination of the regularity of patterns

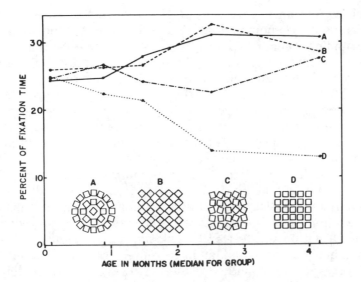

Figure 4.6   Changes with age in visual preferences (Section III-B-1) relative to each of four arrangements of 25 ½-inch white squares on blue felt background, based at each age on percentage of response for each subject given to that pattern out of the total fixation time of the four patterns during exposures in all pairings. Differentials among the four were significant for the three older groups. [From Fantz & Nevis, 1967a.]

can also reveal form perception abilities, and it is this aspect that is of concern here.

Contrary to some experiments, our own findings have usually been in accord in showing a preference for irregular over regular pattern arrangements after several months of age. Let us begin, however, with a result that violates this generalization. In Figure 4.2, a regular circular pattern (B1) elicited a low, but significant, differential over an irregular arrangement of the same elements (B3). In seeming contradiction, a highly reliable preference was shown for the irregular over the regular arrangement of straight elements (B4–B2). This illustrates the value of finding the subject's own categorizations of stimuli (Section II-B), since from the experimenter's view the two irregular patterns were similar to each other, as were the two regular patterns, compared to a striking irregular–regular difference. The attentional responses among the B patterns in Figure 4.2 indicated a strong interaction between the two variables of curvature and regularity, so that the preferential ranking of the regular pattern as highest or lowest of the four patterns depended on whether it was curvilinear or rectilinear. It is difficult to find an explanation of this in terms of either stimulus dimensions or phenomenology. But these findings do extend the earlier findings on curvilinearity versus rectilinearity: this stimulus difference is important not only in the form of individual contours, but also in the overall configuration. In a further result, the lack of differential between B1 and B5 (the latter having the same elements flipped over to disrupt the circularity) also supports the prepotency of a *regular* configuration of *curved* elements for eliciting attention, but indicates no requirement for this configuration to be *circular,* in agreement with other results in Figure 4.2.

The C patterns in Figure 4.2 gave bidimensional variations in regularity (horizontal pairings) and in size–number of elements (vertical pairings). The size–number comparisons are not pertinent to this section (the low differentials are a result of a marked shift in preference within the 9- to 19-week age range, similar to results reported in Section IV, and, as in those results, this shift showed a close correspondence with PM age). However, the interaction of size–number with regular–irregular is relevant in that the preference for the irregular pattern of the two regular–irregular pairs is of different strength and showed a different course of development: with patterns of 64 ⅜-inch elements (C1–C2) a strong preference for the irregular pattern developed between 6 and 10 weeks, while with patterns of 16 ¾-inch elements (C3–C4), the irregular arrangement was about as much or more preferred at 6 weeks as at 10 weeks; for both pairs the preference decreased at later ages.

These results with the C patterns verify the discrimination and selection of irregular over regular linear arrangements as shown in this chapter (B4–B2 in Figure 4.2, and Figures 4.6, 4.18, and 4.22) and in previous studies (Fantz, 1965a, Figure 6; Fantz & Nevis, 1967a, Figure 11). The absence of a similar preference for irregular or random over regular patterns in some other experiments (Section IV; Karmel, 1969b; McCall & Melson, 1969; Moffett, 1969) is probably related to the demonstrated interaction of this variation with other stimulus variations and with age. The strength and developmental course of irregularity preference for the C patterns depended upon the size and number of elements in the patterns, while for the B patterns the direction of the regular–irregular differential depended upon the form of the elements and the resulting configuration. Thus a broad generalization on the relative attention value of regular and irregular pattern arrangements is not supportable. Further research at various ages is needed to find specifications of the stimuli that might bring more order to these various findings. But relative to form perception capabilities, some irregular versus regular pattern arrangements can be discriminated as early as the second month of age.

3. DIFFERENT REGULAR–LINEAR ARRANGEMENTS

The preference by the third month of age for the pattern of touching diamonds over the lattice pattern of nontouching squares (B versus D in Figure 4.6) was extended (Fantz & Nevis, 1967a, Figure 9) to a strong preference by 7 weeks for a checkerboard pattern over a lattice pattern, shown here as D1–D2 in Figure 4.2. The D series of Figure 4.2 further analyzed the relevant stimulus factors by varying both location of the centers of the ¼-inch squares (top three versus bottom three patterns) and of the degree of tilt of the squares around these centers (left versus middle versus right pairs of patterns). The results given in Figure 4.2 are based on total fixation of each pattern when presented in all possible pairings, converted to percentages for each subject, and averaged for 42 term subjects over 9 weeks.

Neither element location nor element orientation were effective overall. Response did not differ for the upper three compared with the lower three patterns or for the left, middle, and right pairs of patterns. And yet the differential among the six patterns was highly reliable, owing to an interaction of these variations that makes sense from examination of the patterns. Similarity in configuration is present for the two preferred patterns (D1 and D6, with connected corners of squares), for the two least preferred patterns (D2 and D5, with separate and linearly arranged squares), and for the two patterns (D3 and D4) that were intermediate in preference. Apparently the phenomenological similarities for the experimenters agreed in this case with those of the subjects, with "checked" patterns preferred and "lattice" patterns nonpreferred, regardless of whether the elements were in upright or diagonal orientations. Developmentally, a 60% to 70% preference for D1 and D6 over D2 and D5 was present at all PN age levels beginning at 6 weeks for term infants, but not until 14 weeks for preterms. When graphed by PM age the term and preterm groups were in better agreement.

4. OTHER RELATED FINDINGS

A subsequent testing program included further experiments analyzing the stimulus basis for the preference for checked over lattice arrangements of squares. The sample included 40 pairs of twins, each tested as many as eight times, with intervals of at least 2 weeks between tests, again in the mobile laboratory (Figure 4.1). Infants were not selected for gestation and so included few preterm subjects at most age levels, preventing a good comparison of term and preterm development. By inspection the groups were more in agreement by PM age, and so this age scale was used for the combined data. The two twins of a pair were given different stimulus presentation sequences that showed no difference in the results.

The checked and lattice patterns (D1 and D2) were again used, along with patterns composed of circles instead of squares, but in the same spatial positions (D9 comparable to D1, D10 comparable to D2). The checkerboard pattern was again preferred to lattice (Figure 4.7, top), although not until about 52 weeks PM age. With circles instead of squares, the pattern comparable to the checkerboard was also significantly preferred at both 52 and 56 weeks, but

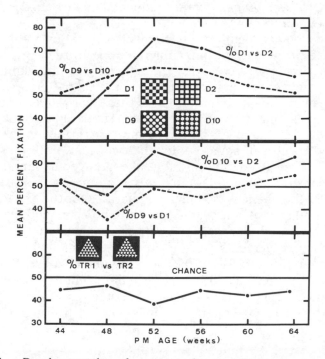

Figure 4.7 Developmental preference results on pattern arrangement, with infants grouped on the basis of postmenstrual age (Section III-B-4). Each curve is based on percentage of fixation to one pattern of the total for both when paired together.

with less strength. The lower differential for patterns of circles suggests some importance of the touching corners for the checkerboard preference. The moderate differential present even with circles is more surprising, and suggests attention to some stimulus difference in addition to touching or nontouching of corners, such as the higher linearity and redundancy of the lattice pattern (D2) that is somewhat maintained with circle elements (D10). Taken by themselves, the results for D9 versus D10 are interesting in showing perhaps the most difficult or subtle form discrimination so far evidenced during the first 6 months of life.

Further interaction between the shape and the arrangement of elements is shown with the same four stimuli by pairings of comparable arrangements of squares and of circles (Figure 4.7, middle). Circles were not preferred to squares in a checkerboard arrangement (D9–D1) but they were moderately preferred (significant at 52 and 64 weeks) over a lattice arrangement (D10–D2). Perhaps a preferred aspect of the checkerboard pattern, such as touching of corners, counterbalanced a preference for curved elements that was evidenced when the squares were not touching.

Another pair of stimuli gave further information on the stimulus basis of the checkerboard over lattice preference. Stimulus D1 differs from D2 most obviously in that corners of the squares touch. But it also differs in that it is less linear–regular: Straight lines connecting edges of elements alternate between light and dark areas for D1, but are more homogeneous for D2. In two arrangements of triangular elements (Figure 4.7, bottom), these two stimulus features of possible attention value were opposed. In TR1 the triangles touch at the corners as in the checkerboard. But also in TR1 black lines along edges of triangles are more continuous than in the lattice pattern of squares (D2). The results show, first, less differential responsiveness than for checkerboard–lattice pairings, suggesting that the two arrangements of triangles did in fact oppose preferred stimulus features that were previously compounded. Second, the direction of the weak preference obtained (significant starting at 52 weeks PM age) was not for the pattern with touching elements (TR1), but for the pattern with the less linear and regular arrangement (TR2). Thus, the touching of corners of elements was not essential for preferences between different regular arrangements of elements, in agreement with results for D9–D10. Another implication is that the *absence* of high linearity–regularity can be a potent feature for eliciting attention, as shown previously in other form results.

Finally, this result and others in this section further illustrate how the method of equivalent stimuli (Section II-B) can be used, even with the untrained responses of young infants, for the detailed analysis of relevant stimulus parameters.

C. Form Discrimination via Novelty Response

The results reported in the preceding Sections III-A and III-B depended upon intrinsic selectivity relative to particular stimulus variations for evidence of discrimination. This method gave much information on discrimination capacities and selectivities relevant to form perception, but cannot give information for patterns eliciting no differential response. Another method is the experimental formation of a preference through pre-exposure to a particular pattern that may then be less preferred than a novel pattern (see Chapter 5 by Cohen & Gelber, in this volume). Such an induced preference at the same time gives evidence of short-term memory for form that cannot be obtained otherwise.

Early studies comparing responsiveness to novel and previously exposed targets used stimuli that differed along a number of dimensions, so that implications for form discrimination were not clear. In recent studies, selective fixation of the novel pattern by infants from 16 to 30 weeks of age was shown with three different arrangements of four squares (Fagan, 1970, Experiment I), or of 25 squares (Fagan, 1973; Experiments I and IV), and with circular versus checkerboard arrangements of squares (Miranda & Fantz; see Section VI-E-3 in this chapter). These studies verify the discriminations among different pattern arrangements shown at an earlier age by intrinsic preferences, as well as evidencing subsequent recognition memory of such configurational differences.

The response to novel over previously exposed face photographs is relevant to form perception, although such stimuli do not allow as good control of nonconfigurational differences as abstract pattern arrangements. Two further procedures have given better stimulus control. Fagan (1972, Experiments I, III, and V) found that discrimination and recognition memory was shown at 20–24 weeks between upright face photographs, but not between the same photographs when upside down, indicating the differentiation depended upon previous perceptual learning from everyday exposure to faces that are usually in upright orientation. And of most relevance here, features discriminated in upright faces, but obscured by inversion, are probably subtle configurational differences possibly similar to those involved in facial recognition at later ages. The second procedure that allows control of nonconfigurational differences is use of upright and inverted versions of the same face photograph as novel or previously exposed stimuli, a procedure that has resulted in discrimination at about 16 weeks (Fagan, 1972; McGurk, 1970).

We recently obtained additional results with upright and inverted faces as well as with two different configurations of the same pattern elements. Both novelty tests were included for infants over 12 weeks PN age at the end of the testing session for which preference results were given in Section III-B-4. In the familiarization phase, a given pattern was projected for 80 sec simultaneously in three positions: right, middle, and left. On each week of testing, one twin of each pair was familiarized with one stimulus, the other twin with the other stimulus, with results for the two averaged. The two 10-sec test exposures paired the novel and previously exposed stimuli, reversed in right and left positions for the second exposure.

For the upright–inverted comparison, the photograph was the face of a woman (Fantz & Nevis, 1967a,b, stimulus 8B). The results showed a 58% preference for the novel orientation by the two oldest groups of 60 ($p < .001$) and 64 weeks ($p < .01$) PM age. Intrinsic visual preference tests were also given earlier in the same session. Preference was shown for the upright over the inverted orientation, but also only at 60 and 64 weeks, both at about 60% ($p < .01$). Thus different orientations of a face were discriminated toward the end of the first 6 months as shown both by intrinsic preference for the upright face and by experimentally induced preference for the novel orientation. The second recognition problem used the B1 and B5 patterns of Figure 4.2 except that the common center circle was omitted. The results showed a low preference for the novel pattern (55% to 59%), but one that was significant ($p < .05$) at 56, 60, and 64 weeks PM age, indicating discrimination by novelty response for patterns similar to those that had not elicited an intrinsic preference.

These results support previous evidence of discrimination of different orientations of faces during the latter part of the first 6 months of life. They extend previous results from two different configurations of the same elements, in that the patterns differed only in having each element flipped over to give another regular–concentric configuration. It is of interest that a differential response to the novel of several pattern arrangements has not been shown until a month or two later than intrinsic preferences have been shown with similar patterns (Section III-B), suggesting an advantage of intrinsic preferences for studying the development of such configuration discriminations. Another implication is that recognition memory for pattern arrangement develops later than the ability to discriminate and select relative to these differences, as well as later than recognition memory using simpler, multidimensional problems (Sections VI-C-4, and VI-E-3).

Memory is as important as discrimination and selectivity for form perception; information on the development of one of these functions cannot substitute for information on the others. In this instance, the different ages of development of form discrimination–selectivity and of form memory may be of special value for understanding early perceptual–cognitive development, as will also be suggested by differences between Down's Syndrome and normal infants in memory for pattern arrangements (Section VI-E-2).

D. Newborn Form Preferences

Previous studies of the visual responses of newborns to patterns or forms (Fantz, 1963, 1965a; Fantz & Nevis, 1967a,b; Hershenson, 1964; Hershenson, Munsinger, & Kessen, 1965; Miranda, 1970a; Miranda & Fantz, 1971; Nelson & Kessen, 1969; Salapatek, 1968; Salapatek & Kessen, 1966; Stechler, 1964; Stirnimann, 1944) used stimuli that differed in the presence, location, or quantity of patterning or in other variables that do not give definitive evidence for form discrimination. A recent study (Fantz & Miranda, 1975) does give clear evidence of form discrimination and selection by term subjects under 7 days of age. Testing was done at University Hospitals using the apparatus and general procedures previously described (Section II-D-2). Reliability of measurement of the differential-fixation response was shown in simultaneous recordings by two observers of 64 pairs of stimulus exposures for 19 subjects: The correlation between the two recorded fixation times for the stimulus on the left was .80, for the stimulus on the right, .87, and for the percentage of time given to one of the two stimuli, .89.

The main stimulus pairs are shown in Figure 4.8. Each pair was exposed for two 10-sec periods with reversed right and left positions. The number of subjects varied among the pairs because of incomplete data from nonalert subjects or the frequent lack of fixation of either member of certain pairs. Furthermore, some pairings were added and others omitted in successive phases of the experiment to obtain adequate data or to try additional stimulus variations. Each phase included 4 to 6 stimulus pairs shown in one of a number of random sequences. The results in Table 4.1 give mean length of fixation of a stimulus pair, the mean difference in fixation time between the curved and straight members of the pair, and the percentage of total time that was given to the curved member.

The main finding based on either measure of differential fixation (Table 4.1, right two columns) was the significant preference for the curved member of the upper pairs of Types I, II, and III. A supplementary finding was the significant curvature preference in another pair that differed from the pictured upper Type I only in

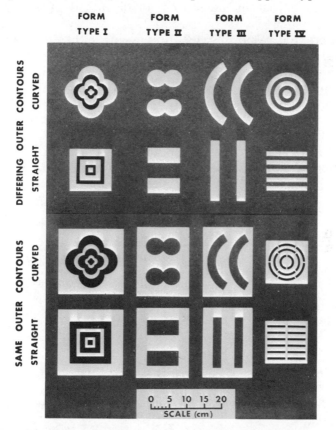

Figure 4.8   Curved versus straight-contoured stimulus pairs used in newborn form study (Section III-C) and presented to the subject in right–left arrangements. Stimuli were constructed of white cutouts (or black on white) glued to blue felt (represented by textured gray) matching test chamber lining. Area of black and of white and total contour were equated in each pair. [From Fantz & Miranda, 1975.]

that the curved form was rotated 45° to give more similar horizontal and vertical dimensions of the two patterns. The two members of each of these four pairs were equal in area of black and of white, in total contour length, in number of elements, and in number of angles (except for four versus eight angles in Type II). In contrast to results for the above pairs, no reliable differential response was elicited by the lower pairs of Types I, II, or III, with the same variations in form of contours as the corresponding upper pairs, but with reversed figure–ground relationships that resulted in equal outer rectangles for the two members of the pair. This implies a special importance of the outer contours for differential response to form of contour by newborns as discussed in the following section.

No differential response was shown with either of the Type IV pairings, in concurrence with previous newborn experiments using the same stimulus pairs (Fantz & Nevis, 1967a,b; Miranda, 1970a). Lack of discrimination of the lower Type IV pair, as with the other three lower pairs, is sufficiently explained by the equal outer contours. The two members of the upper Type IV pair did differ in outermost contours, but they also differed widely in angularity (0 versus 20 angles) and somewhat in number of elements (3 versus 5). The preference by newborns for patterns with more angles and elements (Section IV-A) would be expected to be in opposition to

TABLE 4.1   NEWBORN INFANT FIXATION RESPONSES TO STIMULUS PAIRS OF FIGURE 4.8[a]

Stimulus pair	N	Fixation of pair (in seconds)	Curved–straight difference (in seconds)	Percent for curved
Differing outer contours				
Form Type I	45	16.1	4.4[b]	61.4[c]
Form Type II	43	6.6	1.6[c]	66.4[b]
Form Type III	44	11.3	2.7[b]	60.7[b]
Form Type IV	28	13.8	−0.3	47.8
Same outer contours				
Form Type I	56	12.1	1.1	55.2
Form Type II	46	6.2	−0.4	49.2
Form Type III	39	6.3	1.0	56.0
Form Type IV	30	17.0	−0.6	47.3

[a] From Fantz and Miranda, 1975.

[b] $p < .005$.

[c] $p < .05$ using two-tailed t test based on chance value of 0 for difference scores and 50% for percentages.

the preference for curvature and thus could result in equal response to a curvilinear pattern with no angles and a rectilinear pattern with many angles. The effects of this and other oppositions of two preferred dimensions is further evidenced in Section V-C (Figures 4.16 and 4.17) and is discussed in Section VII.

E. Form Summary and Interpretations

1. Newborn versus Older Subjects

The preceding results give clear-cut evidence of form of contour discrimination in newborn infants. These results also raise two questions when compared with results from older infants. The first concerns the apparent requirement for newborns that the difference in form be present in the outermost contours of the patterns. This is not the case for older infants, as shown by the differentials for E3–E4 and G1–G2 in Figure 4.2, and among the 10 patterns used by Ruff and Birch (1974; Section III-A-3) that had the same square outer contours. Photographic recordings of the scanning of a single stimulus (Salapatek, 1969; Salapatek & Kessen, 1966; Chapter 3 by Salapatek, in this volume) give a cogent explanation. Newborn and 4- to 6-week infants concentrated their fixations on parts of the outer contour of a stimulus pattern, with few excursions into the central area even when contours were present there. In contrast, 8- to 10-week infants more often scanned the patternless central area of a figure, as well as the outline contour, and tended to concentrate their gaze on central contours when these were present. These findings from use of a different technique support and help to explain our finding of a special importance of the outermost contours for form preferences in newborns but not for older infants. This explanation needs more direct confirmation from newborn and older infants' scanning of curvilinear versus rectilinear contours as outer or inner parts of a pattern.

The second question raised by the newborn form preferences is why postneonatal infants (Section III-A-4) have not shown similar preferences until about 2 months of age. Of the 13 curved–straight pairings included in the graphs of Figure 4.3, only three pairs included in the bottom term graph are directly relevant to the newborn results. For F1–F2 in Figure 4.2 (upper Type I in Figure 4.8), a chance response was shown before 10 weeks; for J1–J2 and K1–K2 (upper Types III and II), some curvilinear preference was present for the earliest age level of 5–6 weeks but then increased at later ages. In view of the variability of these results, obtained from different subject samples and testing apparatus than the newborn results, an exploratory experiment was made using the same term subjects and portable testing apparatus at successive weeks of testing from 1 to 11 weeks PN age (*N* of 6 to 11 at various weeks). At close to 1 week of age the curvature preference for each of two pairs was similar to that shown for newborns at the hospital, but then decreased until 4 weeks (more so for upper Type I than for upper Type III forms), and was followed next by an increase to the usual strong curvature preference by 7 weeks of age. These results, now being verified with a larger sample, support both the presence of initial form preferences and some drop in subsequent weeks before the later strong curvature preferences.

Taking the visual selection of curvilinear over rectilinear patterns as the standard result that is evident throughout most of the first 6 months and with a wide variety of stimulus pairings, one might ask why there are exceptions for certain curvilinear–rectilinear pairings at certain ages. But if one considers the many developments in the visual system during the early months, perhaps a more pertinent question is why the same degree of curved over straight selectivity is shown at such differing points in development as, for example in the newborn, the 2- or 3-month, and the 5-month infant, a degree of constancy in visual preferences that is unusual. As a possible answer, the selection of the curved member of a pair may be mediated by different processes at different ages and with different stimuli: The selection of outer curved contours by the newborn, probably based on fixation of a limited section of contour, is quite a different visual performance from the selection by the 2- or 3-month infant of a variety of curvilinear patterns, including some with only inner curved contours and some not equated with the rectilinear pattern in angularity. And the latter performances, based often on long examination of a single stimulus, are in turn different from those at later months involving increasingly shorter fixations of each stimulus, and implying improved information processing, perhaps due to taking in more of a pattern in a single fixation, along with more direct comparisons between patterns. It is not surprising that the preference for curvature and other stimulus features sometimes varies with, or during, the shift between such different phases of oculomotor activity and perceptual-cognitive processing. Nor is it surprising that the more primitive mode by which the newborn attends to a pattern results in less generality of the differential for curvilinear over rectilinear patterns as well as preventing other form differentiations that are later possible with practice and improved modes of attending.

2. FORM DISCRIMINATION SUMMARY

We will briefly review the results in Section III, especially those that appear to indicate discrimination abilities not included in previous reviews by Bond (1972) and Hershenson (1967). Additional relevant findings are given in other chapters of these volumes.

The ability to discriminate between some patterns with curved versus straight contours was evident in newborn infants, whatever visual–motor process was involved and regardless of subsequent changes in degree of preference. The three pairs discriminated by newborn infants (Figure 4.8) allow some generalization of the discrimination between outer curved and straight contours: Type I forms are concentric, while Types II and III forms each have two separate elements, oriented horizontally in one case and vertically in the other. While the curved contours of Types I and II could tend to keep visual scans within the pattern more than the straight contours, this is not the case for Type III. In sum, the three pairs appear to have nothing in common other than the difference in form of contour. Patterns differing in the arrangement of identical elements have not been differentiated by newborns, whether because of limitations in the subjects' abilities or in the experimenters' ingenuity. Certainly the concentration of attention upon outer contours would make more difficult the demonstration of ability relative to pattern arrangement.

For infants over 2 months of age, additional instances were provided of the ability to discriminate regular–curved from regular–straight patterns, including those of equal outer contours (Section III-A; Figure 4.2). A notable exception was the lack of differentiation between irregular arrangements of the same curved or straight elements (B3–B4) that had been discriminated in regular arrangements, suggesting some perception of the overall configuration in addition to the form of particular elements. Further evidence of discrimination on the basis of broad configurational differences was provided, at least by 2 months, from experiments using different arrangements or orientations of the same pattern elements, variations allowing further control of nonconfigurational features and evidencing additional and often more difficult form discriminations. These included discrimination of curvilinearity versus rectilinearity of element arrangement, irregularity versus regularity of arrangement, arrangements of square elements in checked versus lattice configuration, and similar arrangements of round elements that lacked the difference of touching corners present in the checked pattern (Section III-B; Figures 4.2, 4.6, 4.7). Late in the first 6 months of life some of these and other differences in element arrangement, along with different orientations of the entire stimulus pattern, were not only discriminated but also remembered for a short period as shown by differential fixation of a novel and a previously exposed stimulus (Section III-C).

Form perception develops throughout infancy and childhood; many beginning points might be given, depending upon the type of stimulus variation and the response measure by which form perception is operationally defined. The discovery a decade ago of the ability of newborn infants to receive patterned stimulation indicated at least that a basic requirement for form perception was present at birth, and even in premature infants (Miranda, 1970a). The present results for newborns (Section III-D) go considerably further by showing discrimination and selection on the basis of configurational variations that will later be important in form perception: form of contour variations independent of the size or amount of patterning. Whether or not this performance is considered to qualify as form perception, this and the additional discriminations shown at later months are certainly relevant for tracing successive phases of development and for understanding the process of development. It is unlikely that the limits of discrimination abilities pertinent to form perception have been found at any point in infancy, in view of the short period of research on infant perception, a period that has been devoted largely to developing useful techniques or to studying variations in stimulus "complexity" rather than form. Further research should be accelerated by the present availability of a number of discriminative response measures and promising techniques including conditioning (e.g., see Chapter 1 by Maurer in this volume and Chapter 2 by Bower in Volume II). However, the natural visual selectivities of the young infant have revealed some discriminations (e.g., Figure 4.7, top, D9–D10) that might be difficult to obtain even from the trained responses of older subjects. Some additional or finer form or depth discriminations have been obtained (e.g., Bower, 1971) and will increasingly be obtained using techniques not dependent on the presence of untrained visual selectivities; but the latter will continue to give better evidence of what the infant looks at and processes in nonexperimental situations.

3. UNDERLYING MECHANISMS

Results showing newborn differential responsiveness to variations in pattern and form indicate some initial degree of function of
optical, oculomotor, retinal, geniculate, and cortical parts of the
visual system. Evidence from other disciplines has verified this
initial function, even though showing incomplete development and
imperfect functioning of most parts (Kessen, Haith, & Salapatek,
1970; Chapter 2 by Karmel and Maisel, Chapter 1 by Maurer, and
Chapter 3 by Salapatek, in this volume). The visual areas of the
cerebral cortex are known to be critical for pattern vision in
mammals and especially in primates, and are known through
electroencephalographic recordings to be functional in newborn
and premature infants (Ellingson, 1960). It is fortunate that a source
of more detailed information on the function of these areas has been
provided by the development of techniques for electrical recordings
from individual neural cells. The outstanding findings are those of
Hubel and Wiesel, obtained from the recordings of the response of
cells in the visual cortex to visual figures stimulating specific retinal
areas of anesthetized monkeys (1968), cats (1965), and young,
visually inexperienced kittens (1963). A summary of some of the
most pertinent findings is taken from a section on implications for
perception:

> In the striate area, cells respond to the contours of a form . . . . A portion of
> the boundary of a figure will activate that population of complex cells whose
> receptive fields are not only crossed by the boundary but also oriented in the
> direction of the boundary. A segment of a curve will activate a complex cell best
> if the tangent to the curve does not greatly change its direction within the
> receptive field. . . . Hypercomplex cells are still more selective. From these cells
> continuous straight boundaries . . . evoke no response. There must be discon-
> tinuities such as interruptions of a line or changes in direction. A simple image
> like a square activates only hypercomplex cells whose fields include the
> vertices . . . . The hypercomplex cell can, in a sense, serve to measure
> curvature; the smaller the activating part of the field, the smaller the optimal
> radius of the curvature would be [Hubel & Wiesel, 1965, pp. 285–286].

These findings show some unlearned, neurological basis for form
perception in the selective response of certain complex cells to line
stimuli of a certain figure–ground type, orientation, size, and
location (Dodwell, 1971; Graham, 1965). This neurological basis has
been extended to additional aspects of form with the more recent
discovery of hypercomplex cells—presenting possibilities that have
been insufficiently explored by behavioral scientists. Most perti-

nently, these findings give a possible neurological mechanism for the discrimination between curved and straight contours in that complex cells are selectively activated by continuous straight contours, while hypercomplex cells are selectively activated by discontinuities in lines such as angles and curves. This similarity in the neural-activating properties of angles and curves could account for the importance of equating elements and angles for eliciting curved–straight differentials in the newborn infants. But with elements and angles equated, the activation of a higher number of hypercomplex cells could serve as a neurological "detector" of curved contours.

The behavioral *selectivity* of curved over straight contours requires further speculation than is required for *discrimination* between them. To begin with, any patterned surface is presumably more "neurally stimulating" than an unpatterned surface that elicits few responses from any known type of visual–cortical cell, and perhaps accounts for the high visual–motor-stimulating effect of patterned surfaces. Such a gross explanation is not sufficient for preferences among different patterned surfaces. One hypothesis is that the hypercomplex cell, being at a higher neural level and receiving the output of a number of complex cells with different receptive properties, may have more direct efferent connections with centers related to visual–motor responses. This could result in selective visual fixations of patterns with either more line discontinuities, more angles, or more contour curvature. And with discontinuities and angles equated, the pattern with more curvature would then receive more visual fixation. An additional hypothesis is that a pattern with many redundant straight contours, simultaneously activating many complex cells sensitive to lines of the same type, size, and orientation could produce "hypersynchrony" in neural activity, resulting in less fixation tendency or even avoidance. The latter hypothesis could account for the demonstrated visual preferences for irregular over regular–linear element arrangements, and perhaps for checked over more linearly redundant arrangements.

Such hypotheses may even now be replaceable by others that are more appropriate or specific, based on further neurological advances. But in such further attempts to relate visual responses to underlying neural mechanisms, the direction of visual response will remain as important as the ability to discriminate: Neural responses, like visual–motor responses, are selective in nature. It is also likely that visual perception can more easily be related to visual–cortical mechanisms in young infants, prior to the later increasing dominance of cerebral areas beyond the striate cortex or (in different terms) the increasing effects of experience and higher cognitive processes upon the direction of gaze at later ages.

IV. QUANTITATIVE PATTERN VARIATIONS

Most of the stimulus dimensions varied in infant studies of response to "complexity" or response to the amount of information in a pattern might be described as "quantitative" pattern variations, including size of element, mean contour length, total contour, number of elements, and number of angles or intersections. Such variations contrast with the more "qualitative" pattern variations considered in the results on form (Section III), including variations in element arrangement (redundancy or regularity) that have often been classified as complexity variations. Another, more systematic, classification of different stimulus variations will be presented in Section VI-A. In this section, however, we are concerned with the distinction between two different types of quantitative pattern variations that are simply described as number and size of elements.

A. Number versus Size: Newborn Results

An initial experiment (Miranda & Fantz, 1971) used the bidimensional design discussed in Section II-B and the hospital apparatus and general procedures (Section II-D-2). The stimuli (Figure 4.9) were black-and-white nonglossy photographs measuring 8.5 by 4.5 inches. The subjects were 22 infants with a mean age of 3 days and mean gestation of 40 weeks. The six patterns were presented in pairs for 6 sec in each of the 15 possible combinations, in random sequence and left–right positions. The relative attention value of the six patterns was measured by totaling fixation times over the 15 pairings.

Results in Figure 4.9 show highly preferential attention both to larger pattern elements of the same number (along the rows) and to more elements of the same size (down the columns), but with little differential along the diagonals inversely varying size and number. These results were further analyzed by taking the time scores for the 15 pairings separately, each transformed into percentage of total response to one of the pair. Each of the four size pairings

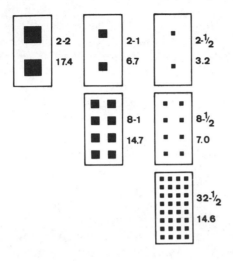

Figure 4.9   Stimulus patterns and results for the newborn number–size experiment (Section IV-A). Top pair of numbers beside each pattern indicate number of squares and size of each square in inches. Bottom numbers are mean fixation time during paired exposures totaling 30 sec. [From Miranda & Fantz, 1971.]

showed a significant preference for larger over smaller elements of the same number, with a mean of 80% for larger size. Each of the four number pairings showed a significant preference for more elements of the same size, with a mean of 77% for higher number. Along the diagonals, the mean of the four pairings was 59% for fewer, larger elements; the preference for the 2–2 pattern over the 8–1 and 32–½ patterns was significant only with results for the two pairs combined.

The size of elements and number of elements were both important stimulus determinants of attention in newborns; when these two variations were put into opposition, size tended to be dominant. But we must also consider the covariation of both size and number with total area of black and therefore with overall reflectance. Area of black did not vary along the diagonal of the array which, nevertheless, indicated some preference for the pattern of two large elements, similar to other results from neonatal infants using patterns equated in area of black (Brennan, Ames, & Moore, 1966; Hershenson, 1964; Miranda, 1970a). And results from a further pairing, given after the main 15 pairings, provided supplementary evidence against a difference in area of black as being related to the differential responsiveness. The 2–½ pattern, containing only ½ square inch of black compared to 38 square inches of white, received 83% of fixation time when paired with a plain white rectangle—a degree of preference comparable to that shown between patterns having large differences in area of black and in reflectance. This highly significant preference for a patterned over a plain stimulus also demonstrated visual resolution of the smallest size of element used, and so eliminated absolute pattern threshold as a determinant of the results. While total contour length also increased with both the size and the number of elements in the pattern, contour was equated in the pairing of 2–2 with 8–$\frac{1}{2}$, and yet 88% of fixation time was given to the 2–2 pattern. Thus the number and the size of elements were the only apparent stimulus variations eliciting differential responses.

B. Number versus Size: Developmental Results

A more extensive experiment (Fantz & Fagan, 1975) used the same bidimensional stimulus design as the newborn experiment, but with the array of Figure 4.9 extended to include another column of stimuli with still smaller ($\frac{1}{4}$-inch) pattern elements. Also another array of nine stimuli was used (Figure 4.10) differing only in that the arrangement and orientation of elements were random instead of centered within a segment of the total pattern area, both to give more generality to the results from the regular patterns, and to see if there would be differences between the two sets. Such differences were not found, probably due both to the lack of direct pairings of regular versus irregular patterns and to the small differences in arrangement as compared with those already considered (Section III-B-2). We will consider here only the combined results from regular and irregular patterns for each of the two twins of a pair, who received different random stimulus sequences and responded similarly.

Tests were given at 5, 10, 15, 20, and 25 weeks of age, and when possible, to the same subjects at several ages. At each postnatal age level, 22 term infants were tested as well as 22 preterm infants that averaged 5 weeks less in postmenstrual age. This careful selection of subjects permitted comparison of term and preterm groups at either the same PN age or the same PM age. Exposures of 6 sec were given with each of 72 possible permutations of the 9 size–number cells; half using the regular patterns and the other half, with reversed right–left positions, using the irregular patterns.

When the age of both term and preterm groups was measured from birth, an analysis of variance showed a strong interaction between the term–preterm variable and the age variable in determining differential fixation among the nine patterns. But in another analysis of variance a postmenstrual age scale was substituted, thus juxtaposing a given preterm group with the 5-week younger term group that had 5 weeks longer gestation and thus an equal total developmental period (PM age). In this analysis, the interaction between gestation and age disappeared: Term and preterm groups of the same PM age did not respond differently. Further analyses of the data showed a high similarity between term and preterm infants when matched for PM age, both in overall responsiveness and in differentials among the patterns, compared with a marked disparity when matched for PN age. Consequently, the results in Figure 4.10 are based on the PM age scale, combined for term and preterm

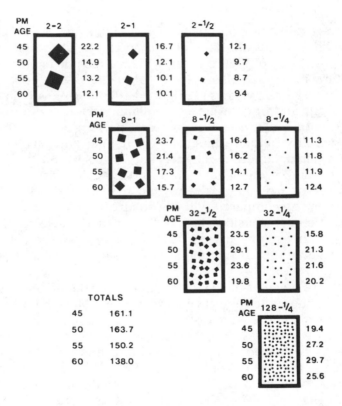

Figure 4.10   The array of irregular patterns used in the developmental number–size experiment (Section IV-B), along with combined results for irregular and comparable regular patterns and for term and preterm infants, including PN ages of 5, 10, 15, and 20 weeks for term and 10, 15, 20, and 25 weeks for preterm subjects. Numbers are seconds of fixation of that pattern in pairings with each of the other eight patterns for a total of 96 sec of exposure. Totals for the nine patterns are for 432 sec of exposure during the testing session.

groups at each of the four age levels at which both groups were tested.

Relative to stimulus determinants, we will first consider number versus size of elements that were the basis of the bidimensional design. Patterns of larger size (toward the left side of rows in Figure 4.10) elicited at 45 weeks much higher fixation times, but usually with successive decreases in the differentials at 50, 55, and 60 weeks. Number variations, pictured vertically, initially elicited high differential fixation for patterns of more elements; this differential often became still larger with age—most markedly in the right column containing the pattern of 128 elements that was by 55 weeks PM age preferred to all others.

The developmental changes for size and number are more succinctly contrasted in different analyses of the data. Seconds of fixation to the two patterns of a pair presented together were converted to percentages of response for the pattern with larger elements or with more elements. Average percentages were then computed for the seven pairings varying size and holding number constant. Similarly, averages were computed for the seven pairings varying number and holding size constant. Analysis of variance based on these data again showed no term–preterm effect, but strong effects for both PM age and for size versus number, as well as a strong interaction between these two factors that is apparent in Figure 4.11. Size preferences start high but decrease with age while number preferences start somewhat lower but reach a higher level beginning at 50 weeks. In spite of these changes in the *relative* attention value of size and number, both preferences are reliable: Of the seven separate size pairings and seven separate number pair-

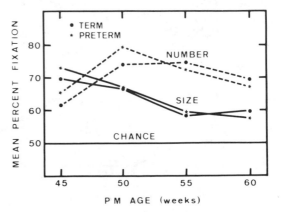

Figure 4.11   Comparison of the development of number and size preferences (Section VI-B), based on the average of percentages for the pattern of more elements or larger elements in the seven such pairings in each case. [From Fantz & Fagan, 1975.]

ings, all elicited a significant preference for the pattern with larger or more elements at each of the four age levels, with the exception of three of the size pairings at 55 or 60 weeks. Further decrease in the size preference was shown at 65 weeks by term infants not included in this analysis.

Since total contour increases with both number and size of elements, the number–size comparison cannot show the effect of length of contour. The results of three pairings of patterns equated in total contour are graphed in Figure 4.12. All three start with a significant preference for the pattern with fewer, larger elements, a preference that subsequently drops out and is reversed for one pairing (32–¼ versus 8–1) to a significant preference for the pattern with more, smaller elements. Clearly length of contour was not the sole determinant of the obtained differential responses; but it cannot be excluded as a possible contributing factor as will be discussed in Section IV-C-2).

Incidental variations in area of black and in consequent overall light reflectance were concomitant with the pattern variations in size, number, and contour length. But area of black was equal along each of the three diagonals of the array of Figure 4.10. The pattern with more numerous but smaller elements was significantly preferred with few exceptions in the pairings along the diagonals at 50, 55, and 60 weeks PM age. At 45 weeks the differentials were generally weaker but in one case (8–1 versus 128–¼) indicated a significant preference for the pattern with fewer, larger elements,

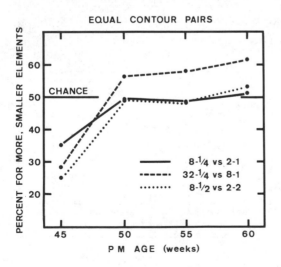

Figure 4.12 Developmental number–size results for the three pairings in Figure 4.10 for which total contour length was equal for the two members of the pair. [From Fantz & Fagan, 1975.]

concordant with the above results from newborns of 40 weeks. As in the results with newborns, variations in amount of black or overall light reflectance cannot here account for the differential responsiveness.

C. Interpretation of Present and Previous Results

1. Opposed Number and Size Variations

A series of checkerboards used in previous studies can be compared with the patterns along the diagonals of Figure 4.10 in that light–dark ratio was constant but the number of squares increased as their size decreased. Some of the results are also comparable. For newborns (Figure 4.9), the pattern of two squares of 2 inches was preferred to patterns with more numerous smaller elements, just as checkerboards of a few large squares have been preferred (Brennan *et al.*, 1966; Hershenson, 1964). For the developmental study (Figure 4.10), a further analysis included only the data for the 12 permutations of the four patterns along the main diagonal; total seconds of fixation were graphed in Figure 4.13 for each of the four patterns. Term and preterm groups again re-

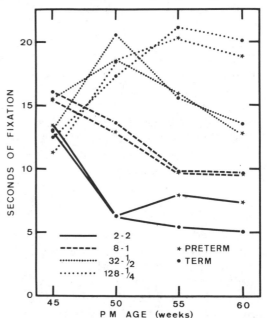

Figure 4.13 Developmental changes in visual responsiveness to each of the four number–size patterns along the main diagonal of Figure 4.10 based on results for all pairings of these four patterns, including 36 sec of exposure of a given pattern (Section IV-C-1). [From Fantz & Fagan, 1975.]

sponded similarly at each postmenstrual age level. At 45 weeks the 8–1 pattern was preferred with 32–$\frac{1}{2}$ a close second. At 50 weeks, pattern 32–$\frac{1}{2}$ was preferred with 128–$\frac{1}{4}$ close behind. At both 55 and 60 weeks the pattern 128–$\frac{1}{4}$ was clearly preferred. Results with checkerboard patterns have shown similar changes with age (Brennan *et al.*, 1966; Greenberg & Weizmann, 1971).

If our patterns had been limited to those along the main diagonal of the stimulus array, the most reasonable interpretations would have been similar to those in previous studies: an increase with age in the preferred or "optimal complexity" or in the quantity of detail (information) that can be assimilated. These interpretations are shown to be erroneous or misleading by the fact that even newborn infants looked longer at more complex patterns containing more information (elements, angles, and contour) when the initially more prepotent variable of size, that has never been included among the complexity variables, was equated; and by the fact that developmental changes during the early months were due largely to a shift in the relative attention value from size to number of pattern elements rather than to an increase in the amount of detail that was preferred or could be assimilated.

2. NUMBER VERSUS CONTOUR LENGTH

The three quantitative variations that can be separated in the results are size of element, number of elements, and to some degree, total contour. Size alone cannot account for the findings, since responses were usually for more elements of the same size; number is insufficient since there were differential responses especially at early ages for larger elements of the same number; contour is insufficient since patterns of equal contour differed in attention value (Figure 4.12). For an adequate description of the data, two of these three variations are needed. During the early ages, the prepotent size variable must be one of these two. This leaves either contour or number as the complementary variation that best describes the data. In Figure 4.14 the responses to the nine patterns are plotted, related both as to number of elements (left) and to total contour (right), with lines connecting patterns of a given size of element. At 45 weeks PM age the responses are a function of both number and contour in equal-size curves, but the strong effect of size is evident in differences among these curves for both number and contour plots. At 55 weeks the responses among all nine patterns are better related to both number and contour. At 65 weeks

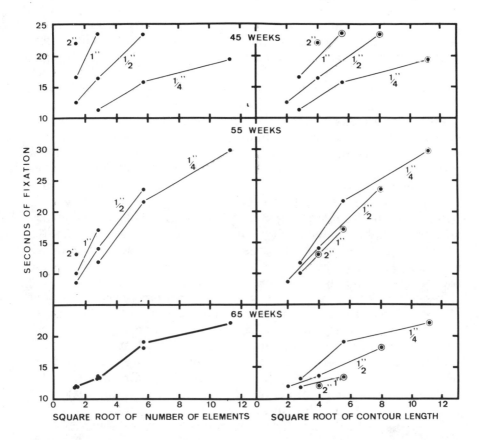

Figure 4.14   Plots of length of fixation of each of the nine number–size patterns (Section IV-C-2), as related to number of elements in the patterns on the left, and to total contour length on the right, with line patterns of equal element size. Data used are from Figure 4.10 for 45 and 55 weeks (PM), and for 65 weeks are from term infants (25 weeks PN age) not included there. Encircled points on right plots are for patterns in the main diagonal of Figure 4.10. [From Fantz & Fagan, 1975.]

the responses are slightly more dispersed than at 55 weeks along the scale of contour length; while along the scale of number, patterns with differing size and contour are closely enough grouped to give a single curve connecting the points with increasing number of elements in a pattern.

If it were necessary to describe the data in terms of a single variable, length of contour might be best over all ages studied, perhaps because it is correlated with both size and number of elements. In the absence of any apparent value of such a compromise unidimensional solution, the two variables of size and number —changing in relative importance with age—provide a much better description of the stimulus determinants.

3. CHECKERBOARDS VERSUS OTHER CONFIGURATIONS

We used patterns of unconnected elements to allow the separate variation of size and number that is not possible with checkerboard patterns of constant overall size. A side benefit was the generalization of previous results from checkerboards to the different but comparable sets of patterns: i.e., those along the diagonals of our arrays. In Figure 4.14, right, the encircled points represent the four patterns along the main diagonal of Figure 4.10 that inversely vary size and number of elements. The changes with age in relative attention to these four patterns are similar to those found in experiments using checkerboards: By drawing curves through the four points at each age level one might obtain a set of curves fitting the set of curves of Karmel (1969b) for responses to sets of checkerboard patterns, with increasing amount of contour preferred at successively higher ages. But the limited value of such a set of curves based only on contour length is evident from the fact that the remaining five points in each plot of Figure 4.14, right, do not fit the curves derived from the results from the diagonal patterns, due to the competing influence of size at 45 weeks and number of elements at 65 weeks.

Other experiments have gone beyond the checkerboard configuration with the aim of giving wider generality to the findings. Karmel's (1969b) set of curves included his results from random as well as checked configurations of squares. His conclusion that visual response was a function of length of contour in an intricate interaction with age was based in part on the similarity in response to checked patterns and to random patterns of equal total contour, but with the random patterns described as having more smaller squares. However, the manner in which Karmel derived his random patterns resulted in conglomerations of squares that were larger and fewer than the individual squares in the checkerboard from which it was derived, as well as having less contour. As a result, random and checked patterns that received similar responses, attributed by Karmel to equal length of contour, appear by inspection (Karmel, 1969b, Figure 1) to be also roughly similar in size and in number of parts. Certainly size and number were confounded with contour length in Karmel's random patterns as much as in his checkerboards, although not as objectively measurable in the random patterns.

Greenberg and O'Donnell (1972) also sought to generalize earlier results from checkerboard configurations. They used three levels of complexity in sets of patterns composed of checks, stripes, or dots, and found with each set a shift in highest fixation time from the middle level of complexity at 6 weeks of age to the high level at 11 weeks, a finding interpreted to support the theory of increasing optimal complexity with age. However, each set of patterns confounded variations in size, in number, and in contour just as much as a set of checkerboards. The results of Greenberg and O'Donnell, as well as of Karmel, can be explained in terms of age-shifts in the relative strength of size preferences and number preferences similar to those shown in our experiment that separated the effects of size and of number.

A more interesting finding of Greenberg and O'Donnell (1972) was the difference in response to checks, stripes, and dots patterns of a given complexity level, in spite of the similarity in contour length. This departure from a contour interpretation was challenged in a reply by Karmel (1974), who corrected for omission of border contours and adjusted for the difference in distance and in overall pattern area from his and other experiments, under the reasonable assumption that the most appropriate variables for comparing different studies are the visual angles subtended by elements, and the contour density within a certain visual-angle of the stimulus rather than the absolute contour length. However, graphs drawn from Karmel's adjusted contour measures are similar to Greenberg's and O'Donnell's (1972) original graphs, and quite different from the *hypothetical* curves given by Karmel (1974, Figure 1) based on the responses to Greenberg's and O'Donnell's patterns that would be *predicted* if related only to contour density. Thus Karmel ignores the actual differences in response to the three sets of patterns, differences interpreted by Greenberg and O'Donnell as due to variations both in number of elements and in configuration at each complexity level. The data give support in particular for one configurational interpretation: the attention given to patterns of dots increased considerably relative to checks or stripes at each level of contour density or complexity from 6 to 11 weeks of age—an age range during which marked increases in preference for patterns with curved over those with straight contours was shown in Section III-A.

Moffett (1969), using still different configurations, gave support for the prepotency of number of elements rather than contour density for infants 9 to 19 weeks of age. In one experiment, fixations increased with the number of horizontal lines in a pattern. But when vertical lines were added, the response was higher when more spaces (elements) were formed by crossing lines than for the same number of lines in one direction and with the same total contour length.

4. UNDERLYING PROCESSES

Possible underlying processes might be divided for convenience into those concerning cognition, and those concerning more strictly sensory processes. Cognitive interpretations of results based on size–number variations are largely based on the supposition that obtained changes with age are due to the ability or tendency to process patterns with increasing informational content at increasing ages (e.g., Greenberg, 1971). This supposition was questioned by the results previously discussed in which patterns with the most information (elements and angles) were strongly preferred even by newborns when size was equated (Section IV-A). It will be further questioned in Section VI-D-2 by the similar size and number preferences obtained from Down's Syndrome infants and from normal infants. These findings do not however argue against the more general expectation that information-processing abilities or preferred levels of information increase with age. For example, a ceiling effect may have occurred from the use of patterns too simple in number of details or in configuration for even newborn or Down's Syndrome infants to show optimal response at an intermediate level of information content.

Response to patterning depends both on ocular image-focusing mechanisms and on neural stimulation evoked by the patterns that then affect eye movements and fixations. High neural stimulation from patterned in contrast to unpatterned stimulus areas is known to be present at all neural levels of the visual system, and especially in the visual cortex (Hubel & Wiesel, 1963; Section III-E-3). But this general interpretation applies equally to many dimensions of patterning and to all ages. Increased neural stimulation could result from any of the marked developments in the visual system shown during the early months of life (Chapter 1 by Maurer, in this volume; Kessen et al., 1970). Oculomotor and neural developments are the two categories most likely to be involved in the response changes shown earlier in this section. In the first category, improved ability quickly to find even a small pattern detail, to hold foveal fixation with both eyes, and to explore successively the many details available might all increase neural stimulation and hence fixation times given at successive ages to patterns with many details, as well as decreasing the importance of large size.

But various considerations favor the category of neural developments as the primary cause of changes in preferences relative to size and number of pattern details. The most marked improvements in oculomotor coordinations occur in the early weeks, whereas the most marked attentional changes have been found later. Also, the attentional changes within our array of stimuli were a function of total developmental period rather than of the postnatal portion that gave the preterm groups some extra weeks for oculomotor practice. More direct evidence for neural maturation as the critical factor underlying changes in size–number preferences is given from recent recordings of electrical activity in the visual cortex evoked by a patterned light source. Both Harter and Suitt (1970) and Karmel, Hoffman, and Fegy (1974) found that the peak amplitude of evoked potentials changed with age among a series of checkerboard patterns, shown in flashes too short for oculomotor activity or accommodation to enter in. The changes were similar to those shown in studies measuring fixation times—that is, patterns of more numerous but smaller squares became optimal at successive ages during the early months. This was interpreted either as related to acuity improvements (Harter & Suitt) or to decreasing size of the receptive fields of neurons in the visual system (Karmel *et al.*), but in both cases with the assumption that decreasing size of element was the developmentally relevant feature, in contrast to the increasing amount of information (details or contour) emphasized in behavioral studies including that of Karmel (1969a) with similar patterns and results. These discrepant dimensional interpretations were possible only from the confounding of size, contour density, and number of elements in electrophysiological as well as behavioral studies using checkerboards. It seems likely that, as for the fixation results discussed earlier (Section IV-B), visually evoked cortical potentials are influenced by both the size and the number of details but with a shift in relative dominance to produce at increasing ages preferences for patterns of more smaller elements when the two dimensions vary inversely. This interpretation is not opposed to an influence of acuity development that is likely correlated both with a decrease in size preferences and a shift in dominance to number preferences. But any interpretation based only on results from checkerboard or other patterns with size and number inversely varied cannot specify either the relevant stimulus dimensions or the underlying developments.

The various findings in this section on quantitative variations have proved the importance of several such variations, interacting strongly with age, and have suggested neural maturation as the primary underlying factor. An implication for concepts and methods is the futility of describing the fixation responses of young infants simply as a function of "pattern complexity," even if precisely defined. Through the use of a bidimensional design, we were able to show the strong influence of the size dimension confounded in one such "precise" definition of complexity (the number of intersections in a checkerboard). And when the shape and configuration of elements are allowed to vary, as in Greenberg and O'Donnell (1972), precise quantitative measures could not predict the responses, a fact that may also account for discrepancies obtained in complexity results using other patterns (e.g., random polygons necessarily varying configuration as in Hershenson *et al.,* 1965). Quantitative variations in patterning clearly influence the attention of infants and can provide useful information if they are not assumed to be the only important variables—an assumption amply refuted in Section III relative to configurational variables, and in Section V relative to additional stimulus variations.

V. OTHER STIMULUS VARIATIONS

A. Pattern Contrast

Over the years we have increasingly used stimuli with a high degree of contrast between figure and ground, both to make differences among patterns more visible and because such patterns tended to elicit more attention. Thus pattern contrast was important in arriving at optimal experimental conditions.

Pattern contrast was first considered as a stimulus variable in its own right as a result of an incidental finding from the weekly testing of groups of home and institution infants using 18 pairs of stimulus targets, for which group differences are summarized in Section VI-A. This finding (Fantz, 1970; Fantz & Nevis, 1967b) was longer attention during the first 2 months of life to each of eight pairs that included black-and-white patterns than to any of the remaining 10 pairs, even though both the black-and-white pairs and the remaining pairs differed widely among themselves. For example, even the least fixated of the black-and-white pairs, patterns having two black circles on a white oval, was fixated longer than pairs of stimuli including more or larger elements, bright colors, subtle shading, solidity, movement, or a flickering light. After 8 weeks of age the response to most black-and-white pairs decreased rapidly relative to various other types of stimuli. In the same experiment, the highest preference (80% to 90%) for one or the other member of a pair during the early weeks of life was for a black-and-white schematic face pattern over a face photograph with much less feature–ground contrast and sharpness of contours. Results with the same pair of targets for full-term newborns and for premature infants of 35 weeks PM age (Miranda, 1970a) indicated a similar high preference for the black-and-white pattern. Incidental results from newborns are provided in the form experiment already described in Section III-D: In total responses for a pair (Table 4.1), the two pairs of highest fixation time were black and white. And in an additional pair of the same forms as the lower Type II pair (Figure 4.8) but with the inner forms black instead of blue, the black-and-white pair received reliably longer responses. Finally, in an early study of the visual attention of newborns to cards of different colors (Stirnimann, 1944), supplementary tests made with two colors on the same card showed more response than to either color alone, an effect that was most marked when the two colors contrasted in brightness, even when the two (yellow and black) had received lowest responses of the colors presented individually.

The preceding results in this section were from experiments not initially designed to study pattern contrast. Brightness differential between figure and ground was more directly varied by comparing black and gray crosses, each on a white square; exploratory results from newborn infants showed much longer fixation of the more contrasting pattern. Another way of decreasing pattern contrast is to make the contour less definitive while keeping the same overall brightness difference between figure and ground. This was done by out-of-focus photographing and printing of an irregular, jagged white form on black ground (Figure 4.15, top left) and pairing it with the original pattern. Developmental testing as part of the experiment described in Section III-B-4 resulted in a strong preference for the more contrasting pattern at 45 and 47 weeks (Figure 4.16, top), which then decreased to equal response to patterns with

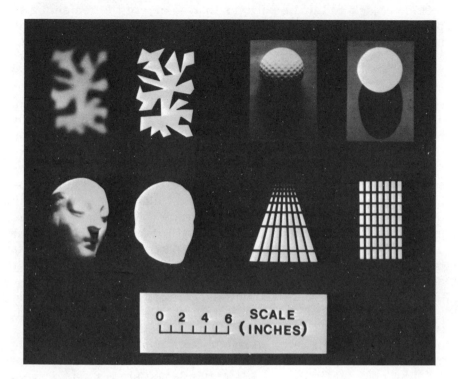

Figure 4.15   Photographs of four pairs of projected stimuli varying in pattern contrast and/or depth cues (Section V-A-B).

sharp or blurred contour. Pattern contrast might be operationally varied in still other informative ways, although it is difficult in this as in other stimulus areas to isolate a single stimulus dimension. For example, the black versus gray cross patterns varied figure brightness as well as figure–ground contrast. And the blurring of the contour of a pattern gave curvature and the impression of depth to the stimulus, perhaps increasing at later ages its attention value relative to that of contour sharpness and angularity, just as some of the stimuli labeled in the following section as having "depth" and preferred after the early months also had less pattern contrast or definition.

The various results in this section have agreed regarding the early attentional prepotency of pattern contrast, however defined. One obvious interpretation is that this is related to early deficiencies in sensory or visual–motor abilities that are known to show rapid development during the early months. Experimental information is available on the early development of one related visual ability. Doris, Casper, and Poresky (1967) varied the degree of brightness difference between the alternating light and dark stripes of a moving field used to elicit optokinetic nystagmus. Nystagmic movements of the eyes were obtained with less light–dark contrast in infants several months of age than in newborns, indicating a decrease in differential-brightness threshold with age, and suggesting that patterns with little contrast, such as photographs, might be seen as unpatterned areas by the very young infant and, therefore, receive little attention (see Section VII-A-1).

B. Depth or Representations of Depth

In previous studies (Fantz, 1966; Fantz & Nevis, 1967b), infants by 2 to 3 months of age preferred a sphere to a disk, but only when both were textured to emphasize the pattern variations accompanying depth. Similarly, a solid head model, with features visible only by shading from directional lighting, was strongly preferred to a flat outline form. In both cases some earlier preference was shown for the flat form, perhaps due to the higher overall reflectance or to the higher contrast of the outer contour against the background. And in both cases, the later solidity preference was shown with one eye covered, indicating that binocular vision was not essential, although not excluding other three-dimensional cues.

Depth cues were limited to those available from two-dimensional patterning in three stimulus pairs presented in the experiment already described in Section III-B-4, using projected stimuli. One (Figure 4.15, bottom left) paired photographs of the solid head model and of the outline form described in the preceding paragraph. And the results (Figure 4.16, second graph) were similar, showing an initial significant preference for the flat form followed by a strong preference for the head model photograph beginning 4 weeks later. In the second pair (Figure 4.15, top right), solidity was emphasized by the texture and directional lighting of a golf ball, while its schematic representation eliminated depth cues but gave high contrast. In the results (Figure 4.16, third graph), the early preference for the flat contrasting stimulus did not shift to a significant solidity preference until 51 weeks PM age. In the third pair (Figure 4.15, bottom right), stimulus differences unrelated to

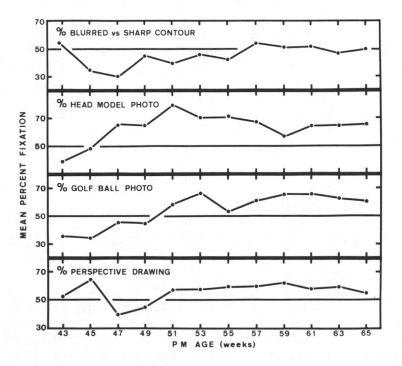

Figure 4.16   Developmental preference results for each of the four pairs of stimuli in Figure 4.15, with percentage based on the left stimulus of the pair.

depth were eliminated as much as possible by using two patterns of equal area of light and dark, equal contour length and contrast, and equal number of elements, but with only one pattern having line perspective representing a surface receding in depth, corresponding schematically to a stimulus pair that previously elicited a preference for a slanting patterned board over a vertical patterned board (Fantz & Nevis, 1967b). After early variable response (Figure 4.16, bottom), a small but consistent preference for the pattern with depth perspective developed that was significant at the .01 level for the 55-, 57-, and 59-week groupings and at the .02 level at 63 weeks.

From one viewpoint, this last differential response to "depth" involved the best control of stimulus variations and the best exclusion of peripheral visual abilities of any relevant visual preference results, and therefore might be considered the best evidence of depth discrimination. From another viewpoint, this differential response provides further evidence of early development of abilities to discriminate configurational differences, possibly related to the preference for an irregular over a regular–linear pattern arrangement (Section III-B-2). Actually the two viewpoints are not in opposition. Depth perception ordinarily involves objects also differing in configuration, while form perception ordinarily involves objects differing in three dimensions. The convenient but arbitrary separation of form perception and depth perception can interfere with our understanding of perceptual development as argued by Gibson (1966). Certainly the development of a discriminative response to a configuration that is also representative of a solid object is an adaptive shift in the stimulus features determining direction of gaze (Section VII).

C. Opposed Stimulus Variations

Many of the results in this chapter have paired stimuli differing in two separable dimensions, with each stimulus being at certain ages toward the preferred end of one of these dimensions. This is illustrated by opposing size and number dimensions along the diagonals of the arrays (Figures 4.9 and 4.10) that revealed marked developmental changes. And in the preceding two sections, three pairs (Figure 4.16, upper three) to some degree opposed contrast with depth and revealed a direction of developmental change from the stimulus of higher contrast toward the one with depth cues. Such an opposition might be expected to result in lack of developmental changes or of preferences at any age, due to the canceling effect of inversely varying dimensions. The actual presence of developmental changes in preference can most simply be explained by an increase in preference with age along one dimension and/or a decrease in preference along the other; in other words, the dimension dominant for attention changes with age (Section VII-B). This explanation was proven in the case of the opposition of size and number variations by the decrease in the size preference and the increase in the number preference with age in independent variations of the two. Such a bidimensional test is time consuming and with some variations is not feasible. The expedient of a single pair of stimuli with opposing stimulus variations was used in the following results.

The early lack of preference for bull's-eye over stripes (Section III-A-4; Section III-D) may have been due to the confounded quantitative variations (more angles and elements in stripes). If so, the replacement of stripes with a pattern that accentuates this confounding should further decrease or delay the bull's-eye preference. The E1 pattern (Figure 4.2) was paired with the lattice pattern D2 that had eight times as many elements as E1 and with 100 versus 0 angles, but with total area and contour the same. The results (Figure 4.17, top) showed a significant preference for lattice over bull's-eye at 47 weeks (the age at which a preference for bull's-eye over striped patterns was first significant in Figure 4.4), while the later preference for bull's-eye over lattice was not significant until 53 weeks. This strong opposition of quantitative variations considerably delayed the age of appearance of a bull's-eye preference, but did not decrease the eventual strength of the usual preference for curvature.

In another pair (Figure 4.17, middle), the pattern of large squares tended to be fixated longer initially followed by a shift to the pattern with smaller elements, equal in total contour length but of varied contour forms, that was preferred beginning at 51 weeks PM age. In the final pair, a stimulus with high figure–ground contrast (10 black

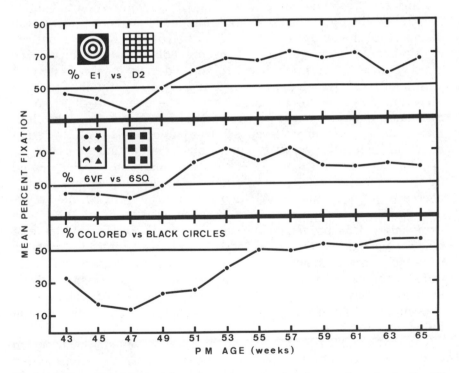

Figure 4.17   Developmental preference curves for three pairs of stimuli with several opposing stimulus dimensions (Section V-C).

circles on white ground) was paired with a stimulus with less contrast but much variety in color and brightness (10 circles of various bright, saturated colors). In the results (Figure 4.17, bottom), the black circles were highly preferred in the early weeks, followed by a chance response. This could be due simply to dropping out of the early dominance of high contrast; more likely it also involves the competing influence of color and variety at later ages.

In summary, these three pairings as well as previous results show developmental changes in visual preferences that involve a shift in the relative dominance of two opposed stimulus variations, due to decreasing attention value of one variation and/or increasing attention value of the other. The psychophysicist might ask what is gained from deliberately adding to the frequently unavoidable confounding of stimulus variables. Indeed, the analysis of particular stimulus dimensions or visual abilities would be better achieved by separating the variations as much as possible, as was attempted through the use of the bidimensional design, the equivalent stimulus approach, and in testing the limits of certain discrimination abilities. But perceptual development involves much more than the improvement in ability to discriminate particular stimulus features; at least equally important is the change in the type and subtlety of stimulus features eliciting attention and thus facilitating learning, presumably moving toward stimulus features that are or will later be needed to direct intelligent behavior. Hypotheses will be presented in Section VII about early phases of such developmental shifts in the direction of attention. In the meantime we will present results for experiments in which the primary aim was neither to oppose stimulus variations nor to specify the stimulus dimensions discriminated and selected, but rather to use whatever stimulus variations might best differentiate among selected groups of subjects and thereby give information on the underlying developmental influences or processes.

VI. VARIATIONS IN SUBJECT SAMPLES

For determining the causes of developmental changes in visual preferences, comparing two samples of infants differing in known ways may reveal the importance of certain factors or processes (Section II-C). One simple population comparison is males versus females—a comparison that could be informative relative to other findings suggesting, for example, earlier development in girls of social or cognitive abilities. Similar differences have sometimes been shown in early attentional or memory development in previous studies (Chapter 5 by Cohen & Gelber, in this volume; Fagan, 1972). But none of the studies reported earlier in this chapter revealed any reliable difference between boys and girls in the course of development of differential visual response.

The following sections are arranged in chronological order. First, an institution sample was compared with a home-reared sample differing in cognitive potential as well as in early experience. Then, experience was varied alone by perceptual enrichment of half of the institution subjects. A fortuitous outcome of this study was the suggestion that another way of varying early experience was by determining the effects of the extra period of postnatal experience available to infants born before term. Length of gestation then became a major variable in a number of experiments. Soon thereafter we began comparisons of Down's Syndrome and normal infants in an attempt to identify a genetically determined cognitive component in visual preference development.

A.   Institution-Reared versus Selected Home-Reared Infants

Many of the early studies of the senior author used subjects at a home for infants of unwed mothers. This population was first used for comparative purposes in the experiment of Fantz and Nevis (1967a,b), in which 10 institution infants were compared with 10 home-reared infants of university faculty fathers or mothers. Weekly tests during most of the first 6 months of life used 18 pairs of stimulus targets. Each pair was exposed for two 20-sec periods in varied right and left positions.

The age-preference curves for the home and institution samples were usually similar in shape, suggestive of a basic developmental change. But the two curves were often displaced from each other along the age scale, indicating a developmental difference that significantly favored the home infants for a number of individual pairs and in the mean for all pairs. Changes shown earlier or more markedly by the home group included differential attention to configuration variations such as bull's-eye versus stripes and irregular versus regular arrangements of squares, and decreased attention to nonconfigurational dimensions such as size, color, brightness, and movement. The home group was also several months ahead in the development of response to a novel pattern over one that was exposed repeatedly during the experimental session—a response requiring short-term recognition memory of a multidimensional pattern difference.

The reason for the differences in preference development between the two groups is not certain since the groups were selected so as to differ widely in several respects. The institution sample had a presumably inferior early environment and may have also had inferior prenatal conditions (although mean birth weight was the same). In addition, the home sample had a higher expectation for cognitive achievement, based on method of selection, on superior performance at 4 and 5 months on an infant development scale, and on the fact that in follow-ups at about $3\frac{1}{2}$ years of age the Stanford-Binet IQ of eight of the home infants then available averaged 135. While the presence of some group differences in preferences at early weeks also argues for congenital differences, the effects of early experiences cannot be excluded.

B. Perceptual Enrichment of Institution Infants

The importance of early experience for behavior development has received much experimental support in recent years (Newton & Levine, 1968; Young & Lindsley, 1970). Indirect support is given by the findings presented in this and other chapters, since early perceptual abilities and attentional propensities show the infant to experience, and at least potentially be affected by, many features of the environment. Determining effects of different experiences on young human infants is difficult since experimental manipulations of experience that are large or could have deleterious effects are not permissible, and since it is difficult to find reliable response measures to assess the effects of small experiential variations at early ages.

The approach in one experiment (Fantz, 1970) was to provide extra visual experiences to every other incoming neonatal infant at a home for infants of unwed mothers, and to assess the effects by giving both enriched and control infants a series of visual preference tests weekly as long as they remained at the institution. The enrichment, from 1 to 10 weeks of age, consisted of patterns and pictures attached outside the plastic sides of the cribs, a mobile hanging above the crib, an interesting color-patterned cloth covering the bottom pad of the crib, and, usually, (after 3 to 4 weeks of age) daily exposures to black-and-white television and to a "merry-go-round" of varied objects. Systematic observations in the cribs, in varying sequence among infants, showed that the enriched infants were more often awake and either quiet or active at 9 of the 10 weekly observations and less often crying or fussy at 8 of the 10 weeks. These data confirmed the impressions of institution personnel that infants were more often quiet and attentive while in the enriched environment. But the data could not show whether there was any persisting effect outside of this environment. Scores on a developmental scale were at most weeks of age about the same for the enriched and control groups. An effect of the enrichment was more likely to be revealed in tests of perception and attention, especially those involving stimuli taken from the enriched environment.

Starting at 5 weeks, weekly visual preference testing was given by individuals who did not know whether the subject was from the enriched or the control group. Results are restricted to infants staying at the infant home long enough to receive at least four tests; this included, at various ages, from 10 to 25 enriched subjects and 11 to 32 control subjects. In three of the stimulus pairs, a stimulus present on the sides or bottom of the crib of the enriched infants was paired with an unfamiliar but comparable stimulus; in each pair, at certain weeks the enriched group tended to fixate longer than the control group the stimulus to which they had been familiarized; but the group differences varied considerably with age and among the three pairings, giving no basis for a clear conclusion on such specific experience effects.

As a second intergroup condition, *both* stimuli of two stimulus pairs were exposed daily to the enriched group (and to the control group only in weekly tests given to both groups). One of these pairs (Figure 4.18, top left) elicited essentially the same preference development for an irregular over a regular arrangement of black squares from both groups, despite the fact that for the control infants both patterns were novel while for the enriched infants the same two patterns had appeared side-by-side on the cribs throughout the first 10 weeks of life, and were reported by institution personnel to receive a high proportion of the infants' visual attention. For the other pair (Figure 4.18, bottom left), the enriched group, which had had daily exposures of both members of the pair on the "merry-go-round," showed an earlier increase than the control group (group difference significant at 9 weeks) in the response to a patterned cylinder over a similarly patterned but flat

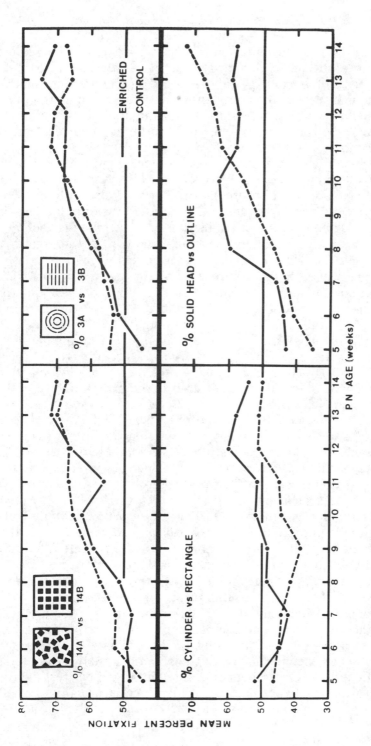

Figure 4.18 Developmental preference results for infants at an institution who were given perceptual enrichment compared with those who were not (Section VI-B). For the left two graphs, both stimuli of the pair were stimuli of the pair were exposed to the enriched group; for the right two graphs, the stimuli were equally unfamiliar to enriched and control infants.

rectangular board. The latter group difference might be related either to the specific experience with these stimuli or to more general effects of visual experiences in the enriched group relative to variations in depth. The latter effect was suggested as the more likely possibility by other results from stimulus pairs that were unfamiliar to both groups. In one case, an unfeatured head model and a flat outline of it were paired. The enriched group gave a higher response than the controls to the solid object (Figure 4.18, bottom right), significant at 8, 9, and 10 weeks (the later reversal, based on fewer subjects, was not reliable). Another pair also unfamiliar to both groups and varying in depth also favored the enriched group, to a lesser degree than the previous pair, in preference for solidity. In contrast to these depth variations, among 11 other pairs of stimuli, again equally unfamiliar to both enriched and control groups, earlier or stronger preference was suggested more often for enriched than for control infants, but for only one pair did the difference at any week of age reach significance. In particular, three form variations similar to some shown in Figure 4.2 (D1–D2, E1–E2, G1–G2) gave no suggestion of earlier development by the enriched group; results are given in Figure 4.18, top right, for G1–G2 (here labelled 3A–3B), the pair that had given the most marked indication of earlier development for the selected home sample than for the institution sample (Section IV-A).

The outstanding finding was that the visual enrichment had so little demonstrable effect, aside from quieting the infants while in the enriched situation. In the testing situation, the group difference was usually small and unreliable, even for pairings that used a part of the environment to which the enriched group was given intensive exposure. Less specific effects of the enrichment, in the form of earlier discrimination and hence earlier differential attention, resulting from ample opportunity for examination and comparison, were expected but not found in two other pairs of enrichment stimuli. Specifically, for the stimulus pair examined most intensively by the enriched group (Figure 4.18, upper left), no group difference was present in development of a configurational preference, just as in the case of pairs equally unfamiliar to both groups (e.g., Figure 4.18, upper right), suggesting that the development of such form preferences does not depend on learning to discriminate the difference between the pair members. Only in the area of depth discrimination was an effect of the enrichment suggested in preference testing. But this effect was equally present for two depth variations (Figure 4.18, bottom), one of which had been exposed to the enriched group for short daily periods and the other equally unfamiliar to both groups, suggesting a more general learning effect, such as from the "merry-go-round," seen only by the enriched infants, of objects of varied and continuously changing three-dimensional aspects.

Overall, the results of this experiment argue against a strong influence on the development of perceptual discrimination and selectivity by such early additions to the visual experiences as were practical with human infants at a home in which relatively varied visual stimulation was initially present. With this qualification, we believe that the enrichment we provided was optimally suited for accelerating the development of discrimination and selective fixation between stimuli. The lack of evidence of such an influence, except in the area of depth, points to maturation of the eye and brain, along with the visual experiences common to various lighted environments, as predominant causes of visual preference developments; even though such lesser experiential variations as our enrichment procedures may have had additional effects not detectable by our measures or at such early ages.

C. Length of Gestation

1. Introduction and Depth Variation

While analyzing the data of the preceding experiment varying early experiences, we realized that both enriched and control groups varied in length of gestation and that this variable was also relevant to the effects of experience (Section II-C). As a first attempt to make use of these different lengths of gestation as a natural variation of experience, those enriched and control infants for whom an estimate of gestation was available were divided into a preterm group of 36, 37, or 38 weeks (N of 5 to 9 at various weeks of PN age), a term group of 39 or 40 weeks (N of 11 to 27), and a postterm group of 41 or more weeks (N of 9 to 14).

For the pairing of a solid head model versus flat form pictured in Figure 4.15, the development of preference was in better agreement for the three groups when graphed by postnatal age than when graphed by postmenstrual age (Figure 4.19), suggesting that development was more a function of duration of opportunity for visual experience than of duration of maturation, both prenatal and postnatal. This suggests a parallel with results from the same pair unfamiliar to both enriched and control groups, but showing earlier development for enriched infants (Figure 4.18), even though in one

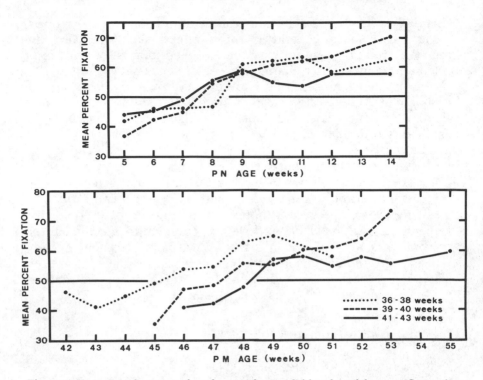

Figure 4.19   Development of preference for a solid head model over a flat outline form; percentages are for head model (Section VI-C-1). In top graph, institution infants of three estimated lengths of gestation are plotted separately, using a postnatal age scale. In the bottom graph the same results are plotted according to postmenstrual age (gestation plus age from birth).

case the variation was duration of postnatal experience and in the other case the amount or type of postnatal experience. The effects of longer postnatal experience are also supported by results from monkey infants reared in darkness to varying ages (Fantz, 1965b, 1967), showing some weeks of unrestricted experience to be necessary in particular for the development of visual preference for solid over flat objects. Other relevant results from human infants were obtained from projected photographs of the same solid head model and outline form, presented in a preceding section (Figure 4.16) as a single developmental curve based on a PM age scale. When graphed by PN age, instead, the small preterm group showed later development of the solidity preference than the term group, indicating no effect of premature experience in development relative to two-dimensional depth cues, and suggesting that the effect of experience on development of solidity preference depended on three-dimensional cues such as those given by binocular vision or movement parallax.

For most of the other stimulus pairs of the enrichment experiment, the analysis based on gestation either was ambiguous or suggested that development was more a function of total maturation (PM age); these results will not be reported since many of the same stimulus pairs appeared in later studies (summarized later in this section) with wider and more verified differences in gestation.

This discovery that the comparison between infants differing in length of gestation is another way of studying the role of early visual experience in the development of visual preferences led to experiments in which length of gestation was systematically varied. These experiments used twins, providing a wide range of postmenstrual ages, with prematurity often due to twinning and less often due to fetal or maternal abnormalities than in premature singletons. Infants were excluded if there was any ambiguity in date of onset of the mother's last menstrual period or if they had birth measurements that deviated markedly from expectations for the length of gestation as determined in this conventional way.

2. FORM VARIATIONS

In the first experiment (Section III-A-1), the twin pairs were selected with priority for those of short gestation to provide sufficient preterm subjects (under 38 weeks) to compare with a similar number of term pairs, using either postnatal or postmenstrual scales. There were variations in responses among the stimulus pairs, but overall the age of development of form preferences for term and preterm groups was in better agreement when plotted by PM age than by PN age, as illustrated by the two groupings of curvilinear versus rectilinear patterns in Figures 4.3 and 4.4. Thus there was no indication that the "extra" experience of preterm subjects accelerated the development of form perception. But even the plots by PM age at some ages suggested lower differentials for the preterm group, thus bringing to mind the higher risk of mental or perceptual retardation that has sometimes been found to be associated with prematurity. This possibility would apply particularly to the more preterm subjects; but exclusion of those with less than 35 weeks gestation gave no better match between term and preterm groups. And results from other samples and other stimulus variations did not support a retardation of preterm subjects when measured by total development (PM age).

3. QUANTITATIVE VARIATIONS

In the developmental experiment on variations of size and number of elements in a pattern (Section IV-B), subjects were carefully selected at 5-week intervals and with 5-week differences in gestation between term and preterm infants, so that data for the same groups could be plotted on either a PN or a PM age scale and could be analyzed statistically to test which scale gave the best data description. The postmenstrual age scale was far better; there was no indication that the development of size, number, or size versus number preferences were influenced by age from birth. However term–preterm comparisons at earlier postnatal ages would be desirable in view of the hypothesis (Section IV-C) that the developmental change, at least the decreasing differential response to large pattern elements, is due to improved ability to fixate small details— an ability that would presumably improve with oculomotor practice in the early weeks of experience.

While size preferences were hypothesized to be related to unperfected visual abilities, the sizes involved were all above threshold visibility. Visual performances more clearly related to pattern visibility were obtained by differential-fixation measures of minimum-separable or minimum-visible acuity (Section III-A-5). To reduce response variability and provide an overall developmental analysis, percentages were averaged for each infant for three widths of black-and-white striations, four widths of separated horizontal lines, and four widths of separated curved lines—each paired with an unpatterned stimulus of similar reflectance. The results (Figure 4.20) show better agreement between term and preterm infants when grouped and plotted by PM age than by PN age, thus failing to show any effect of the extra weeks of experience of the preterm infants. However, as for the size–number experiment, the PM ages did not extend low enough to reveal any difference in performance between preterm infants having had a few weeks of visual experience and oculomotor practice and term infants of the same PM age but with very little experience. Such experiential effects would be of theoretical importance even if, as was suggested by the results given here, the advantage to preterm subjects is only temporary.

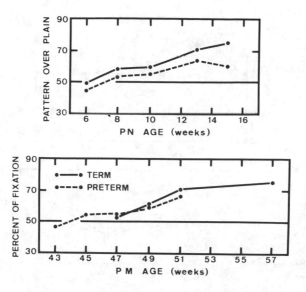

Figure 4.20 Visual acuity development (Section VI-C-3), based on combined results for various widths and types of pattern detail, each paired with a plain target. In top graph, results for term (38 weeks or longer gestation) and preterm infants are plotted according to postnatal age. In bottom graph, same results are plotted according to postmenstrual age.

4. RESPONSE TO NOVELTY AND RECOGNITION MEMORY

Prior to testing form variations and acuity (Section III-A-1), the same subjects were given 100-sec familiarization periods with one of two abstract multidimensional black-and-white patterns, followed by 10-sec exposures of both patterns in each right–left arrangement (Fagan, Fantz, & Miranda, 1971). The development of longer fixation to the novel pattern of the pair was similar to that shown in other studies. To determine whether this developmental trend could be adequately described in terms of postnatal age, results for term and preterm groups were compared (Figure 4.21, top). The term group reached a reliable preference at 11 weeks, the preterm group not until about a month later. In a second analysis, comparing the performance of the two samples as a function of PM age (Figure 4.21, bottom), the curves for the two samples are quite similar. Both show an initial chance level of response followed by a rapid rise to a reliable novelty preference at about 51 weeks of PM age.

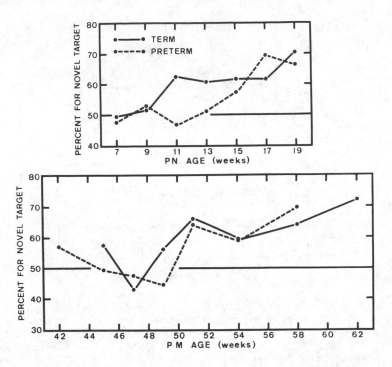

Figure 4.21   Development of preference for a novel over a previously exposed multidimensional pattern (Section VI-C-4), with results plotted by either postnatal age (top) or postmenstrual age (bottom).

5. INTERPRETATION

The development of visual preference and discrimination relative to form, to size and number variations, to the development of visual acuity, and to the development of response to novelty and short-term recognition memory have all been found to be primarily a function of age from conception or total period of maturation. The extra weeks of visual experience of the preterm infants had no noticeable accelerating effect on these developments. But this of course does not mean that visual experience has no importance. For example, results from monkey infants (Fantz, 1965b, 1967) with severe initial visual deprivation showed grossly abnormal development of visual preferences as well as other visual performances even after the deprivation period. Apparently our human infant subjects had adequate visual experience at a sufficiently early age, whether starting at or before the usual time of birth, to allow the development of perceptual–attentional processes to proceed normally. From an evolutionary viewpoint it would not be surprising if birth usually occurs at the stage of neural maturation at which visual experience can be assimilated, and that at an earlier stage the experience might have little or no developmental benefit. Is the use of birth as a starting point in developmental studies then justified only by the ease and objectivity of its determination? This is questioned by the fact that a 1-month preterm infant 1 month after birth is distinguishable observationally from a full-term newborn infant. This experiential advantage would be expected to continue in subsequent months for social and some other behaviors. The comparison of infants of varying gestation provides one way of experimentally testing this expectation and of specifying such experience effects, just as the above results indicated that visual response to three-dimensional variations in depth was related to both the duration and the nature of postnatal experience, even though response to variations in the patterning of two-dimensional stimuli revealed no clear experiential influence even for test stimuli continuously exposed in the cribs of some subjects (Section VI-B).

D. Down's Syndrome versus Normal Infants: Visual Preferences

The comparison of institution-reared with selected home-reared infants (Section VI-A) confounded experiential and organismic factors. These factors were better controlled in subsequent studies. Possible influences of experience on preference development were researched by the comparison of enriched with nonenriched institution infants (Section VI-B), and of preterm infants with term infants equated for PM age, and thus varying in length of postnatal experience (Section VI-C). Organismic factors were instead investigated in the studies to be reported next by comparing normal infants and infants with Down's Syndrome (DS) or mongolism. Down's Syndrome can be diagnosed at birth and almost invariably leads to later retarded cognitive performance. Therefore, abnormalities in the development of visual preferences in DS infants not attributable to sensory or motor abnormalities are presumably due to cognitive deficiencies.

1. COMPARISON AT EIGHT–NINE MONTHS

In the first experiment (Miranda and Fantz, 1973), 20 DS infants (mean PN age 34 weeks) were compared with 20 normal controls (mean PN age 32 weeks). All infants lived at home, where they were tested (Section II-D-2). The stimuli were selected primarily from those that showed a difference between institution-reared and selected home-reared infants (Section VI-A). For 6 of 13 pairs of stimulus targets the normal group showed significantly higher preferential fixations for one member of the pair. One of the group differences was preference of normal subjects, but not by the Down's Syndrome group, for a face photograph over a schematic face, perhaps suggestive of the normal group's greater ability to assimilate information from the environment. Two additional group differences, plus a third suggestive one, indicated higher preferences for solid over flat stimuli by the normal group. One solidity pair was the solid head model versus flat form for which an effect of experience was indicated in other results (Sections VI-B and VI-C-1). It is not surprising that visual preferences dependent on experience in normal infants would be retarded in infants congenitally predisposed toward mental deficiency, a deficiency that must include impaired ability to utilize experience.

The remaining three stimulus pairs eliciting DS–normal differences showed preferences by normals for patterns of curved contours over patterns of straight lines. These patterns were similar to G1–G2 (Figure 4.2), with the two members of each pair being equated in length of contour and in black–white ratio. However, the number of segments and angles was higher for the linear pattern in one of the pairs and higher for the circular pattern in the remaining two pairs, thus suggesting that "form" rather than "complexity" was the relevant stimulus difference. The influence of differing visual capacities was contraindicated by the fact that the width of line ($\frac{1}{4}$ inch) was the same for circular and linear patterns and was wider than those discriminated by both groups in acuity pairings ($\frac{1}{32}$ inch). Also, DS infants were not deficient in fixation response abilities, as shown by higher total response time to the stimuli. The results of this comparison at 8 months indicated the desirability of an extensive longitudinal study, to be discussed next.

2. LONGITUDINAL DS–NORMAL COMPARISON

Over a period of 4 years we were able to use 31 Down's Syndrome infants, each at a number of biweekly tests during the first 8 months, with from 9 to 21 subjects included in each test. These subjects were approximately matched with 28 normal controls in gestation, race, number of siblings, and parental education, of which from 8 to 16 were included at each biweekly test. The normal subjects were healthy infants with no known visual defects. The DS subjects were free from diagnosed visual defect and from active central nervous disease or other illness at the ages of testing. All subjects lived at home and were tested there using the portable equipment (Section II-D-2). Details of procedure and additional results are given elsewhere (Fantz & Miranda, in preparation). Stimulus variations included those that have shown marked developmental changes in normal infants as well as those that had elicited differences between DS and normal subjects at 8–9 months.

One emphasis was on variations in form. Five stimulus pairs had bull's-eye versus striped configurations; the combined results are given in Figure 4.22, top. The initial development of bull's-eye preference was 2 to 4 weeks later for DS than for normal subjects, with a significant group difference for the five pairs combined at 7 weeks. Also the preference subsequently decreased for DS infants, showing significant group differences after 27 weeks, similar to those found in the 8 to 9-month study previously discussed. For four of the five individual pairs, the bull's-eye preference was shown at least 2 weeks earlier by normal than by DS infants. The degree of group difference was not related to particular characteristics of the pair—whether it was more similar to E1–E2 or to G1–G2 in Figure 4.2, whether the lines were $\frac{1}{2}$-inch or $\frac{1}{4}$-inch wide, or whether the bull's-eye had less, equal, or more elements and angles than the striped pattern of the pair. That curved versus straight contour was the critical stimulus difference was further suggested by similar group differences for pairs F1–F2 and J1–J2 in which a different approach was used to vary curvilinearity versus rectilinearity. Figure 4.22 (middle) gives results for F1–F2, in which the preference was shown 4 weeks later by DS subjects and the group difference was significant at 7 and 9 weeks of age. In another form variation (Figure 4.22, bottom), significant group differences were shown at 7 and 11 weeks and after 6 months in the preference for an irregular over a regular element arrangement.

Other stimulus pairs with more widely varying stimulus differences yielded in some cases larger group differences. One of particular interest was the schematic face versus face photograph pair used in the 8- to 9-month study. The normal group showed an early preference for the schematic face that decreased and was reversed at 5 months to a significant preference for the photograph. The DS group showed a preference for the schematic patterns that was significantly higher than that of the normal group on the first 10 testing sessions and, while also decreasing with age, never was

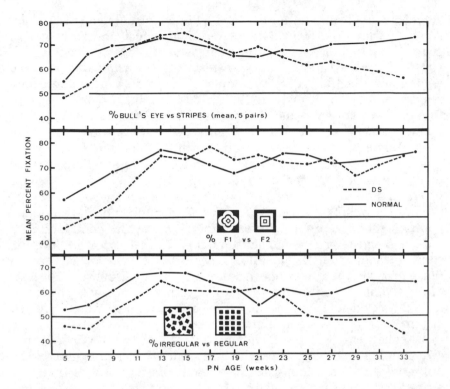

Figure 4.22   Form preference development curves from longitudinal study of Down's Syndrome and normal samples (Section VI-D-2). Top graph is mean for five different pairs of targets with similar form variations; other graphs are for single pairs of targets. For middle graph, outer black areas of targets representing blue felt background, measured 6 inches across; in bottom targets the white squares measured 4½ inches.

reversed. The possible role of sensory functions for this pairing was examined by concurrent acuity testing. In pairings of stripes of either ⅛ inch, 1/16 inch, or 1/32 inch with gray, DS infants were, respectively, 2, 5, and 4 weeks later than the controls in resolving the patterning. In contrast, the decrease in preference for the schematic face by DS infants lagged 2 to 4 months behind that of normal subjects, indicating that the degree of retardation in acuity development in DS infants is not sufficient to account for the large group difference for this pairing. Two stimulus differences that could be relevant instead were pattern contrast and facial resemblance. The black-and-white schematic face has been highly preferred over the photograph by newborn and premature infants

(Miranda, 1970a). But a decrease with age in preference for this and other patterns of high contrast toward patterns with less contrast but with more subtle stimulus features such as depth cues, brightness and texture gradients, and variety of patterning has been shown often by normal infants (Section V-A-B). The later development of selective attention to such features essential in later visual perception (Section VII) may be indicative of retardation in perceptual–cognitive development in DS infants. In addition, the stimulus with the subtle features also presented a more realistic representation of a human face. Similar face photographs have been shown by Fagan (1972) to be recognizable by 5 months when in the ordinary upright position (Section III-C). Also, in results to follow (Section VI-E-2; Figure 4.24), DS infants of 17 to 29 weeks did not show recognition memory for face photographs while normal subjects did. So lack of development of preference for a face photograph by DS infants could indicate retardation of social recognition as well as the more general retardation suggested earlier.

The remaining results we will report here are interesting for the lack of DS–normal differences rather than for their presence. The stimulus variations were similar to those used in the number versus size experiments (Section IV), but included only a three-stimulus array. For the pair varying only in size of four elements (Figure 4.23, top), the similar initial size preference dropped out earlier for normal than for DS infants, with group differences at 11 and 13 weeks. For the pair varying only in number of $\frac{1}{2}$-inch elements (Figure 4.23, middle), the number preference was initially equal for both groups but then increased some and later dropped less for DS infants, although the group difference was reliable only at 27 weeks. For the pair opposing four 1-inch squares with 16 $\frac{1}{2}$-inch squares (Figure 4.23, bottom), similar curves were shown for DS and normal infants with no reliable differences.

The comparison of results for quantitative variables with those for form variables is of particular interest. The lack of retardation in DS infants in the development of preference for patterns with more elements and angles and contour (Figure 4.23, middle and bottom) supports the interpretation (in Section IV-C) that changes with age in preference for number of elements in a pattern were likely related to the maturational and experiential perfection of elementary optical, oculomotor, and neural mechanisms for pattern reception and visual-motor response—developments not retarded in DS infants—and not to increasing information-processing capacity or cognitive development that would be expected to be retarded in DS

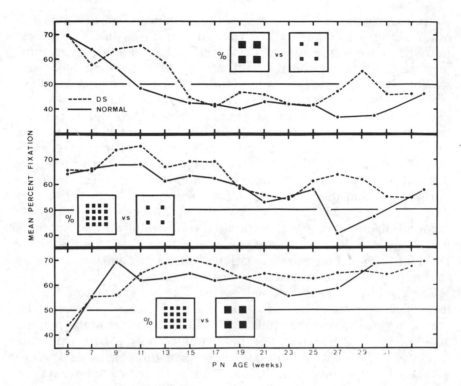

Figure 4.23   Number–size preference development curves from longitudinal study of Down's Syndrome and normal samples (Section VI-D-2). The three targets presented in three combinations included either 1-inch or ½-inch black squares on 5-inch white cards.

infants. In contrast, DS–normal differences were shown with another type of variation—form—that later becomes essential in the adaptive use of visual perception for intelligent behavior. The potential significance of DS–normal differences relative to form preferences is increased by the fact that the group difference was usually greater in later months than in the initial appearance of the curvature preference. This possibly suggests less effect of the genetic defect of DS on early developments than on later developments, perhaps involving higher neurological levels and more influence of experience. Some results in both the 8- to 9-month and longitudinal studies were, in fact, suggestive of deficient utilization of experience by DS infants.

A clear conclusion from DS–normal comparisons is that early

visual preference development reflects more than the development of basic sensory capacities; it reflects higher processes that could be described at least as perceptual and likely cognitive, as will be further evidenced in the next section.

E. Down's Syndrome Infants: Recognition Memory

Selective attention to novel over previously exposed targets has shown that the normal infant by 2 to 3 months of age has the ability to take in and store information from a visual stimulus that allows him to recognize that target as familiar at some later time (Sections III-C and VI-C-4; Chapter 5 by Cohen & Gelber in this volume). This method has high potential significance, since studies have shown that retarded children are inferior in various aspects of memory when compared with children of average intelligence (e.g. Belmont & Butterfield, 1969; Fagan, 1968, 1969) and the latter are similarly inferior when compared with children of superior intelligence (e.g. Fagan & Binzley, 1970; Fagan, 1972). Therefore we explored the usefulness of infant tests of recognition memory for studying early cognitive functioning; again DS infants provided a population with future retardation certain without waiting for IQ tests.

1. INITIAL STUDIES

In the first results, Miranda (1970b) reported that immediate recognition memory for abstract black-and-white patterns varying multidimensionally is present for both normal and Down's Syndrome infants at 34 weeks of age. Fagan (unpublished manuscript) extended the testing of Down's Syndrome infants down to a median 22 weeks of age. His procedure consisted of presenting three novelty problems during a single session, and testing for both immediate and delayed (1 to 7 min) recognition memory. The stimuli were again abstract black-and-white patterns differing in many features. The 18 DS infants performed about the same as normal infants (the subjects in Fagan, 1971). The DS subjects showed reliable preferences for novelty on immediate recognition tests for each of the three novelty problems and no reliable decline on delayed testing.

We interpreted these results to mean that immediate and delayed recognition memory for stimuli varying multidimensionally is a relatively simple performance that can be accomplished even by Down's Syndrome subjects by 5 months of age, therefore resulting in "ceiling" effects. If so, then either younger subjects or more difficult recognition memory problems might reveal differences in functioning between normal and DS infants, as was tested in the following study.

2. VARIATIONS IN AGE AND STIMULI

In an experiment by Miranda and Fantz (1974), 16 DS and 16 normal subjects were used at each of three age groupings: 8 to 16 weeks, 17 to 29 weeks, and 30 to 40 weeks. At each age level three problems of expected differing difficulty were given. Problem 1 included patterning and color as independent novel features—that is, after presenting a given one of four stimuli for familiarization, this stimulus was paired successively with a different pattern of the same color and with the same pattern in a different color, so that, in effect, recognition of two stimulus features was tested in one problem. The two patterns varied multidimensionally; the colors (red versus blue) were highly saturated and contrasted against the white ground. Problem 2 used nonglossy photographic prints of a baby's face and of a woman's face (taken from Fagan, 1972). In the third problem, 25 black $\frac{3}{8}$-inch squares were arranged on a white card in either circular or checkerboard configuration. The technique was to present duplicates of a stimulus target in both right and left positions for a 60-sec familiarization period, followed by two 10-sec testing periods in which the previously exposed target was paired in alternate right and left positions with a novel stimulus; or for Problem 1, it was paired alternately in four testing periods with either the novel color or novel pattern.

Figure 4.24 shows the percentage of fixation paid to the novel target in each age grouping. Differences are evident among the problems for normal subjects, indicating that the problems indeed varied in difficulty. And for each of the four stimulus variations, the normal group showed differential response at an earlier age than did the DS group. For the pattern variation of Problem 1, the novelty preference of the normal group began at 8–16 weeks, but not until 17–29 weeks for DS infants. For Problem 2, the preference first attained significance at 17–29 weeks for the normal infants but not until 30–40 weeks for DS subjects. Problem 3 was reliably solved by both middle and older normal groups but not by any DS group. The color variation of Problem 1 elicited a reliable novelty preference only by the oldest normal group. While the wide age groupings prevent a close estimation of the degree of developmental

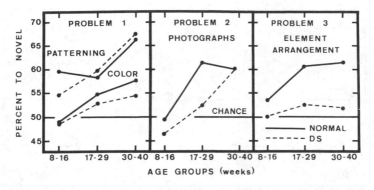

Figure 4.24 Preference for novel over previously exposed targets by Down's Syndrome versus normal infants in three age groupings (Section VI-E-2) indicating development of recognition memory relative to four types of stimulus variation, including the two variations in Problem 1. [From Miranda & Fantz, 1974.]

lag of DS infants in recognition memory, a DS–normal developmental differential of at least 2 months was suggested for each of the four stimulus variations.

3. LONGITUDINAL STUDY

The course of development of recognition memory for a multidimensional pattern variation was shown better in another experiment included in the longitudinal visual preference study (Section VI-D-2). The stimulus patterns and procedure were the same as those used in the comparison of novelty response of institution and selected home infants (Section VI-A). Instead of a single familiarization exposure, one of two patterns (alternating in successive test weeks) was exposed during each interval between exposures of a long series of stimulus pairs; at the middle and end of this series the repeatedly exposed pattern was paired with the other (novel) pattern for recognition testing. Figure 4.25 gives the mean percent for the novel pattern for these two recognition tests. The novelty preference was significant beginning at 9 weeks for normals (about as early as in any study), but not until 17 weeks for DS infants. The retardation of DS infants in the initial development of recognition memory and response to novelty suggested in the multidimensional pattern variation of the preceding experiment was verified, with about a 2-month difference in development for DS and normal subjects. But, as in previous studies, at later months of age there

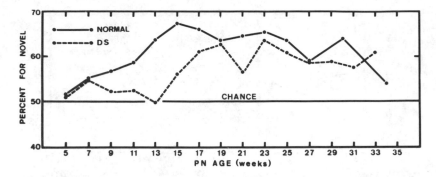

Figure 4.25   Novelty preference development curves from longitudinal study of Down's Syndrome and normal samples (Section VI-E-3). The two targets, differing multidimensionally in patterning, were given repeated pretest exposures on alternate test weeks for each subject.

were few group differences in degree of response to the novel of two patterns differing in many features.

4. DISCUSSION

Down's Syndrome infants were retarded in development of response to a novel over a previously exposed target. But this retardation was evident only at a certain age level for a particular stimulus variation. The dependence on age suggests a basic developmental process common to both groups, but slower for DS infants. The retardation for DS infants was not primarily in either selective attention per se, or in pattern discrimination ability, since pairs of patterns differing in more restricted ways than the present pairs were differentiated by DS infants at earlier months in visual preference tests not requiring memory (Figure 4.22). In particular, checked and lattice arrangements of squares were differentiated by DS infants as early as 9 weeks of age, while checked and circular arrangements (Problem 3) did not elicit novelty preference for DS infants at any of the three age levels.

This retardation shown by Down's Syndrome infants, attributable not to discriminative deficiency or to general unresponsiveness to novelty, gives further evidence that the developmental changes evidenced in this section are related to cognition. In principle this would have been assumed from the known relation of memory to the development of intelligence. But more than this principle is needed: Responsiveness to novel multidimensional patterns by infants over 4 months of age provided no indication of abnormal

performance even for DS infants. Age and stimulus variations are
critical for the study both of response to novel over previously
exposed patterns and of intrinsic stimulus preferences. With both
techniques, stimulus differences in form or configuration appear to
be related to expected subsequent cognitive development, provided
that the age range is wide enough to include the age of onset of
differential response for both groups. But results on one stimulus
variation at one age level could lead to false conclusions.

VII DISCUSSION AND THEORY

A. Classification of Stimulus Variations

On the basis of visual preference experiments extending over
many years, using hundreds of stimuli and thousands of infants, we
are here presenting a classification of the stimulus variations
relevant to visual attention during the first 6 months of life. In the
next section suggestions are included on how the variations are
ordered developmentally. The stimulus domain is restricted to
nonmoving surfaces or objects of limited extent. Furthermore, the
first three categories are limited to the patterning of flat surfaces:
the *presence* of patterning (definition or prominence), the *amount* of
patterning, and the *kind* of patterning (configuration). Interpretations for each category will be sought in terms of both underlying
mechanisms and adaptive value.

1. PATTERN DEFINITION

High pattern definition is given by sharply defined contours, high
figure–ground contrast, large elements, and wide lines. Also relevant is the absence of texture, of brightness gradations, and of other
subtleties that might interfere with the visibility of the most
prominent parts of patterning, especially at early ages. At one
extreme of any specific dimension varying in definition, the patterning will no longer be visible; but even among suprathreshold
patterns, the *relative* visibility or prominence has been an important
determinant of attention value. Black-and-white stimuli with sharp
contours were attended to most by newborns (Section III-D) and by
infants during the first 2 months (Section V-A), with subsequent
decrease in their prepotency. Large elements were also strongly
preferred by newborns (Section IV-A), with markedly decreasing
strength after the first few months (Sections IV-B and VI-D-2).

This developmental similarity is one reason for including variations in size in the same category as variations in sharpness of contour or figure–ground contrast. The other reason is that both of these variations make the existing patterning more easily fixated and discriminated. The hypothesis follows that the early prepotency of these variations is due to early incomplete development of such visual processes as accommodation and other optical factors; fixation, convergence, and other oculomotor abilities; maturation of the retinal fovea and of other neural centers for vision; and resulting behavioral skills such as visual acuity and visual scanning patterns. A corollary is that the decreasing prepotency of pattern definition and prominence during the early months of life is due to perfection of these visual mechanisms to the point that attention can be easily directed to other stimulus variations (e.g., form of contour and number of elements) that may have been earlier obscured by the primary requisite of clearly defined, prominent, large patterning.

The early selective visual responses to well-defined and prominent patterns, while likely attributable to the immature state of the visual system, even so may be quite adaptive, since these responses concentrate attention on stimuli that are most effective for the practice of visual skills and that provide the most readily assimilated information. Such selective responses, while operationally termed "visual preferences," are obviously of a different nature from those in which a selection is made between equally processible stimuli. Therefore, unless the purpose is to test early visual or oculomotor abilities, it is usually desirable to exclude stimulus variations in the category of pattern definition.

2. PATTERN QUANTITY

"Quantitative pattern variations" was proposed (Section IV) as a term preferable to "pattern complexity" for variations not involving the form, arrangement, or meaningfulness of features. The results of experiments presented there suggested that one quantitative variation (i.e., size) differs markedly from other quantitative variations in the course of development. In addition, arguments were given in the preceding section for putting size of element in the category of pattern definition or prominence, for which the early prepotency was attributed to immaturity of basic visual skills. The variations remaining in this new category of "pattern quantity" include number of elements and angles, contour length, contour density, or other measures of the amount as distinct from the type of patterning. These measures are related to amount of information in the pattern; but so are nonquantitative aspects, such as form and depth variations, that at later ages give most of the information for visually directed adaptive behavior. Amount of information is even involved in the preceding category of pattern definition, if one is talking not about potential information, but about information actually available to the immature infant. Hence "pattern quantity" is a better description than "amount of information."

In the size–number experiments (Section IV), high pattern quantity (number of elements and angles) was preferred for attention throughout the first 6 months beginning with newborn infants. The preference tended to increase in strength until 50 or 55 weeks of PM age and then decreased slightly. This relatively small influence of age on the preference for more patterning was highly dependent on the exclusion of other variations, as is shown in the following two cases. When size varied inversely with number, the initial preference tended to be for patterns of fewer large elements over those with higher pattern quantity. Subsequently, a preference for patterns of more elements, angles, and contour appeared and increased with age. In contrast, when form variations were confounded with pattern quantity (Figure 4.17, top), the pattern with considerably more elements, angles, and contour was slightly preferred at early ages, while the pattern with three circular elements, no angles, and much less contour was later strongly preferred. Thus the direction of the developmental change relative to pattern quantity was opposite in these two cases, depending on whether the confounding variation was in the above category of pattern definition or in the next category of configuration. This suggests a developmental hierarchy in the influence of the three categories of pattern variations upon infants' attention, to be discussed further in the following sections.

As discussed previously (Section IV-C-3), in terms of mechanisms the selective fixation of patterns with more elements, angles, and contour can be accounted for at any age by greater stimulation of neurons in the retina and especially in the visual cortex, while various developmental changes in preference might occur from perfection of such visual abilities as oculomotor coordination or scanning patterns. In terms of behavioral adaptation, there is a definite value for the infant to look at and learn from stimuli with more of such informational features as contour, elements, and angles that are necessary (though not sufficient) for most later perceptual performances.

3. PATTERN CONFIGURATION

Among the unlimited variations in configuration or form, those so far found to influence visual responsiveness in early infancy include shape of contour, regularity, concentricity, orientation, and several aspects of the arrangement of elements in a pattern (Section III). As was the case for pattern quantity, even newborn infants showed selective attention to configuration under optimal circumstances— that is, for form of contour when varied in the outermost contours of a stimulus, with equated pattern quantity and with pattern definition high and equated.

Selective attention to configurational variations is more important for behavior in the older infant, the child, and the adult than the preceding stimulus categories. It is essential in the development of such performances as object recognition, spatial orientation, social responsiveness, and reading. The possible adaptive value of the particular directions of preference, such as curved over straight contours and irregular over regular arrangements, is less obvious, but deserves further investigation. A possible underlying mechanism for form discriminations (Section III-E-3) is the highly-selective activation of "hypercomplex" cells in the visual cortex to allow "detection of any change in direction (curvature) of the contours [Hubel & Wiesel, 1968, p. 238]."

4. DEPTH AND PATTERN SUBTLETY

Findings presented in Section V-B and elsewhere are in agreement in that the developmental trend is toward visual preference for a solid object or a representation of a solid object over a comparable flat object (the latter usually with better definition), and that a reliable solidity preference is shown sometimes at about 2 months and sometimes later. The value of attending to solid stimuli that often are of special behavioral importance and that provide opportunity for further development of depth perception is evident. In the perfection of the necessary skills, at least for three-dimensional depth variations, visual experience was suggested to be important (Sections VI-B, VI-C).

For this stimulus category, the difficulty lies not in knowing its adaptive value but in specifying the relevant stimulus variations, since actual solid and flat objects present a wide variety of stimulus differences. Projected stimuli (Figure 4.15) excluded such depth cues as binocular and movement parallax, but still varied in such two-dimensional features as figure–ground contrast, texture, brightness gradients of shading and shadows, and configurational differences (especially in drawings with and without perspective). These variations later on are all involved in depth perception and so are functionally in a single category for the child and adult. This cannot be assumed to be true for the young infant: The perfection of depth perception must be a complex and prolonged process, even though Bower (Chapter 2 in Volume II of this work) has shown beginnings of it at early ages. A safer assumption is that the discrimination and preference for a stimulus conveniently described as having solidity or depth initially may at first involve only one or several of the many stimulus dimensions that are later integrated phenomenally and behaviorally into what we term "a solid object."

Prominent among the features of solid objects or their photographs is the presence of brightness and texture gradients and other subtle variations that cannot be adequately described as low pattern definition, as high pattern quantity, or as a type of form. The developmental trend during the first 6 months has been toward a stimulus with this subtlety of patterning (Figure 4.16), whether or not it is representative of depth; but the presence or strength of such preferences appeared to depend on the degree to which the paired stimulus contained opposing stimulus features that were highly preferred in the early months, especially high pattern definition and contrast. So preference changes were probably due both to decreasing attention value of these confounded variations and to the emergence of attention value for other more subtle pattern variations. Both processes involve the perfection of abilities to assimilate the less sharp and obvious aspects of patterning—aspects that will eventually be of critical importance for behavior, including, as well as depth discrimination, social and object recognition, and many other behaviors.

5. VARIETY WITHIN A STIMULUS

This category might be considered an extension of the variation of irregular versus regular patterns to include, along with differences in arrangement, differences among details in form, color, brightness, size, etc. It is thus related to a decrease in "redundancy" as used in information theory, although including variations that would be difficult to order in amount of information. Like the preceding category of pattern subtlety, it is not easily defined. It is included here to suggest some of the additional kinds of stimulus variations that at later ages must elicit selective attention for vision to become such an efficient sensory modality. The included results most pertinent to this category are developmental trends from a pattern of the same forms to one of smaller but varied forms, and away from black circles on white toward circles with less contrast but of varied colors (Section V-C).

6. RESPONSE TO NOVELTY

Response to novelty is a unique category of stimulus variation. It depends on the natural tendency to attend more to a novel visual stimulus, but this in turn depends on specific previous experiences that make another comparable stimulus familiar. Another consequent unique aspect of novelty preferences is that since they depend upon the recognition of the previously seen stimulus, they show visual memory as well as discrimination and selectivity. This memory ability is clearly related to cognition. Memory is also clearly of adaptive value, as is the attention to novel stimuli that facilitates wide exploration of the environment and perceptual learning. In spite of these uniquely advantageous aspects, the preference for a novel over a familiar pattern depends upon the discrimination and attention to certain intrinsic stimulus differences between the two patterns—differences that must be large and multidimensional to be retained as early as 2 or 3 months of age, but at later ages may be increasingly smaller or unidimensional, such as different arrangement of pattern elements or different face photographs (Sections III-C and VI-E). Apparently there exists a developmental hierarchy within the category of stimulus novelty relative to the stimulus attributes remembered and differentiated at successive ages; how this hierarchy is similar to or different from that given in this section for unfamiliar stimuli could be informative, for example, on the relationship between perceptual and memory processes.

B. Interpretation of Developmental Changes

In experiments varying both size and number of elements in a pattern (Section IV), the strong developmental trend toward patterns of many small elements over those with large elements was best explained by decreasing preference along the size dimension accompanied by increasing preference along the number dimension. In terms of the preceding classification, this means a developmental shift in relative attentional prepotency from pattern definition to pattern quantity. And the initial absence of preference for a bull's-eye pattern over stripes was suggested to be due in part to the confounding variation of more angles and elements in the stripes (Section III-D), an interpretation supported by other results (Figure 4.17, top) that showed a reversal from pattern quantity to pattern configuration as the prepotent variation.

These two cases illustrate a proposed general hypothesis: There is a developmental ordering or "hierarchy" in the relative prepotency of different stimulus dimensions for maximal influence on visual attention. Whether one or another dimension determines the preferential response at a given age is also dependent on the specific stimuli used; for example, in the number–size arrays, pairs of patterns can be found for which more numerous but smaller elements are preferred even by newborns (Figure 4.9, 32–$\frac{1}{2}$ over 2–1), but the increase with age in preference for such patterns (Figure 4.10) still indicates a *relative* change in prepotency from size to number.

The first three categories, that is, pattern definition, pattern quantity, and pattern configuration, have previously been listed according to this proposed developmental ordering. From the limited evidence available for the other categories it would seem that, without attempting to put them in any order, variations in depth, pattern subtlety, variety within a stimulus and response to novelty all reach their maximal attention value at later ages than any of the first three categories. Among the findings that led to this ordering, the size–number experiments clearly indicated a shift from pattern definition to pattern quantity. Other results (Section V-A) have shown the initial prepotency of pattern definition, as well as a decrease during the early weeks and months in favor of other stimulus categories, including those with depth and subtle patterning (Figure 4.16) and those with variety within a stimulus (Figure 4.17). A shift in prepotency from pattern quantity to pattern configuration was also shown in Figure 4.17, top.

This developmental ordering in the relative prepotency of categories of stimulus variations leads to the prediction that in further experiments comparing the attention given to stimuli that oppose preferred stimulus features in two categories, there should be a shift with age toward the stimulus having the preferred feature in the higher-ranking category. A converse prediction is more hypothetical: A marked developmental change in preference or other measure of visual attention, especially when there is a reversal in direction of response among stimuli, indicates that the stimuli oppose dimensions at different levels of this developmental hierarchy. In other words, a reversal or a large change in visual preference with age is likely attributable to a shift in the relative prepotency of different dimensions rather than a change in the preferred point along a single dimension. For example, earlier experiments using a series of checkerboard patterns did not, as was thought, indicate progressive shifts with age in the preferred point along a "dimension of complexity," or even shifts along size or number dimensions separately, since both larger elements and more elements in a pattern were preferred at all ages. Thus the checkerboard results were instead due to a shift in *relative* prepotency from size to number. But this example also suggests that a marked developmental change in degree of preference may, for stimuli differing in relative visibility, be caused by improvement in visual abilities. This brings up one reason for categorizing and ordering the stimulus variations that are prepotent for visual preferences at various ages: to aid in finding the relevance of particular preference developments to particular aspects of visual or psychological development.

Visual preferences show both discrimination and selective attention among stimuli. If one of the stimuli had previously been exposed, then the preference for the novel one also shows memory, a function known to be related to intelligence, at least at older age levels. But what do the visual preferences between equally novel stimuli indicate relative to later development? The type of stimulus variation is one way of answering this question. The appearance with age of the selective fixation of finer pattern details and the decrease with age in the importance of high contrast, sharp contours, and large elements, are all likely related to the perfection of pattern fixation, scanning, and resolution abilities. On the other hand, visual selectivity to form of contour and of configuration, including subtle configurational differences, and including equivalent responses to different stimulus variations that have in common a configurational invariant (Section III), is related to development of form perception, a function that requires higher levels of the nervous system than the detection of fine pattern details and a function that is more critical for the later use of vision in intelligent behavior.

As a complement to stimulus variations, variations in the selection or treatment of subjects can clarify the meaning of various visual preferences and discriminations. In particular, the comparison of infants with Down's Syndrome with normal infants verified that the development of form preferences, as well as novelty preferences and the accompanying recognition memory, are related to processes that we term "cognitive." In contrast, the Down's Syndrome versus normal results gave no indication of cognitive relevance for variations in size or number of elements or length of contour in a pattern. These examples illustrate what can be discovered by varying population parameters along with stimulus parameters.

Visual selectivities and discriminations thus can reveal the development of both sensory and cognitive abilities and so provide a means for the experimental study of a wide variety of processes during the early months of life. One of these processes is perceptual learning: Visual selectivities and discriminations determine what parts and aspects of the environment are experienced and provide the opportunity for oculomotor practice or for receiving and retaining specific information about the environment—as examples of two quite different learning processes that occur during early infancy. And in both cases, visual selectivity is a causative factor in early perceptual learning simply by determining, along with the surroundings, the opportunities for learning. In the following section three phases of this developmental process will be suggested that incorporate the classification of stimulus variations in the preceding section, the developmental ordering of these categories in the present section, and knowledge or conjectures on what is learned by the young infant in successive phases, supplemented by relevant information from older children and from monkey infants.

C. Phases of Visual Selectivity and Learning

A requisite for learning about a part of the environment by the young infant, as by any organism with highly specialized central areas of the retinas, is to *look at* that part of the environment (aside from minor learning that might occur through peripheral vision). Visual fixation provides the *opportunity* for learning from the environment, through whatever little-understood processes this occurs. These opportunities, and therefore what is available to be learned from, change when the infant consistently selects different parts or aspects of the environment for attention. Hence one approach to tracing early perceptual–cognitive development is to trace changes in predominant visual selectivities, such as those shown in Sections VII-A and VII-B during the early months, but also going beyond this period. Changes in visual selectivity cannot give a complete picture of early development any more than can the changes in sensory, motor, and other abilities tested in developmental scales. At least, it is another approach to an area in which previous approaches have not been sufficient. At most, it is an approach that can show the changes in actual information acquisition and retention, and in the resulting cognitive development, at successive ages. It is an approach that was supported by the success in differentiating groups with later differences in intelligent behavior (Sections VI-A, VI-D, VI-E). The following proposal of three broad phases of visual selectivity in early development is a modification and extension of the analysis in Fantz (1970).

The initial phase of visual selectivity is dominated by various immaturities of the visual system that make it difficult to find, to maintain fixation of, and to resolve small details, fuzzy contours, or subtle pattern variations. The result is initial restriction of attention to stimuli high in the first listed category (Section VII-A) of "pattern definition," with a secondary basis of attraction being in the category of "pattern quantity" (the more parts in a pattern of high definition, the better the chance of the immature infant's finding and fixating some part of it). This patterning that is most easily visible often provides little information to direct more active and adaptive behaviors in a natural environment, but such behaviors are not required in the early months of human life. However, in preparation for the time when precise, adaptive, visually directed behavior becomes important, oculomotor practice and other benefits from using the initial sensory abilities are facilitated by concentration on patterns with large, sharply defined details that can be more easily fixated and processed by the immature visual system. Though rarely containing patterning of such high definition as our simple black-and-white stimuli, any natural visual environment contains some features that are sufficiently prominent relative to the background to hold the attention of the infant. For example, the human face has many subtleties of patterning and coloring, but for a face close to the infant there are always certain features such as the outer contour, the hairline, the eyes, and the open mouth that will attract and hold the gaze enough to assist in this "visual practice" phase of perceptual development (whether or not more specific information about faces can then be processed and even retained).

If selectivity was *not* shown among the unlimited features of a natural environment, and if *all* the features were resolvable, the infant during the early weeks of life would indeed be faced with a "great blooming buzzing confusion." But the high acuity threshold, poor oculomotor coordination, and lack of accommodation for different distances in the early weeks all reduce considerably the amount of visible patterning and actually *aid* early development by restricting attention to limited salient features of the surroundings. Thus through highly selective attention, assisted by initial poor visual abilities, the visual world of even the newborn infant is not likely either chaotic or lacking in processible information.

The second proposed phase of selectivity and learning overlaps the first but is predominant starting at about 2 months of age. Developments during the first phase have multiplied the features in the surroundings that are visible to the infant and have improved the oculomotor skills and scanning techniques important for visual exploration and processing of these features. Of further aid in this phase is the tendency to attend to the same stimulus for a prolonged period. This is another way of preventing visual chaos and facilitating instead the slow, piecemeal examination and processing of selected parts and aspects of the environment. It also gives optimal conditions for *learning by looking* when presented with an unfamiliar stimulus. The theoretical framework most appropriate here is the "differentiation" viewpoint of the Gibsons as presented in E. J. Gibson (1969): learning not by "enrichment" through association or conditioning of the visible features, but by differentiating "distinctive features" of the pattern looked at. Our second phase of development would seem ideally suited for the intensive visual examination needed for the successive differentiation of new and more subtle distinctive features.

What is learned during this second phase of development (as distinct from the process) is again suggested by the visual selectivities that determine the learning opportunities within a given environment. Visual selectivities related to form or configuration, to variety of patterning, to depth cues and other pattern subtleties, and to novel patterns, become stronger and more persistent, even over patterns with higher definition and quantity. The importance of configurational features does not suddenly emerge at 2 months, as was evidenced by certain newborn form differentiations, but it is usually obscured earlier, in part by the primary requirement for high pattern definition, size, and contrast; and differentiation of configurational features does not suddenly disappear in later months or years of age, even though visual selectivity for differences among flat patterns decreases during the following third phase of selectivity.

For the adaptive use of visual perception in active responses to the environment, what is learned from visual exploration alone is not sufficient. The first alternative to looking as a response for exploring the environment comes through the gradual development of reaching, grasping, and manipulation of objects. After 3 or 4 months, visual attention increasingly shifts toward "graspable" objects of the environment as a prelude to manual contact, even if the object cannot be reached or successfully manipulated. This is evidenced in preference testing by increased looking at solid objects (including parts of the apparatus), often accompanied by reaching movements. The stimuli that had elicited differential attention to solidity in earlier months differed prominently in configurational cues of depth, but by 4 to 5 months a head model with painted features was preferred to its photograph that had essentially the same configurational indications of depth (Fantz & Nevis, 1967b). Other results (Fantz, 1970) show preference after 5 months for a lighted globe over a flat but highly patterned stimulus that had been preferred from 2 to 4 months.

Better information on the third phase as well as support for the other phases is given by an experiment with rhesus monkey infants reared from birth with or without visual deprivation (Fantz, 1965b, 1967). Visual preference testing used procedures comparable to those for human infants. In the early weeks of life, with visual experience allowed only during testing, preferences were shown for patterned over plain stimuli and for a bull's-eye over a striped pattern, but not for solid over flat stimuli, comparable to human infant first-phase results. After the monkeys were moved to a lighted room, preference increased during the early weeks for patterned over plain stimuli, emerged during the early months for solid over flat stimuli, and was maintained for concentric patterns. However, this was true only for monkeys that had been reared for short periods under visual deprivation: In contrast, none of these configurational preferences were shown by monkeys that had undergone 2 or more months of visual deprivation, that instead showed increased preferences relative to color, reflectance, or size. Hence, these results emphasize the importance of visual experience for maintaining and further developing initial pattern and form abilities and selectivities. The similarity between rhesus monkeys and human infants in initial visual selectivities and their early development is of interest in suggesting primate communalities in visual and neurological functions as well as in general experiences and behavior development.

Later tests of the monkeys at about 15 months, using a modified Wisconsin General Test Apparatus go beyond our results with human infants. Initial tests with either stimulus block rewarded showed more selectivity for three-dimensional form differences than for the pattern, size, or color brightness of flat plaques. And in subsequent discrimination training, the only 7 of 24 pairs that received as many as 20 correct responses in a session of 30 trials all differed tactually in form, texture, solidity, or size, even though the choice was made visually. Few monkeys discriminated to criterion in one session flat stimuli such as checkerboard versus plain and black versus white—discriminations shown by intrinsic preferences in the early weeks of life. By contrast, much more subtle, but "palpable," discriminations such as blocks with smooth versus finely textured surfaces or a segment of dowel rod versus a comparable segment of a tree branch painted the same color were discriminated to criterion by most of the subjects in a single session.

Our third postulated phase of visual selectivity and perceptual development, in which manual and other active exploration possibilities begin to influence selectivity beginning in human infants late in the first 6 months, was clearly dominant for monkeys at about 15 months. They shifted their predominant attention, both without and with training, to "palpable" stimulus features that were most relevant for behavior, and had apparently *learned to ignore* previously dominant features not relevant to adaptive behaviors such as manipulation or locomotion. Other studies of monkeys have shown fine discriminations in the patterning of flat plaques after more intensive training that resulted in renewed attention to such variations. A similar change is shown by human infants even without such training: After many months of attention directed mainly by stimulus features indicating objects or surfaces that can be manipulated or that support crawling, climbing, or walking, the child again shows more interest in flat patterns such as pictures representational of real objects, and eventually even abstract, symbolic patterns. While this is a much later phase of perceptual selectivity than we have been concerned with in the research of this chapter, it depends upon previous experiences, including those in the second phase that give intensive opportunity for learning about configurational differences. More generally, it supports, along with the monkey results, the proposal of successive changes in visual selectivity as facilitating first, early oculomotor practice, and much later, such behaviors as reading and precise movements relative to the visual surroundings.

D. Epilogue

For such a new field of experimental inquiry as infant perception, general agreement on the facts or on their interpretations would not be expected, while agreement on specific methods would restrict future progress. Our closing comments will circumvent these differences by taking broader epistemological and historical perspectives.

The *difficulty* of studying young infants was emphasized when methods developed for older humans or for animals were not found to be applicable. Now that various testing methods and conditions are available for infants of any age, an emphasis on the *advantages* of studying young infants is more appropriate. Young infants are truly "naive" subjects, whose responses can be expected to be related to the stimulus situation and to early stages in processing of information from that situation, without expectations or preconceptions. Given a natural response such as visual exploration by a quiet but alert infant, there is even more reason to expect a direct relationship to sensory or perceptual processing. But the new methods appropriate for young infants also call for new techniques of stimulus selection. Since the relevant stimulus dimensions cannot be *specified* by instructions or training, they must be *discovered*. In this discovery process, the experimenter has two handicaps. He himself has had several decades or more of perceptual learning and development that have given a visual world that is likely to be quite different, phenomenally and behaviorally, from that of the young infant. This may lead the experimenter to choose stimulus variations that are not distinguishable or not relevant for visual exploration by the young infant. In addition the experimenter has had years of specialized education that have probably instilled certain preconceptions about infant perception, derived perhaps from findings with children, adults, or animals, from theories based on uncontrolled observations of infants, or from preliminary experimental findings (e.g., the senior author's early experiment with schematic versus scrambled face patterns influenced much subsequent research, with the neglect of other areas that have proven more fruitful).

A preconception that discouraged experimental research on infant perception until the last decade or so was the idea that the visual field of the young infant was a formless blur. This preconception was derived either from the known immaturity and assumed nonfunctioning of various parts of the visual system, especially the cerebral cortex; or from the theoretical supposition that learning, requiring further motor development, was necessary for development of pattern perception. After its experimental rejection, the idea of a complete lack of pattern vision was replaced by new erroneous preconceptions, such as that the infant's differentiation among patterns could be adequately explained by or reduced to preferences along some dimensions of "complexity". An early preconception of the senior author was not lack of pattern vision, but that visual preferences were of value *only* for showing the early *presence* of pattern vision. For example, it was many years before the bull's-eye over stripes preference found in the first experiment, as an indication of discrimination between certain patterns, led to the research described in this chapter, showing a wide generality of selectivity for curved-regular forms, but dependent both on maturational age and on expected future intelligence. And many more years may be needed to find out what the infant learns from early intensive experience in "just looking" at such environmental features, and how this experience facilitates later shifts in attention to more subtle features essential for adaptive visually directed behavior.

REFERENCES

Amiel-Tison, C. Neurological evaluation of the maturity of newborn infants. *Archives of Disease in Childhood*, 1968, *43*, 89–93.

Attneave, F. Criteria for a tenable theory of form perception. In W. Wathen-Dunn (Ed.), *Models for the perception of speech and visual form.* Cambridge, Massachusetts: MIT Press, 1967. Pp. 56–67.

Belmont, J. M., & Butterfield, E. C. The relations of short-term memory to development and intelligence. In L. P. Lipsitt, & H. W. Reese (Eds.), *Advances in child development and behavior.* Vol. 4. New York: Academic Press, 1969. Pp. 30–83.

Berlyne, D. E. *Conflict, arousal and curiosity.* New York: McGraw-Hill, 1960.

Bond, E. K. Perception of form by the human infant. *Psychological Bulletin*, 1972, *77*, 225–245.

Bower, T. G. R. The object in the world of the infant. *Scientific American*, 1971, *225*, 30–38.

Brennan, W. M., Ames, E. W., & Moore, K. W. Age differences in infant's attention to patterns of different complexity. *Science*, 1966, *151*, 335–356.

Brunswik, E. *Systematic and representative design of psychological experiments.* Berkeley: Univ. of California Press, 1949.

Dodwell, P. C. (Ed.) *Perceptual processing: Stimulous equivalence and pattern recognition.* New York: Appleton, 1971.

Doris, J., Casper, M., & Poresky, R. Differential brightness thresholds in infancy. *Journal of Experimental Child Psychology*, 1967, *5*, 522–535.

Ellingson, R. J. Cortical electrical responses to visual stimulation in the human infant. *Electroencephalography and Clinical Neurophysiology*, 1960, *12*, 663–677.

Fagan, J. F. Short term memory processes in normal and retarded children. *Journal of Experimental Child Psychology*, 1968, *6*, 279–296.

Fagan, J. F. Free recall learning in normal and retarded children. *Journal of Experimental Child Psychology*, 1969, *8*, 9–19.

Fagan, J. F. Memory in the infant. *Journal of Experimental Child Psychology*, 1970, *9*, 217–226.

Fagan, J. F. Infant's recognition memory for a series of visual stimuli. *Journal of Experimental Child Psychology*, 1971, *11*, 244–250.

Fagan, J. F. Infant's recognition memory for faces. *Journal of Experimental Child Psychology*, 1972, *14*, 453–476.

Fagan, J. F. Infant's delayed recognition memory and forgetting. *Journal of Experimental Child Psychology*, 1973, *16*, 424–450.

Fagan, J. F. Recognition memory in normal and Down's Syndrome infants. Unpublished manuscript.

Fagan, J. F., & Binzley, V. Free recall in children of superior, average, and retarded IQ. Paper presented at the Gatlinburg Conference on Mental Retardation, Gatlinburg, Tennessee, March 12, 1970.

Fagan, J. F., Fantz, R. L., & Miranda, S. B. Infant's attention to novel stimuli as a function of postnatal and conceptional age. Paper presented at Society for Research in Child Development Meeting, Minneapolis, Minnesota, April 4, 1971.

Fantz, R. L. A method for studying early visual development. *Perceptual and Motor Skills*, 1956, *6*, 13–15.

Fantz, R. L. Pattern vision in young infants. *Psychological Record*, 1958, *8*, 43–47.

Fantz, R. L. Pattern vision in newborn infants. *Science*, 1963, *140*, 296–297.

Fantz, R. L. Visual perception from birth as shown by pattern selectivity. In H. E. Whipple (Ed.), New issues in infant development. *Annals of N.Y. Academy of Science*, 1965, *118*, 793–814. (a)

Fantz, R. L. Ontogeny of perception. In A. M. Schrier, H. F. Harlow, & F. Stollnitz (Eds.), *Behavior of nonhuman primates*. Vol. 1. New York: Academic Press, 1965. Pp. 365–403. (b)

Fantz, R. L. Pattern discrimination and selective attention as determinants of perceptual development from birth. In A. H. Kidd, & J. F. Rivoire (Eds.), *Perceptual development in children*. New York: International Universities Press, 1966. Pp. 143–173.

Fantz, R. L. Visual perception and experience in early infancy: A look at the hidden side of behavior development. In H. W. Stevenson, E. H. Hess, & H. Rheingold (Eds.), *Early behavior: Comparative and developmental approaches*. New York: Wiley, 1967. Pp. 181–224.

Fantz, R. L. Visual perception and experience in infancy: Issues and approaches. In F. A. Young, & D. B. Lindsley (Eds.), *Early experience and visual information processing in perceptual and reading disorders*. Washington, D. C.: National Academy of Sciences, 1970. Pp. 351–381.

Fantz, R. L. Visual preferences as a function of age, gestation, and specified variations in form, in preparation. (a)

Fantz, R. L. Visual acuity tests of infants as related to pattern preferences and gestation, in preparation. (b)

Fantz, R. L., & Fagan, J. F. Visual attention to size and number of pattern details by term and preterm infants during the first six months. *Child Development,* 1975, *16,* 3–18.

Fantz, R. L., & Miranda, S. B. Newborn infant attention to form of contour. *Child Development,* 1975, *46,* 224–228.

Fantz, R. L., & Miranda, S. B. Longitudinal development of visual selectivity and perception in Down's Syndrome and normal infants, in preparation.

Fantz, R. L., & Nevis, S. Pattern preferences and perceptual-cognitive development in early infancy. *Merrill-Palmer Quarterly,* 1967, *13,* 77–108. (a)

Fantz, R. L., & Nevis, S. The predictive value of changes in visual preferences in early infancy. In J. Hellmuth (Ed.), *The exceptional infant.* Vol. 1. Seattle: Straub & Hellmuth, 1967. Pp. 351–413. (b)

Fantz, R. L., Ordy, J. M., & Udelf, M. S. Maturation of pattern vision in infants during the first six months. *Journal of Comparative and Physiological Psychology,* 1962, *55,* 907–917.

Fantz, R. L., & Sockel, I. Apparatus and mobile laboratory for visual preference and other experiments with young infants, in preparation.

Gibson, E. J. *The senses considered as perceptual systems.* Boston: Houghton Mifflin, 1966.

Gibson, E. J. *Principles of perceptual learning and development.* New York: Appleton, 1969.

Graham, C. H. (Ed.) *Vision and visual perception.* New York: Wiley, 1965.

Greenberg, D. J. Accelerating visual complexity levels in the human infant. *Child Development,* 1971, *42,* 905–918.

Greenberg, D. J., & O'Donnell, W. J. Infancy and the optimal level of stimulation. *Child Development,* 1972, *43,* 639–645.

Greenberg, D. J., & Weizmann, F. The measurement of visual attention in infants. *Journal of Experimental Child Psychology,* 1971, *11,* 234–243.

Harter, M. R., & Suitt, C. D. Visually-evoked cortical responses and pattern vision in the infant: A longitudinal study. *Psychonomic Science,* 1970, *18,* 235–237.

Hershenson, M. Visual discrimination in the human newborn. *Journal of Comparative and Physiological Psychology,* 1964, *58,* 270–276.

Hershenson, M. Development of the perception of form. *Psychological Bulletin,* 1967, *67,* 326–336.

Hershenson, M., Kessen, W., & Munsinger, H. Pattern perception in the human newborn. In W. Wathen-Dunn (Ed.), *Models for perception of speech and visual form.* Cambridge, Massachusetts: MIT Press, 1967. Pp. 282–289.

Hershenson, M., Munsinger, H., & Kessen, W. Preferences for shapes of intermediate variability in the newborn human. *Science,* 1965, *147,* 630–631.

Hubel, D. H., & Wiesel, T. N. Receptive fields of cells in striate cortex of very young, visually inexperienced kittens. *Journal of Neurophysiology,* 1963, *26,* 994–1002.

Hubel, D. H., & Wiesel, T. N. Receptive fields and functional architecture in two nonstriate visual areas (18 and 19) of the cat. *Journal of Neurophysiology,* 1965, *28,* 229–289.

Hubel, D. H., & Wiesel, T. N. Receptive fields and functional architecture of monkey striate cortex. *Journal of Physiology,* 1968, *195,* 215–243.

Karmel, B. Z. Complexity, amount of contour and visually dependent behavior in hooded rats, domestic chicks, and human infants. *Journal of Comparative and Physiological Psychology*, 1969, *69*, 649–657. (a)

Karmel, B. Z. The effect of age, complexity, and amount of contour on pattern preferences in human infants. *Journal of Experimental Child Psychology*, 1969, 7, 339–354. (b)

Karmel, B. Z. Contour effects and pattern preferences in infants: A reply to Greenberg and O'Donnell (1972). *Child Development*, 1974, *45*, 196–199.

Karmel, B. Z., Hoffman, R. F., & Fegy, M. J. Processing of contour information by human infants evidenced by pattern-dependent evoked potentials. *Child Development*, 1974, *45*, 39–48.

Kessen, W., Haith, M. M., & Salapatek, P. H. Infancy. In P. H. Mussen (Ed.), *Carmichael's manual of child psychology*. (3rd ed.) New York: Wiley, 1970.

Kluver, H. *Behavior mechanisms in monkeys*. Chicago: Univ. of Chicago Press, 1933.

McCall, R. B., & Kagan, J. Attention in the infant: Effects of complexity, contour, perimeter, and familiarity. *Child Development*, 1967, *38*, 939–952.

McCall, R. B., & Melson, W. H. Attention in infants as a function of magnitude of discrepancy and habituation rate. *Psychonomic Science*, 1969, *17*, 317–319.

McGurk, H. The role of object orientation in infant perception. *Journal of Experimental Child Psychology*, 1970, *9*, 363–373.

Miranda, S. B. Visual abilities and pattern preferences of premature infants and full-term neonates. *Journal of Experimental Child Psychology*, 1970, *10*, 189–205. (a)

Miranda, S. B. Response to novel visual stimuli by Down's Syndrome and normal infants. *Proceedings*, American Psychological Association, Miami Beach, Florida, 1970. (b)

Miranda, S. B., & Fantz, R. L. Distribution of visual attention of newborn infants among patterns varying in size and number of details. *Proceedings*, American Psychological Association, Washington, D. C., 1971.

Miranda, S. B., & Fantz, R. L. Visual preferences of Down's Syndrome and normal infants. *Child Development*, 1973, *44*, 555–561.

Miranda, S. B., & Fantz, R. L. Recognition memory in Down's Syndrome and normal infants. *Child Development*, 1974, *45*, 651–660.

Moffett, A. Stimulus complexity as a determinant of visual attention in infants. *Journal of Experimental Child Psychology*, 1969, *8*, 173–179.

Nelson, K., & Kessen, W. Visual scanning by human newborns: Responses to complete triangle, to sides only, and to corners only. *Proceedings*, American Psychological Association, Washington, D.C., 1969.

Newton, G., & Levine, S. (Eds.) *Early experience and behavior*. Springfield, Illinois: Thomas, 1968.

Riggs, L. A. Visual acuity. In C. H. Graham (Ed.), *Vision and Visual Perception*. New York: Wiley, 1965. Pp. 321–349.

Ruff, H. A., & Birch, H. G. Infant visual fixation: the effect of concentricity, curvilinearity, and number of directions. *Journal of Experimental Psychology*, 1974, *17*, 460–473.

Salapatek, P. H. Visual scanning of geometric figures by the human newborn. *Journal of Comparative and Physiological Psychology*, 1968, *66*, 247–258.

Salapatek, P. H. The investigation of geometric pattern by the one and two month old infant. Paper presented at AAAS meeting, Boston, Massachusetts, December 1969.

Salapatek, P. H., & Kessen, W. Visual scanning of triangles by the human newborn. *Journal of Experimental Child Psychology*, 1966, *3*, 113–122.

Spears, W. C. Assessment of visual preference and discrimination in the four-month old infant. *Journal of Comparative and Physiological Psychology*, 1964, *57*, 381–386.

Spears, W. C. Visual preference in the four-month old infant. *Psychonomic Science*, 1966, *4*, 237–238.

Stechler, G. Newborn attention as affected by medication during labor. *Science*, 1964, *144*, 315–317.

Stirnimann, F. Über das Forbenempfinden Neugeborener. *Annales Paediatrici*, 1944, *163*, 1–25.

Young, F. A., & Lindsley, D. B. (Eds.) *Early experience and visual information processing in perceptual and reading disorders.* Washington, D. C.: National Academy of Sciences, 1970.

chapter 5: Infant Visual Memory[1]

LESLIE B. COHEN
University of Illinois

ERIC R. GELBER
University of Arizona

I. INTRODUCTION

The study of memory, and infant memory is no exception, involves much more than the examination of the nature of the memory trace. It also must take into account attention, perception, encoding and retrieval processes, as well as information on the structure of the storage mechanism itself. In fact, memory cannot be isolated from the entire set of mechanisms and events through which the organism processes information; that is, memory must be viewed within the context of an entire cognitive system. This same point has been made by others in reference to adult memory models. Reitman (1970), for example, concludes that "Memory behavior does not depend solely upon a memory subsystem; it reflects the activity of the human cognitive system as a whole. In this view simple models are of limited use as aids to a general understanding of memory [p. 490]." Understanding the ontogeny of

[1] Preparation of this chapter and much of the research conducted by the authors was supported in part by research grant HD 03858 to L. B. Cohen from the National Institute of Child Health and Human Development.

memory may be even more complex, since the cognitive systems involved are themselves undergoing qualitative changes which might be reflected in the organization and processes of memory. Recent data bearing on this point provide rather startling evidence that children's recall of seriated arrays may actually improve over time, presumably because the memory code evolves so as to become consistent with the child's current, more advanced operational level of functioning (Piaget & Inhelder, 1973).

The adult memory literature, with its emphasis on verbal aspects of memory, is of limited value to one interested in infant memory. For example, how could the study of infant memory be elucidated by models which rely on such processes as rehearsal strategies, scanning and search operations, naming processes, verbal encoding, decision processes, and intentional forgetting? What, if any, are the infant memory counterparts of the above processes?

The emphasis on verbal aspects of adult memory is no doubt due to the great difficulty of obtaining reliable and valid data on nonverbal features of memory from organisms with a highly developed and efficient verbal system. It is extremely difficult to avoid the confounding effect of the verbal system even in studies which use "meaningless" visual stimuli (e.g., Glanzer & Clark, 1962). Just as nonverbal memory is complicated by the presence of a powerful linguistic system, the study of verbal memory is similarly affected by other nonverbal systems as evidenced, for example, by the observed facilitating effects of imaginal mnemonics (e.g., Paivio, 1969). The point is, then, that any model of adult human memory is incomplete to the extent that the interaction between verbal and nonverbal memory is ignored.

There are, however, many issues and distinctions referred to in the adult memory literature that are relevant to the study of the ontogeny of memory. Interesting questions can certainly be posed regarding those characteristics which infant and adult memory systems have in common, and regarding the development of those characteristics which differentiate adult and infant memory function. After all, although one might expect numerous qualitative and quantitative differences in the nature of infant and adult memory, an account of the sequence of events by which those differences are eventually overcome is an ultimate goal of a developmental theory.

One of the major issues in the memory literature concerns the number of different types of memory storage. Is there only one storage system in which traces are set down and, through repetition, gradually increase in strength? Or, on the other hand, are there two (or more) separate storage locations—a limited capacity short-term memory in which items are held for only brief periods of time, and a high-capacity long-term memory in which items are complexly coded thereby greatly reducing information loss due to forgetting or retrieval failure? Related questions pertain to whether or not repetitions produce increments in memory strength by adding to the clarity of existing traces or by increasing the quantity of equal strength traces. While these questions are yet to be resolved in the adult literature, they have received little or no attention in the infancy literature. Does the infant come equipped with the same storage structures as the adult? Do infants have long-term memory? Surely they are capable of recognizing stimuli after long intervals (as will be discussed later); however, most conceptualizations of long-term memory contend that information is transferred into this store only after the original perceptual code is transformed into an essentially verbal code by some kind of labeling process. Does this imply completely different long-term memory systems in the infant and adult?

Another major distinction to be found in memory research is that between recall and recognition memory. There is still some controversy as to whether recall and recognition are measures of the same or of different memory systems. The literature on adult memory, in addition to dealing primarily with verbal stimuli, has been concerned mainly with recall memory. The limited investigations of infant memory, on the other hand, have used procedures which are analogous to those used for assessing recognition memory. This state of affairs is primarily due to obvious methodological difficulties in working with organisms with limited overt response repertoires, but it also represents a major departure between adult memory models and data on infant retention. Questions about the origins and development of recall have, therefore, received little attention, although one might consider differential response production in operant paradigms as instances of motor recall.

II. QUALITATIVE CHANGES IN MEMORY DEVELOPMENT

An issue raised in relation to all areas of cognitive development is whether or not developmental changes represent qualitative shifts, changes in kind, or whether they merely represent quantitative differences, changes in the degree to which a certain cognitive mode of functioning is represented in behavior. In this regard, Bruner (1964) has postulated three representational modes, or ways of constructing models of one's environment, which are said to be acquired in a fixed developmental order. Each successive mode represents a qualitative change in the primary way in which the child processes information. The first of these cognitive styles is referred to as *enactive representation;* past events are represented in terms of the motor responses appropriate to them. The second mode, *iconic representation,* is most closely linked to what is referred to as image or perceptual memory. The final stage is marked by the onset of *symbolic representation,* and is of less relevance to infant memory since it deals primarily with ways in which information is represented in terms of the verbal system. These three modes of representation do not merely replace one another, but rather enhance and are integrated with one another to form an efficient information processing system.

There is little direct experimental evidence with infants to support Bruner's developmental sequence. Corsini (1971) reports pilot data with 4-year-olds that are consistent with the claim that young children are more likely to utilize enactive encoding than iconic encoding when a choice is available. The task was a discrimination problem in which position and picture cues were both relevant and redundant. A transfer task was then presented in which the child was given a choice of responses, one of which would indicate that the child had been performing on the basis of position (enactive) cues while the other would indicate responding on the basis of picture (iconic) cues. The results revealed a preference for the enactive over the iconic mode of representation. Devising an analogous task for testing infants would seem to be feasible, and, from Bruner's developmental sequence, one would expect the enactive mode to be extremely strong.

Bruner's postulated sequence is very reminiscent of Piaget's theory of intellectual development. Piaget's period covering the months of infancy, the sensorimotor period, begins with the child's representing his world in terms of the actions which he performs upon objects, and ends when the child is first capable of symbolic thought. A relevant concept, and one that might be considered an initial focal point for those interested in infant memory, is what Piaget refers to as recognitory assimilation (Piaget, 1952). Upon encountering a familiar object, the infant who has reached the stage of secondary circular reactions will make certain movements that are abbreviations, or outlines, of the responses which the infant has made to the object in the past. "Everything takes place as though the child were satisfied to recognize these objects or sights and to make a note of this recognition, but could not recognize them except by working, rather than thinking, the schema helpful to recognition [Piaget, 1952, p. 185]." Whether or not the validity of the concept of recognitory assimilation holds up under empirical test, the observations and hypotheses of Piaget and Bruner suggest that a major focus of infant memory study should be on motor performance and motor skills. Given the limited evidence and observations which suggest that the infant does process information and represent his environment in terms of his overt motor responses, additional research in this domain would be expected to be quite fruitful (see Volume II, Chapter 3 by Gratch, on object permanence tasks.)

An additional area of research that has some bearing on infant enactive memory, although not usually conceived of in those terms, is infant operant conditioning. Several recent reviews of the infant learning literature (e.g., Reese & Lipsitt, 1970) indicate that very young infants can be operantly conditioned. In these tasks, reinforcing a particular response on early trials usually increases the infant's tendency to repeat that response on later trials. While some information from the earlier trials must carry over (i.e., be remembered) to influence performance on later trials, it is not at all obvious what that information is. Whatever is stored, though, must include some information about the appropriate response and therefore may be an instance of enactive memory.

Although there is evidence for enactive memory at an early age, there is also evidence that the very young infant is capable of storing perceptual information or using iconic memory. Infants as young as 2 months of age (Fantz, 1964; Wetherford & Cohen, 1973) and perhaps even newborns (Friedman, 1972) will decrease their attention or habituate when the same visual pattern is repeatedly presented and will attend longer to a novel than to a familiar pattern. Since the main difference in behavior toward the novel and familiar stimuli is in the duration of a response rather than the form of the response, one would have difficulty arguing that the infant was storing the information motorically rather than perceptually. In fact, as will be discussed later in this chapter, the assumption of a perceptual storage mechanism in young infants becomes a valuable tool for explanations of infant visual attention and recognition memory.

While present evidence seems to indicate that in the first few months of life the infant is capable of both enactive and iconic representation, these primitive storage mechanisms are not necessarily fully developed at birth. However, rather than assuming as Bruner does that enactive and iconic storage represent different developmental stages, it would seem more fruitful to assume that both systems are present early in life and both become more precise or sophisticated as the infant becomes older. The research task then becomes one of designing experiments to assess the encoding, storage, and retrieval properties of each system as well as how these properties change developmentally.

Instead of assuming a qualitative developmental shift from enactive to iconic memory, one could argue that the more important shift is from independent enactive and iconic systems to an integration of the two. Evidence is scanty on this point, but Cohen (1973) reported a series of experiments in which 4-month-old male infants quickly habituated to a repetitive pattern but did not easily learn to turn their heads to the pattern. Four-month-old girls, on the other hand, habituated very little but did learn to turn more rapidly or slowly depending upon the pattern's attractiveness. Although the reasons for these sex differences are unclear, Cohen has hypothesized that males were storing information about the physical characteristics of the pattern (i.e., iconic information) while females were storing more about the response (i.e., enactive information), or the contingency between response and reinforcement. It certainly would be unreasonable to conclude from these results that 4-month-old males have iconic and 4-month-old females have enactive memory. However, the data are consistent with the notion that in the particular type of habituation task used by Cohen, some infants store more iconic and others more enactive information.

While one can relatively easily demonstrate operant conditioning or habituation in 2- to 4-month-old infants, discrimination learning appears to be a more difficult task. One reason may be that such a task requires retention and integration of information about both the nature of the stimuli and the appropriate response.

One study suggesting this integration between iconic and enactive representation has been reported by Gelber (1972b). In the first phase of the experiment 4-month-old infants were repeatedly shown two simple geometric patterns. In the second phase either these same patterns or two new ones were used as positive and negative stimuli in a two-choice simultaneous discrimination problem. If the infant looked at the positive stimulus it remained on and a light blinked on and off for 5 sec. If the infant looked at the negative stimulus, it went off and no stimulation occurred for 5 sec. In general Gelber found that males habituated more than females in the first phase of the experiment, and females learned more than males in the second.

This result is similar to the one reported earlier by Cohen, namely that in a habituation task males habituated more (and presumably stored more iconic information) while females learned to turn their heads and eyes toward the source of stimulation (and presumably stored more enactive information). One important difference between the Cohen and Gelber tasks, however, is that the latter involved making a discrimination while the former did not. If learning a discrimination requires both iconic and enactive representation, then only those subjects capable of both should be able to solve it. Support for this hypothesis comes from Gelber's additional finding that females who had previously shown habituation were more likely to learn the discrimination. For females a significant correlation of +.65 was found between percent habituation and number of correct responses. For males, however, the correlation was only +.06. Although most males habituated, few, if any, learned the discrimination. What this pattern of results suggest is that most 4-month-old females are capable of storing enactive information and those also able to store iconic information can solve a discrimination. On the other hand, 4-month-old males seem to be more likely to store iconic but not enactive information, and hence are less likely to learn a discrimination problem. Admittedly, this hypothesis of a shift from separate to integrated memory systems is still very tenuous. A careful study is needed that independently assesses iconic and enactive memory in each infant and then examines performance on a discrimination problem to see if those who store both are the ones that learn. The few studies available at this time are promising enough to warrant such future research.

III. BEHAVIORS IMPLYING INFANT MEMORY

Much of an infant's behavior indicates that he can remember, and many investigations of infant development involve tasks that require some type of memory for solution. Imitation, object permanence, attachment, conditioning, and preference for novel stimuli all imply the infant is remembering something, but what it is that is stored, how long it is stored, or whether it is recognized or recalled are questions not usually asked.

In order for an infant to imitate the behavior of a model, some information about the model's actions or the stimulation produced by those actions must have been stored by the infant. Obviously, the infant's imitative response does not match the model's behavior exactly. For example, when a mother speaks to her infant, he may attempt to reproduce the phonemic and intonation pattern he has just heard but will probably not reproduce the fundamental frequency of his mother's voice. However, if she lowers her voice noticeably the infant is likely to lower his voice also. Certainly no explanation of infant imitation is complete without an analysis of how the infant selects from and interprets the multitude of information provided by the model. Imitation is usually defined as making the same response as a model, but the meaning of "same" is rarely examined. Yet, that is, perhaps, the most intriguing issue for one interested in the development of perception, information processing, or memory.

Object permanence tasks also require some memory on the part of the infant. When the infant finds a toy which has just been hidden under one of several cloths, he must be remembering something about the location of the toy, the type of cloth under which it was hidden, or both. Several chapters in these volumes discuss object permanence, and the one by Gratch (Chapter 3, Volume II) in particular includes a few studies on the role of memory. Nevertheless, very little is currently known about how the developing memory ability of the child influences his performance on object permanence tasks. One interesting line for further inquiry might be based upon Piaget's (Piaget & Inhelder, 1973) distinction between recognition, reconstruction, and recall. For example, when an infant retrieves an object which is partially covered, is he simply recognizing the visible part or reconstructing the whole object from the portion he can see? This should be a relatively simple question to investigate. One could partially hide some object such as a doll leaving only its legs exposed. The experiment could be arranged so that on some trials the infant would be able to retrieve the whole doll while on other trials he would be able to retrieve only the legs. Any show of surprise [using Charlesworth's (1969) procedure, for example] when only the legs were obtained, but not when the whole figure was obtained, would provide evidence for reconstruction.

A third area indicating memory is infant attachment. Whether one is considering positive responses to the appearance of a familiar person such as a parent, or negative responses to the appearance of a stranger, some sort of recognition memory is involved. Obviously the parent and stranger may differ in many respects, but to the extent that familiarity is an important factor, so also, by definition, is memory. Chapter 4 by Lewis and Brooks, in Volume II, considers the role of familiarity in some detail so an extensive discussion will not be given here. However, it should be stated that important advances are beginning to be made in infant recognition memory using habituation and novelty preference procedures that could have a direct bearing on our understanding of the development of attachment.

The growing body of literature demonstrating classical and instrumental conditioning with preverbal children can also be viewed as a source of data on infant memory. What follows is a brief discussion of the kinds of memory implied in successful learning procedures and some of the variations in the learning paradigms that should have implications for a theory of infant memory.

In classical conditioning, the eliciting power of an unconditioned stimulus is transferred to a previously neutral stimulus through the systematic pairing of the two stimuli. While it is unclear whether the organism remembers anything of either the unconditioned stimulus or the unconditioned response, the conditioned stimulus must in some way be recognized; that is, it must be perceived as familiar in the context of the conditioning procedure. The demonstration of classical conditioning requires that the conditioned response be shown only to the conditioned stimulus (or to other very similar stimuli) and not to dissimilar, unpaired stimuli. Otherwise such factors as sensitization can not be ruled out as responsible for the conditioned response.

Variations in the nature of conditioned stimuli, then, would be a useful source of information about the kinds of stimuli which the infant is capable of processing. One interesting finding pertaining to this point that has come out of the classical conditioning literature is that apparently infants as young as 26 days are capable of storing temporal information (Fitzgerald, Lintz, Brackbill, & Adams, 1967). A conditioned stimulus consisting of only a 20-sec time interval was used. The time interval alone was found to be as effective as the interval plus an auditory stimulus, and both of these conditioned stimuli were found to be more effective in eliciting the conditioned response than an auditory stimulus presented with a variable intertrial interval.

Examining stimulus generalization within the classical conditioning paradigm can also provide data regarding the nature of information storage. By comparing differences between those stimuli to which the conditioned response generalizes and those to which there is no generalization, one can determine which stimulus features the infant had been attending to and storing.

In a typical operant conditioning paradigm an appropriate response emitted in the presence of a discriminative stimulus is reinforced, thereby increasing the probability that the response will occur subsequently in that situation. Watson (1967) has presented a detailed discussion of the relationship between infant memory and instrumental learning. Since his is the most thorough coverage to date on the topic, it will be worthwhile to discuss the points made in his paper in some detail.

Watson hypothesized that "the reinforcement of a response can be expected to increase the relative probability of emission of that response only if the infant's next response occurs within a period of time during which he is able to remember the preceding response-reward contingency [p. 56]." In the studies reported, 9- to 14-week-old infants were presented either an auditory or visual stimulus contingent on head turns to a predesignated side. The data were analyzed to determine the probability that the response following a reinforced response would be a repetition (i.e., that it would be another turn to the reinforced side). Probabilities were determined for each of several intervals following the previous response. It was predicted that immediately after the reinforced response, the probability of repeating that response would not differ from the probability of repetition during baseline. This followed from the assumption that the contingency itself takes time to be analyzed; responses occurring before the analysis is complete cannot have utilized the contingency information, and thus, should show no increment in repetition probability. Once the contingency has been analyzed, Watson predicted a sharp increase in the probability of repeating the reinforced response. This probability then steadily drops toward baseline as the time interval since the last reinforced response increases and as memory for the contingency decays. The data did resemble the predicted function, showing that responses occurring 5 sec after reinforcement were more likely to be repetitions of the reinforced response than were responses occurring either less than or more than 5 sec after reinforcement delivery. Thus, it was concluded that the memory span of the infants was about 5 sec in duration. Of course, as was noted by the author, the particular estimate of memory span obtained is no doubt greatly influenced by the particular experimental conditions used. For example, the nature of the reinforcing stimulus (its intensity, complexity, etc.) might be expected to affect the memory span value obtained.

In order for an infant to repeat a reinforced response, something must be remembered. This memory could include information about the response, about the nature and location of the reward, or about the contingency between them. It remains unclear from Watson's data exactly what the proposed 5-sec memory span refers to. Although Watson implies that it is the memory for the contingency itself which is first built up and then forgotten, it seems possible that it might be either the motor memory or information about the reward which dissipates. For example, an infant might store the contingency that to look left will produce a red circle, but 5 sec later not remember that the response was turning left. By the same token, after 5 sec he might still remember to look left, but not that the response will lead to the red circle, or even that it will result in something interesting to look at.

One test for whether the infant actually stores specific information about the contingent stimulus might be to compare performance curves for infants who receive the same stimulus on each trial versus those who are shown different but equally reinforcing stimuli on each trial. If information is stored about the properties of the stimulus, the group with only one reinforcing stimulus might show a more rapid extinction of responding because of the reduced reinforcing effect of familiar as compared to novel stimuli. Using a paradigm analogous to the one just described, Caron, Caron, and Caldwell (1971) obtained data suggesting that infants were storing information about the forms, but not necessarily the colors, of contingent stimuli. Other data reported by Cohen (1973) and by DeLoache, Wetherford, and Cohen (1972) also suggest infants store information about the nature of the reinforcing stimulus. In general, however, an operant conditioning procedure is so complex, one has difficulty isolating just what the infant is remembering. Other procedures, described in the next section, appear to be more efficient techniques for the investigation of infant visual information processing and memory.

IV. PAIRED-COMPARISON VERSUS HABITUATION PARADIGMS

Although an understanding of infant behavior in situations as diverse as those involving imitation, object permanence, attachment, or conditioning all seem to require an understanding of infant memory, these situations may not be most suited to examine information processing and memory in infants. The situations are all rather complex. Some involve social interaction, others the presentation of several stimuli and the production of several responses. In some it is difficult to tell whether recognition or recall is involved, while in others it is unclear whether the infant is remembering a stimulus event, a location, or a response. A more practical approach at this early stage of our knowledge would be to employ tasks specifically designed to assess the development of memory and then try to apply what has been learned to these other more complex situations.

A start has been made in the case of infant pattern recognition. We know a great deal more now than we did just 3 or 4 years ago. Most of the studies make one basic assumption: If an infant's response to a familiar pattern is different from its response to a novel pattern, he is remembering something about the familiar one. By systematically varying the similarity between novel and familiar stimuli, one can discover what the infant is remembering; by varying the time from the end of familiarization to the test with novel and familiar stimuli, one can discover how long the infant will remember; and by comparing different ages, sexes, and populations, one can discover developmental and individual differences in memory ability.

Two experimental paradigms have typically been employed to study infant pattern recognition. In one, a paired-comparison procedure is used in which infants are repeatedly exposed to two patterns simultaneously. One pattern is usually to the left, the other to the right of some central point. After a number of familiarization trials in which the same pattern is presented on both sides, two test trials are presented, one with the familiar stimulus on the left and a novel one on the right, and one in which the position of familiar and novel stimuli is reversed. The percentage of time the infant looks at the novel stimulus during the test is taken as a measure of retention.

The second paradigm involves repeated presentations of a single pattern either for a fixed number of trials or until the infant's fixation time habituates. The pattern may be presented either centrally or off to one side. Test trials follow in which novel and familiar patterns are successively presented. A difference in fixation time to these stimuli is considered a measure of retention.

Each paradigm has certain advantages and disadvantages. As

Fagan (1974) has recently pointed out, the paired-comparison procedure can indicate recognition in 5- to 6-month-old infants in a much shorter time than is required to produce habituation. His evidence was based upon the finding that with certain multidimensional patterns, one 5-sec exposure was sufficient to produce a difference in fixation time to novel and familiar stimuli. In defense of the habituation procedure, however, two comments may be made: First it is quite possible (Wetherford & Cohen, 1973) occasionally to substitute a novel stimulus for a familiar one during the familiarization phase of a habituation experiment without disrupting the course of habituation itself. In this way, one can determine just when the preference for novelty begins to appear and how closely it is tied to habituation. Second, some studies of infant habituation have used a criterion, such as less than 3 sec of fixation (McCall, 1972) or less than half of the initial fixation time (DeLoache, 1973), rather than a constant number of trials. Using this procedure it has been found that many infants habituate very rapidly in only a few trials. While a long familiarization period is unnecessary to assess recognition in most infants, it may not be unnecessary for all of them. Presenting the novel stimulus at that point in time when each infant reaches his own habituation criterion might produce the most reliable measure of the infant's ability to discriminate novel from familiar stimuli.

Another possible advantage of the paired-comparison procedure is that it may be more sensitive to subtle pattern differences. Since both novel and familiar patterns are presented simultaneously, the infant can look back and forth and compare the two patterns directly. In the habituation procedure the comparison must be between what is currently being presented and what was seen in the past. In some cases, however, simultaneous presentation of novel and familiar patterns may have its disadvantages. Most infants tend to turn more and look longer to the right than to the left (Cohen, 1972). Therefore, in a paired-comparison procedure in order to counteract this right-turn bias, two test trials must be given, one with the novel stimulus on the right and one with it on the left. In most experiments the novel stimulus is changed on each test trial, while the familiar one remains the same. This means that in the test alone each infant is exposed to the familiar pattern twice as long as he is to each novel one. Any difference in responding to novel and familiar stimuli might not be due to transfer from an earlier familiarization period, but from the longer exposure to the familiar stimulus in the test. The difficulty could easily be overcome, however, either by using the same novel stimulus on both test trials, or by using a between subject design and counterbalancing the left–right position of the novel stimulus on only one test trial.

In some cases the investigator is more interested in changes in infant fixation as a stimulus becomes more familiar than he is in preferences for novel over familiar stimuli. For example, optimal level theories such as those proposed by Hunt (1965), Berlyne (1963), and McCall and Kagan (1967) predict that as a stimulus loses its novelty an infant's fixation to it should first increase and then subside. As will be seen in a later section of this chapter, evidence for this optimal level prediction is somewhat conflicting. However, if one wishes to test for it, the paradigm of choice would be the habituation or successive presentation method. Although in the paired-comparison paradigm one can determine the percent of time an infant attends to a familiar pattern, it is difficult to tell to what extent changes in percent reflect an increasing interest in novel stimuli and to what extent they reflect a decreasing interest in familiar stimuli.

The habituation paradigm is not without difficulties. One major concern is that when an infant decreases his attention to a pattern is he doing so because the pattern is becoming more familiar or because he is just becoming fatigued in the testing situation? Discussions of the various types of fatigue have been given elsewhere (Jeffrey & Cohen, 1971; Cohen, 1973) and so will not be covered here. It is sufficient to note that if, following a decrease in responding, the infant increases his response to a novel stimulus, fatigue can usually be ruled out.

A more recent problem has arisen with the use of a criterion for habituation, i.e., repeatedly presenting the stimulus until all subjects reach the same criterion response level rather than presenting it for a fixed number of trials. When the criterion is reached, one must be certain the infant has reliably reduced his response and has not just responded less by chance. One way of distinguishing a chance reduction in attention from actual habituation is to continue giving the familiar stimulus to some subjects, while changing the stimulus for others (e.g., DeLoache, 1973). If the response to the familiar stimulus remains low, while the response to the novel one is high, neither a chance reduction nor fatigue can account for the decrease. A second procedure which accomplishes the same goal, but requires fewer subjects is to continue giving all subjects the familiar stimulus for a few trials beyond criterion and then to switch to a novel stimulus. Again, a difference in attention to novel and familiar stimuli would rule out an accidental decrease or fatigue and would be evidence of habituation.

Use of a criterion allows another innovation for investigating habituation, namely backward habituation curves. The argument for using a backward habituation curve is equivalent to the one for using a backward learning curve. Group learning curves do not always reflect the acquisition rate for individual subjects. In retardate discrimination learning, for example, Zeaman and House (1963) have shown that even though a group curve may indicate a gradual increase in performance, once individual subjects begin to learn, they actually solve the problem very rapidly. The gradual slope of the group curve results from individual differences in number of trials before improvement begins, rather than rate of improvement during acquisition. Zeaman and House obtained a more accurate reflection of acquisition rate by constructing backward learning curves, that is, by equating subjects at the point when they reached criterion and then plotting performance on the preceding trials backward from that point.

The typical forward habituation curve also indicates a gradual change in performance over trials, only in this case the change is a decrease rather than an increase. An example of one such curve is given in Figure 5.1. In this particular experiment (reported by Cohen, 1973) 36 infants 4 months old were shown 16 repetitions of a checkerboard pattern. Each infant was allowed one look at the checkerboard on each trial, but that look could be as long as the infant wished. Data from this study were reanalyzed using a criterion measure of habituation. The criterion was three successive trials during which the average fixation time was less than one-half the fixation time on the first three trials. Twenty-four of the 36 subjects reached that criterion, and it is their performance which is shown in Figure 5.1. As can be seen from the figure, infant fixation time gradually drops over the first four or five trials from an initial level of about 7.5 sec to a final one of about 3 sec, and then, although subsequent fixations are somewhat variable, that low level is maintained for the remaining trials. The same data are plotted backward in Figure 5.2. This time the subjects' performances are equated for trials -1, -2, and -3; the trials on which they reached criterion. Since some infants take longer than others to reach criterion, the number of scores making up each point on the graph both before and after criterion varies somewhat, but at least one-half of the subjects are represented at each point. One gets a very different impression of what is going on during habituation

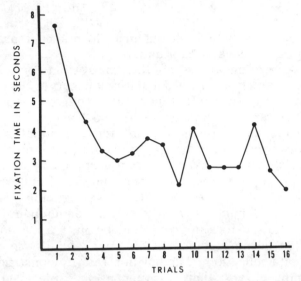

Figure 5.1   A typical forward habitation curve showing a gradual decrease in fixation time over trials. Stimulation in this experiment consisted of repeated presentations of the same checkerboard pattern.

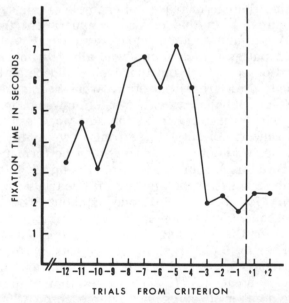

Figure 5.2   A backward habituation curve plotted from the same data as in Figure 5.1. Subjects are equated on trials −1, −2, and −3, the ones on which they reach criterion.

from Figures 5.1 and 5.2. It appears from Figure 5.1 that the infants look at a pattern longest on the first trial, and that they gradually decrease their fixation time to some asymptotic level. However, as shown in Figure 5.2, what the infants actually do is to look moderately at first, then increase their fixation time, and then abruptly, on a single trial, decrease it to a low level. The fact that looking time remains low after criterion has been reached (trials $+1$ and $+2$) indicates that the decrease was not an artifact created by the use of a criterion.

The shape of the backward habituation curve raises several theoretical issues regarding infant recognition memory. For example, from Figure 5.1, one most likely would assume that infants begin processing and storing information about the stimulus on the first trial. From Figure 5.2, however, it is not clear whether they begin storing information on the first few trials or only after their fixation time increases. The decreasing curve in Figure 5.1 would lead one to believe that the infants had a uniform preference for novelty and as the pattern became more familiar the attractiveness of it decreased. The curve in Figure 5.2, on the other hand, is more consistent with optimal level of stimulation theories which predict an inverted-U relationship between attractiveness and familiarity. Finally, most theories of infant memory and habituation assume a comparison between the pattern the infant is currently fixating and some stored representation of the pattern from prior trials. From Figure 5.1 one might assume that as the stored representation gradually becomes more accurate, the comparison becomes more similar, and fixation time decreases. The abrupt decrease in Figure 5.2 would be more consistent with a threshold, or all-or-none type of process. The stored representation may gradually increase in accuracy, but some threshold must be reached before the infant judges it to be the same as what he is currently looking at. Only after that judgment is made does the infant's attention drop.

These and other theoretical issues will be discussed in more detail later in the chapter when additional evidence from other experiments can also be considered. At this point, however, one should be aware that first, backward curves may more accurately reflect the process of habituation than the more typical forward curves, and second, that any theoretical account of infant habituation and recognition memory should attempt to explain the increase in attention to a repeated pattern as well as the subsequent decrease.

The measurement of infant attention also depends on the definition of a trial. In both traditional paired-comparison and habituation paradigms, the length of a trial is determined by the experimenter rather than by the subject. A trial is assumed to begin with the onset of stimulation and to end with the termination of stimulation. Whether a trial is 5 sec or 30 sec, the arbitrariness of this procedure presents certain difficulties. As Cohen (1973) has pointed out, estimates of fixation time depend, to some extent, on where the infant is looking when the stimulus comes on and when it goes off. If, for example, an infant happens to be inspecting his hands when the pattern is presented, he may not turn to look at the pattern at all, on that trial. The infant's fixation time would be scored as zero for that trial. That does not mean if he had looked at the pattern, his fixation time would have been minimal. He might have taken a good long look, if he had noticed there was something to look at.

On the other hand, if an infant had been looking at a pattern for, say, 2 sec when the trial ended, it would not mean that 2 sec was an accurate measure of his attraction to the pattern. He might have looked much longer had he had the opportunity to do so. A better procedure, one used by Cohen (1972) and by Horowitz, Paden, Bhana, and Self (1972), would be to begin a trial when the infant first looks at the pattern and to end the trial when he turns away.

Cohen (1972) described a new procedure that eliminated the problems associated with fixed trial lengths. Each trial began with a light blinking on and off on one side. As soon as the infant looked at the light, it went off and a pattern appeared on the other side. The infant was allowed one unlimited fixation of the pattern. As soon as he turned away, the pattern went off and the light came back on to start the next trial. Although this light-pattern procedure may be an improvement for studying habituation, it is of limited value when applied to paired-comparisons. As mentioned earlier, the main advantage of the paired-comparison paradigm is that it allows the infant to make a direct comparison of the two stimuli presented on each trial. If the infant is allowed only one look at one stimulus, he cannot make that comparison.

This section of the chapter has considered in detail several methodological and measurement issues associated with paired-comparison and habituation paradigms. What began as a simple description of these two techniques turned out to be a complex series of cautions and suggestions. Nevertheless, they are both being widely used today and both have provided valuable information on infant attention and memory. Given the current popularity of the paradigms it would be worthwhile to conduct an experiment that compares the effectiveness of the two procedures. The only investigation on this topic so far has been reported by Greenberg and Weizmann (1971). They were not examining infant memory and so did not familiarize their infants to a single pattern. Instead they were more concerned with whether simultaneous paired-comparison and successive exposure procedures produced the same or different preferences for 2 × 2, 8 × 8, and 24 × 24 checkerboards. Both 8- and 12-week-old infants were tested. In general Greenberg and Weizmann found that the two methods produced very similar results, with older infants looking longer at complex patterns than at simple ones, and females looking longer than males. The only significant effects involving method were that infants looked somewhat less at the 2 × 2 and somewhat more at the 8 × 8 and 24 × 24 stimuli when in the paired-comparison than in the successive exposure procedure, and that this difference was more true of males than of females.

Obviously the same type of study should be run on infant preferences for novelty and familiarity. Yet even without it, as we shall see in the next section, paired-comparison and habituation studies have usually yielded similar results, and either appears to be a viable technique for investigating the development of infant recognition memory.

V. PARAMETERS AFFECTING INFANT RECOGNITION

A. Temporal Parameters

One of the most basic questions about infant recognition memory is how long the infant can remember what he has seen. Is his memory for visual stimuli merely a transitory phenomenon disappearing after a few seconds, or does he have the ability similar to that of adults or older children to store visual information over long periods of time? Adults, for example, have been found to store pictorial information for as long as a year (Nickerson, 1968) and nursery school children for as long as 28 days (Brown & Scott, 1971). In the Brown and Scott experiment, the probability of 3- to 5-year-old children recognizing a twice-seen item after 28 days was still .78. Most explanations of adult memory (Norman, 1970) assume, to a greater or lesser extent, that transfer of information into long-term memory involves verbal encoding mechanisms. But if it can be shown that infants under 6 months of age are also capable of storing pictorial materials over days, weeks, or even months, the necessity of these mechanisms for long-term recognition would appear less persuasive.

A demonstration of long-term recognition in infants would also refute the argument that preferences for novelty are due to sensory adaptation. It could be claimed that during familiarization, the receptors stimulated by the familiar stimulus adapt. Those stimulated by the novel stimulus would not have adapted, and this difference in receptor sensitivity could result in longer fixations to novel stimuli. If, however, a substantial delay occurred between the end of familiarization and the test for novelty preferences, the adapted receptors would have had ample time to recover, and any remaining difference in fixation to novel and familiar stimuli could not be explained by sensory adaptation.

Experiments on infant habituation or preference for novelty began to appear in the 1960s; and although most had methodological shortcomings (see Jeffrey & Cohen, 1971), a few produced results suggesting delayed recognition. McCall and Kagan (1967), for instance, exposed 3-month-old infants to a standard pattern four to six times a week for a month, and then tested the infants with patterns varying in amount of discrepancy from the standard. Since the testing occurred up to 24 hr following the end of familiarization, the experiment could be considered a study of delayed recognition memory. No differences in fixation time were found, but the girls did display greater cardiac deceleration to novel than to familiar stimuli. The results must be interpreted with caution, however, because the authors did not counterbalance the stimuli presented during familiarization.

In a similar experiment (Weizmann, Cohen, & Pratt, 1971) 4-week-old infants were each given a 30-min daily exposure for 4 weeks to a stabile hanging over the bassinet. They were tested at 6 and 8 weeks with novel and familiar stabiles using the paired-comparison procedure. The test occurred anywhere from 12 to 24 hr after the previous day's familiarization. At 6 weeks the infants fixated reliably longer to the familiar stabile, and at 8 weeks, reliably longer to the novel one. Either result indicates recognition and, owing to the interval between familiarization and test, delayed recognition.

Delayed recognition was also found by Caron and Caron (1968, 1969), using a short-term rather than a long-term recognition task. Infants 3½ months old were given a total of 15 trials of 20 sec each.

Multicolored geometric patterns were shown on trials 1–4 and 10–12. On trials 5–9 the same checkerboard pattern (either a 2 × 2, 12 × 12, or 24 × 24) was repeatedly presented, and it was re-presented again on trial 13. Trials 14 and 15 consisted of abstract art photographs. Infant fixation times to the checkerboards habituated during trials 5–9 and remained low on trial 13 even though 60 sec of long fixation times to multicolored patterns had intervened. Apparently, some information about the checkerboard was retained for at least 1 min, even though the pattern had been only briefly presented.

While these early experiments provide evidence for delayed recognition, the first two systematic attempts to vary the recognition interval appeared in the same journal in 1970. In one, Pancratz and Cohen (1970) habituated 4-month-old infants to a simple, colored, geometric pattern by exposing the same pattern for 10 trials of 15-sec each, and then tested for recognition either immediately or after a delay of 5 min. The 5-min interval was filled with repeated presentations of a second stimulus, a black star. Immediate recognition was found, particularly for males. They looked significantly longer at a novel than at the familiar stimulus. Results after 5 min, however, were equivocal, with moderate fixation times to both novel and familiar stimuli.

The other experiment was reported by Fagan (1970). Using the paired-comparison paradigm he gave 4-month-olds a 2-min exposure to a rather complex black-and-white multidimensional pattern, followed by an immediate recognition test and the same test 2 hr later. Infants spent more time looking at the novel pattern in both tests, showing both immediate and delayed retention.

It seems rather curious that two experiments so much alike should produce such a difference in results, with Fagan getting evidence for delayed recognition after 2 hr and Pancratz and Cohen not getting it after 5 min. Fagan (1973) has suggested that the critical difference may be either in the type of paradigm used, habituation versus paired-comparison, or the type of stimuli presented, simple patterns versus complex ones. But, a study by Martin (1973) tends to negate both of these alternatives. In a design similar to the one described earlier by Caron and Caron, he habituated 2-, 3½-, and 5-month-old infants to a simple three-dimensional pattern such as a blue square or yellow cross and then tested for retention after intervals of 1.5 min and 24 hr. A difference in fixation to novel and familiar stimuli was found for the two older groups of subjects at both intervals.

Since delayed recognition in infants can be found by using either paradigm and with simple or complex visual stimuli the explanation for the different results in the Pancratz and Cohen and the Fagan studies must lie elsewhere. One additional possibility has to do with the nature of the stimulation to the infant during the retention interval. In Pancratz and Cohen, the infants were kept in the testing situation and repeatedly shown a second pattern, while in Fagan's study the infants were removed from the apparatus and only brought back when it was time to be retested. Perhaps exposing the infant to a second pattern, in the same setting, right after he has been familiarized to the first one, interferes with later recognition. This argument will be developed further in the next section on interference.

The research presented so far has shown that under certain conditions infants can recognize patterns up to 24 hr after originally seeing them. More recent data (Fagan, 1973) indicate retention over longer intervals. In one experiment 5-month-old infants were able to recognize multidimensional patterns after 48 hr, and in another they were able to recognize photographs of faces after a delay of 2 weeks. The paired-comparison paradigm was used in both experiments including the two-trial test procedure which has been criticized earlier in this chapter for providing differential exposure to novel and familiar stimuli. This argument was countered effectively, however, by Fagan's (1973) report that in both experiments infants preferred the novel stimulus on the first test trial just as much as they did on the second test trial.

In summary, the evidence to date strongly supports the contention that infants can remember visual information over an extended period of time. As early as 6 or 8 weeks of age a long-term exposure will produce recognition 24 hr later, and as early as 4 or 5 months of age an exposure as short as 1 or 2 min will lead to recognition 2 weeks later. The results clearly imply some type of long-term perceptual memory in young infants. But an understanding of this memory system requires information not only on how long an infant can remember, but also on how his memory can be disrupted. That is the topic covered in the next section.

B.   Interference Effects

A persistent question in the memory literature is whether retrieval failure is caused by a decay of memory traces or by interfering effects resulting from the processing of extraneous stimuli prior to the retention test. Evidence of long-term recognition suggests the trace does not decay, at least within 2 weeks, but the possibility of interference still exists. If one were to find similar interference phenomena in infants as well as in adults, the claim that analogous memory processes were involved would be strengthened.

Gelber (1972a) examined interference in infant memory using a procedure which involved habituation and recovery of visual fixation. By presenting 1, 2, 4, or 8 intervening stimuli for either 10 or 20 sec, both the length of the recovery interval and the number of stimuli occurring in the interval were independently varied following habituation to a simple visual pattern. The purpose of the experiment was to determine whether recovery (forgetting) was a function of the passage of time (trace decay) or a function of the number of intervening stimuli (retroactive interference). A significant overall preference for the novel stimuli was found in the test phase, but this preference did not significantly decline over the range of interval lengths or number of intervening stimuli used in the study.

Gelber has assumed that the greater the number of intervening stimuli, the greater the interference. However, in its present form, the assumption is not supported by the evidence. Other habituation experiments mentioned previously by Caron and Caron (1968, 1969) and by Martin (1973) also found no evidence of interference even though the retention intervals were filled with novel, changing patterns. On the other hand, it will be remembered that Pancratz and Cohen (1970) obtained ambiguous results when a single novel pattern filled the interval.

An additional study by DeLoache (1973) sheds further light on this point. Her 4-month-old infants were habituated to a pattern with four geometric shapes each of a different color on a black background. Since the light-pattern procedure was used, infants could take one look on each trial. The criterion for habituation was three successive looks equaling less than one-half the first three looks. Following habituation, infants were randomly assigned to one of three groups for the second phase of the study. The High Discrepancy group was given repeated presentations of a new pattern with four new shapes and colors. The Medium Discrepancy group was given an intermediate pattern containing two old and two new shapes and colors, and the Zero Discrepancy group continued to receive the original pattern. On the first trial of Phase II, fixation times in both high and medium discrepancy groups increased, thereby indicating the infants could discriminate the new pattern from the one used in habituation. The Zero Discrepancy group did not show this increase since they were still seeing the old pattern. The second phase of the experiment continued until the infants either habituated to the new pattern or received a total of eight trials. In the third phase, High and Medium groups were again shown the first pattern as a test for delayed recognition. Both groups dishabituated, looking significantly longer than they had at the end of original habituation. The Zero group, on the other hand, did not show any recovery to the old pattern. Apparently, filling the retention interval with repeated exposures of a second similar stimulus interfered with recognition of the first stimulus.

This interpretation of DeLoache's results also makes some theoretical sense. One could reasonably assume that visual information will be stored accurately in long-term memory only after the infant has spent considerable time attending to it, and, possibly, only when he habituates to it as well. In order for any new information to produce interference, it must enter long-term memory and, therefore, must also be extensively presented. Filling the retention interval with a number of novel stimuli, each exposed for a brief period of time, as in the Caron and Caron (1968, 1969), Gelber (1972a), and Martin (1973) studies, should not be sufficient for any of these stimuli to enter long-term memory and should produce little if any interference. However, filling the interval with the same repeated stimulus, as in the Pancratz and Cohen (1970) and DeLoache (1973) studies, should be more likely to interfere with information stored earlier. The assumption that interference is a function of the number of intervening stimuli might still be correct, but only to the extent that each stimulus is exposed long enough to enter long-term memory.

Exposure time to an intervening stimulus is not the only factor influencing interference. The similarity between original and subsequent stimulation seems to make some difference as well. In an experiment by Fagan (1971) no reliable evidence of interference was obtained when the stimuli in the retention interval differed substantially from the original one, although the decrease in recognition from immediate to delayed test did approach statistical significance. In Pancratz and Cohen, original and interfering stimuli were also quite different and again the results were not clear cut. On the other hand, the interfering stimuli in the DeLoache study were somewhat more similar to the originally habituated one, and better evidence of interference was obtained.

Fagan (1973, Experiment IV) has reported the same effect even more strongly using the paired-comparison procedure and pictures of faces as stimuli. Five-month-old infants were first given a 2-min exposure to photographs of either a man's, woman's, or infant's face. Following an immediate recognition test, they were divided into three groups and each received three 10-sec pairings of intervening material. For subjects in the High Similarity group the stimuli were photographs of new faces closely resembling those they had originally seen. For subjects in the Medium Similarity group these new photographs were rotated 180° and for those in the Low Similarity group line drawings of the new faces, also rotated 180°, were presented. All infants then received the original recognition test once again. Interference was obtained only in the Medium Similarity group. Additional data from the experiment suggested that infants in the High Similarity group probably did not notice that the photographs had been changed, so once again there is evidence that interference effects occur most with stimuli similar to the original one.

Finally, Fagan (1973, Experiment V) has shown it also makes a difference when the interfering material is presented. He tested for recognition both immediately after familiarization to one upright face photograph and 3 hr later. If the intervening stimulation (inverted photographs) followed the first test, interference occurred. If it just preceded the delayed test, there was no interference.

So, within the last few years, it has been shown not only that infants have long-term visual memory, but also that the memory can be interfered with or disrupted. While much remains to be learned about the factors producing interference, some information is already available. If someone, today, wished to know the optimal conditions for disrupting infant memory, the answer would be to expose extensively the interfering material, to present it immediately after exposure to the initial material, and to make it similar to but discriminable from that initial material.

C. Stimulus Parameters

1. Discrimination and Memory

Considerable information about the development of infant visual perception and discrimination can be obtained from an examination of an infant's initial preferences for objects or patterns. Fantz,

Fagan, and Miranda (see Chapter 4 in this volume) describe in detail how these preferences can be used to demonstrate the infant's ability to discriminate such stimulus features as curvature, size, number of elements, and regularity. The basic assumption in this research is that if an infant looks reliably longer at one pattern than at another, he must be discriminating between them. But what if the infant's initial fixation time to the patterns is equal? It does not necessarily follow that the infant can not discriminate. He might just be equally attracted to both.

In such cases two techniques are often used to experimentally establish a preference where none existed before. The first is to make one pattern a discriminative stimulus by pairing it with reinforcement and then to condition the infant to respond to it. Bower (1964) has used this procedure successfully to investigate size constancy in infants, and McKenzie and Day (1971a,b) have used it to study infants' discrimination of patterns and orientation. The main drawback of the technique is the amount of time required, often several training sessions over a number of days.

A second, more efficient technique, requiring only a few minutes at most, is to familiarize the infant to one pattern and then compare his reaction to that pattern versus one that is still novel. Both habituation and paired-comparison procedures have been used successfully in this way to study infant discrimination ability. Consider, for example, an experiment by McGurk (1970) on infants' perception of orientation. As McGurk points out, until relatively recently the generally accepted view was that infants and young children could not discriminate between different orientations of the same form. Using three-dimensional faces and two-dimensional pictures of funnels, he first showed that 6- to 26-week-old infants did not look longer initially at an upright orientation of either stimulus than at the same stimulus inverted 180°. Even though no initial preference occurred, McGurk was able to demonstrate with habituation and paired-comparison procedures that the infants could, none the less, discriminate between different orientations. If infant fixation times were first habituated to a stimulus in one orientation, they recovered when the opposite orientation was presented; and if, following a familiarization period, novel and familiar orientations of the same stimulus were presented side by side, infants spent a greater proportion of time fixating the stimulus in the novel orientation.

This experiment and others like it provide information not only on infant discrimination but on what the infant is remembering as well.

In the case of the McGurk experiment, in order for the infants to have increased their attention when the orientation of the stimulus changed they must have remembered something. Whether the change in stimulation was perceived as the same stimulus in a new orientation or as an entirely new stimulus is unclear. In either case, memory for some stimulus characteristic was indicated. In other studies with similar procedures, infants, by the age of 6 months, have been shown to remember facial features (Fagan, 1972; Cornell, 1973), the arrangement of elements in a pattern (Fagan, 1974; Miranda & Fantz, 1974), and the shape and color of particular elements (Cohen, Gelber, & Lazar, 1971; DeLoache, 1973; Miranda & Fantz, 1974).

Unlike the McGurk experiment, most examinations of the stimulus characteristics remembered by infants have presented several variations of the familiar stimulus during the test for recognition. These variations usually lie on some definable continuum, although what is a continuum to the experimenter may or may not be a continuum to the infant. For example DeLoache (1973) habituated 4-month-old infants to a pattern consisting of four different colored forms (e.g., a red circle, green square, magenta cross, and yellow dumbbell). On the subsequent test either two of the patterns or all four were changed. Both changes produced nearly equivalent recovery of fixation time, although a control group which was still receiving the original pattern showed no recovery. These results demonstrated that the infants were storing something about either the colors or the forms of the elements in the pattern, but they do not indicate which. They also show that regardless of the continuum assumed by the experimenter, the infants may have found a change of four elements no greater than a change of two elements.

The question of just what an infant is remembering when he sees a colored pattern has received considerable recent examination. Saayman, Ames, and Moffett (1964) exposed 3-month-old infants to a simple colored geometric pattern for $4\frac{1}{2}$ min. Independent groups were then shown both the familiar pattern and one differing in color and/or form. The only group to prefer the novel stimulus was the one given the pattern novel in both dimensions. In a similar experiment (Cohen *et al.*, 1971) 4-month-old infants were also familiarized to a simple colored pattern and then tested for recovery with successive presentations of patterns novel in color, form, or both. Although some recovery occurred when a single dimension was changed, it was greatest when both were changed. An additional analysis was also performed that showed that individual infants were, in fact, storing information about both dimensions rather than some remembering only the color and others only the form. Finally, Welch (1973), using more complex patterns and a paired-comparison procedure, reported essentially the same results. Her 4-month-old infants also preferred the pattern when both color and form were novel, but not when only one was novel.

The evidence seems to indicate that by 3 or 4 months of age infants are capable of storing information about colors and forms but do not clearly show it unless both dimensions are changed. By 8 to 12 months of age, however, a change in either dimension is sufficient to produce a reliable preference for the novel stimulus (Collard & Rydberg, 1972; Miranda & Fantz, 1974).

2. COMPOUNDS VERSUS COMPONENTS

Even though infants will store both color and form information, the studies mentioned in the preceding paragraphs do not explain how they do it. If, for example, an infant is shown a red circle, will he store it as a single unitary compound, or will he break it down into its component parts, red and circle, and store each independently? One study (reported in Cohen, 1973) has examined this question. Four-month-old infants were first given alternating trials of two simple geometric forms (e.g., a red circle and a green triangle). For the recognition test the subjects were divided into three groups with the first receiving the same two familiar stimuli, the second, two totally different stimuli (e.g., a blue square and a yellow dumbbell), and the third, the same colors and forms they had seen originally, but now rearranged into novel compounds (e.g., a green circle and a red triangle). If this third group performed like the first one and failed to recover in the test, it would indicate they were responding on the basis of familiar components. On the other hand, if they performed like the second group and did recover, it would indicate a response on the basis of two new compounds. The first and third groups' test data were practically identical. Neither showed any evidence of recovery. Only the second group which received totally novel stimuli increased their fixation times in the test. Apparently the information was stored as separable components rather than as compounds. Even with a change in arrangement, the stimuli were perceived as the same old colors and forms.

Cornell and Strauss (1973) also examined infant memory for compounds versus components, but in their study the components were all within the same stimulus dimension. Four-month-old infants were habituated to a circle and a cross separately, and then tested either with a compound containing both components (the cross embedded in the circle) or a compound with novel components (a triangle overlapping a square). Only the males' fixation time recovered, and then only with the triangle–square compound. These results are also consistent with the view that infants process and store information in component form. If the cross–circle compound were seen as different from the individual components comprising it, recovery should have occurred to that compound as well.

It could be argued that in both the experiment reported by Cohen (1973) and the one by Cornell and Strauss (1973), it need not be assumed that infants break down compounds into their constituent elements. The same results would have been obtained had the infants been attending to and remembering only one of the components. For example, if, when shown a red circle and a green triangle, the infants remembered only the shapes, then later, even though the colors had been switched, the stimuli would still be just a circle and a triangle, and no recovery would be expected. By the same token in the Cornell and Strauss study, if the infants only attended to the circle, then later, regardless of what was embedded in it, it would still be the same circle.

When colored forms are used, the argument that infants attend only to one component is made less tenable by the Cohen *et al.* (1971) finding that individual infants attend to both dimensions. Nevertheless, given the tenuous nature of the results on compounds versus components so far, and the importance of this area to the understanding of how infants process and store visual information, future investigations should include the controls needed to assure that selective attention to a single component is not a viable explanation.

Evidence for infant memory of compounds versus components also comes from one other source in which a different procedure was used. Bower (1966) conditioned infants between 8 and 20 weeks of age to make a leftward head movement whenever a compound CS (conditioned stimulus) composed of a disk with a cross and two dots on it was shown. Following conditioning the infants were tested for generalization with the disk, cross, and dots, as well as with the whole compound. If the infants had been conditioned to (had remembered) the CS as independent components, their number of responses to the compound should equal the sum of their responses to each component. However, if they had been conditioned to (and remembered) the CS as a compound, more responses should be made to it than to the sum of the components. The results implied memory for components up to 16 weeks of age and memory for the compound at 20 weeks.

So far the evidence, although scanty, is consistent with the position that infants up to 4 months of age break down compound patterns into component parts, but by 5 months, the parts are combined into a unitary whole. Obviously, the generality of this evidence depends upon many additional unknown factors. For example, whether or not a pattern is remembered as components may depend upon the dimensions involved. Colors and forms may be separated automatically, but what about hue and saturation, or brightness and size? Would stimulation from two different modalities ever be compounded? One might think not for a geometric pattern and a tone, but what about for a face and a voice? If, as in Bower's experiment, the compound is composed of more than two components, do the infants first remember it as independent elements and then as the whole compound, or is there some intermediate stage in which the elements are remembered in pairs? Although none of these questions has yet been answered, the techniques are available to investigate them, and the answers should tell us a great deal more about how the infant processes and stores information than we know today.

3. The Discrepancy Hypothesis

Most investigators have assumed that the more the test stimulus differs from the familiar one, the more the infant will attend. This assumption is not universally accepted, however. McCall (1971) proposed that infant attention can be best described by an inverted-U-shaped function based upon the degree of discrepancy from a familiar stimulus. Several other theorists have proposed similar performance functions (e.g., Dember & Earl, 1957; Hunt, 1965; McClelland & Clark, 1953). According to this "discrepancy hypothesis," infants should display maximum attention to a stimulus which offers an optimal amount of discrepancy—a stimulus which is sufficiently familiar that it can be assimilated but sufficiently novel that it provides some new information. Stimuli which are either too familiar or too novel should recruit little attention.

In support of the optimal discrepancy hypothesis, McCall and Melson (1969) varied the arrangement of x's and y's in a pattern, and found that infants showed less heart rate deceleration to stimuli judged highly discrepant by adults than to less discrepant stimuli. McCall and his co-workers (McCall, Hogarty, Hamilton, & Vincent, 1973; McCall, Wycoff, Hamilton, & Hogarty, 1974) have also found that under certain conditions, if infants were first familiarized to a linear array of elements, and if the discrepancy involved a rotation of that array from vertical to horizontal, infants would fixate longer on a moderate discrepancy than on a more extreme one. For these data to in fact be supportive of the optimal discrepancy hypothesis one must accept the assumption that the stimuli were, first of all, ordered in terms of discrepancy from the infant's point of view, and second, that they were so discrepant as to be at the postoptimal end of the range of possible discrepancies. The first point seems difficult if not impossible to discover, if one assumes that when an infant responds similarly to two stimuli he does so because they are either very similar or very different from one another. Furthermore, given the extreme range of possible stimuli, it seems difficult to believe that McCall's discrepant stimuli, consisting of either a rearrangement or a rotation of the same elements could be above any optimal level of discrepancy. Evidence against the claim that the stimuli were above optimal discrepancy comes from other similar studies of infant responses to discrepant stimuli including one by McCall and Kagan (1970). Studies mentioned earlier by Saayman *et al.* (1964), Cohen *et al.* (1971), and Welch (1973) have all shown preferences to be an increasing function of discrepancy with color and form changes producing more attention than form or color changes alone. In a specific test of the discrepancy hypothesis, Welch actually varied three stimulus dimensions—color, form, and arrangement—and found an even greater preference for novelty when all three were novel than when only two were novel. McCall and Kagan's stimuli contained three of the following components: a flower, a Christmas bow, a rubber doll, a dog, a clown's face, and a bird. Discrepancy was manipulated by replacing one, two, or all three objects on the familiar stimulus with novel ones. They also found increasing attention with greater discrepancy. What seems to be happening is just the opposite of what one might expect from the "discrepancy hypothesis." When the stimulus change is rather subtle, when it consists of a rearrangement or change in location of the *same* elements, some evidence for an inverted-U occurs. On the other hand, when it is more extreme, when it is interdimensional and when some elements or objects are actually replaced by others, the greater the discrepancy, the more an infant looks.

Even in those instances where the same elements are rearranged, one does not always find moderate discrepancies produce the most attention. In one study (reported in McCall, 1972), for example, two out of eight groups actually showed a U-shaped curve. In another experiment (McCall *et al.*, 1974), rapid habituators showed the inverted-U when the retention interval was 5 sec, but showed a U when the retention interval was 15 sec. In contrast, slow habituators showed greatest attention to the most discrepant stimulus with the 5-sec interval, but an inverted-U relationship with the 15-sec interval. The meaning of these results is not all that clear. What is clear is that there is no way a traditional optimal level of discrepancy theory can explain those instances in which infants look more to the most familiar and most discrepant stimulus than they do to those of moderate discrepancy.

Perhaps at this point it would be well to heed Thomas's (1971) criticism that unambiguous tests of discrepancy theory require specification of a number of parameters which are typically not known. These include the shape of the preference curve, the location of individuals on the curve, the distance between stimuli and individual locations. In addition it is essential that the stimuli are ordered unidimensionally. "In the absence of parameter specification, almost any data may be mapped into or found at variance with the models by making different assumptions about parametric values [Thomas, 1971, p. 253]."

D. Individual Differences in Memory

Obviously, not all infants react the same way when confronted with a novel and familiar stimulus. Some respond more to a familiar stimulus, others more to a novel one. Some habituate rapidly, others slowly or not at all. Age, sex, state, and physical well-being all influence the infant's behavior. The interaction of these subject variables with infant habituation and memory is not, as yet, clear. However, age, sex, and other individual differences in performance occur with enough regularity that no discussion of infant memory would be complete without mentioning them.

1. AGE DIFFERENCES

What is the youngest age at which an infant will habituate or will prefer a novel to a familiar pattern? The answer to this question will vary depending upon who is asked. Friedman and his collaborators (Friedman, Nagy, & Carpenter, 1970; Friedman, Carpenter, & Nagy,

1970; Friedman & Carpenter, 1971; Friedman, 1972a,b) have consistently reported a response decrement in neonates to repetitions of the same checkerboard pattern. In one experiment (Friedman & Carpenter, 1971) they found that infants over 66 hr of age reduced their fixation time more than infants under 48 hr of age. In another with the same two age groups (Friedman, 1972a), recovery to a novel stimulus was greater in the older than in the younger newborns. The generality of these results must be interpreted with caution, since the number of infants completing the experiment is often quite low (it was only 32% in Friedman, 1972a). Nevertheless, the checkerboard patterns were properly counterbalanced, and recovery occurred only on those trials where the pattern was changed. In the light of these results it is difficult to argue with the author's conclusion that ". . . some infants from birth have the capacity to store and process simple visual information as reflected in their ability to detect and respond to change in the immediate environment [Friedman, 1972a, pp. 347–348]."

Other investigators, however, have been unable to get habituation and recovery or differential responding to novel and familiar stimuli before 2 months of age. In all fairness to Friedman, most who have tried have not studied newborns, but have begun their investigations with infants who were at least 4 to 6 weeks old.

The experiment that is perhaps the best known was reported by Fantz (1964). Infants 1 to 6 months of age were simultaneously shown two magazine photographs or advertisements. The stimulus remained constant on one side and was varied from trial to trial on the other. Infants 1 to 2 months old continued to attend to both patterns equally, but those over 2 months gradually came to prefer the novel one, with the 4- to 6-month-olds showing a greater preference than the 2- to 4-month-olds. This preference for novelty beginning at 2 months and then increasing over age has also been reported by Fagan, Fantz, and Miranda (1971) using the more traditional paired-comparison technique.

As might be expected, the results on habituation generally parallel those on preference. Wetherford and Cohen (1973) found no evidence of habituation at 6 or 8 weeks, but did find it at 10 or 12 weeks. Other evidence has indicated that for infants over 3 months of age, the older they are, the more rapidly they habituate (Lewis, 1971; Cohen, 1969a).

Up to this point the discussion has centered on attentional differences associated with chronological or postnatal age. But two infants who are the same chronological age may not be the same conceptional age. Fagan *et al.* (1971) compared premature and full-term infants on preferences for novelty. When the infants were equated on postnatal age a novelty preference first appeared at 10 weeks for the term infants but not until 16 weeks for the prematures. However, when the infants were equated on time since conception, attention patterns in both groups were virtually identical. Preference for novelty first occurred for both groups at about 52 weeks of conceptional age. On the basis of this evidence the authors concluded that no evidence existed of retarded memory in their premature infants. However, Sigman (1973) has reported less novelty preference by prematures than term infants at 58 weeks of conceptional age. The difference between Sigman's results and those of Fagan *et al.* could have resulted from the greater degree of prematurity in Sigman's subjects.

To summarize, the evidence clearly indicates a dramatic change in memory ability occurring somewhere between 2 and 3 months of age. This change is frequently highlighted by the finding that at about 2 months of age infants may actually prefer a familiar stimulus before they prefer a novel one. Wetherford and Cohen (1973), for example, using an experimental design that combined both cross-sectional and longitudinal methods, obtained data that suggest that within a brief laboratory session, 8-week-old infants will show an increase in fixation to a repeatedly presented stimulus relative to varying novel stimuli. Infants of 10 and 12 weeks, on the other hand, tend to demonstrate a preference for the novel stimuli toward the end of the experimental session relative to a stimulus which has been repeatedly encountered. Six-week-old infants showed no consistent preference for either the familiar or the novel stimuli.

Similar results were found by Greenberg, Uzgiris, and Hunt (1970) using long-term exposures to the familiarized stimulus (daily half-hour presentations for a period of 1 month). Here again, 2-month-olds showed a preference for the familiar pattern whereas 2 weeks and 4 weeks later, after additional familiarization, preference was switched to novel stimuli. Weizmann *et al.* (1971) also using long-term exposures, and, in addition, controlling for the effects of repeated testing, found that 6-week-old infants (after 2 weeks of 30 min per day exposure) preferred familiar stimuli, whereas 2 weeks later, after additional familiarization, fixation times showed a shifting preference for novelty. Unfortunately, both of these long-term longitudinal studies confounded amount of familiarization with age. Thus it is not altogether clear whether the shift in preference during the second month was due to age-related changes or simply to amount of stimulus exposure. Regardless, these results taken in conjunction with the Wetherford and Cohen (1973) data do suggest a change in preference somewhere between 6 and 10 weeks from familiar visual stimuli to novel stimuli. Other evidence from Fagan *et al.* (1971) and from Lewis (1971) also tend to show a preference for familiarity preceding a preference for novelty. They did not report, however, whether these preferences for familiarity were reliable. One has difficulty reconciling all the evidence that a developmental change occurs in infant recognition memory at about 2 months of age with Friedman's (1972) report of habituation and recovery to a novel stimulus in the neonatal period. At this point in time one can only hope that Friedman's results can be replicated with stimuli other than checkerboard patterns, and that more investigations will focus on infant recognition memory in the first 2 months of life.

2. Sex Differences

No topic is more confusing, no evidence more contradictory, than that on sex differences in infant attention and memory. Some investigators have found that females habituate more rapidly than males (Caron & Caron, 1968, 1969), and some have found just the opposite (Cohen *et al.*, 1971; Pancratz & Cohen, 1971). Some evidence indicates that sex differences depend upon whether the infant is tested in a novel or a familiar environment (Jeffrey & Cohen, 1971; Weizmann *et al.*, 1971); other evidence indicates the novelty of the environment does not affect the two sexes differentially (Parry, 1972).

Many researchers have obtained sex differences in attention at one time or another, but the differences have not always been consistent even within the same laboratory. For example, in two experiments with newborns, Friedman found females habituating more to a 12 × 12 than to a 2 × 2 checkerboard (Friedman *et al.*, 1970; Friedman & Carpenter, 1971). Yet, in two other experiments using essentially the same procedure and stimuli and with the same age infants, no sex differences were obtained (Friedman, 1972a, b). Another example of inconsistent sex differences occurs in the work of McCall and his associates. In general those studies employing long-term familiarization in the home produced differences in male and female responses to discrepancy (McCall & Kagan, 1967; McCall, 1972), while those employing short-term laboratory familiarization failed to produce sex differences (McCall et al., 1973; McCall et al., 1974). In one short-term experiment, however, a sophisticated statistical analysis revealed a difference between males' and females' attention to discrepancies (McCall & Kagan, 1970).

Somewhat more consistent evidence of sex differences has come out of Cohen's laboratory. Several studies have now shown a greater degree of habituation in 4-month-old male than 4-month-old female infants (Pancratz & Cohen, 1970; Cohen et al., 1971; Cohen, 1973; Gelber, 1972b).

Similarly, a greater tendency for males to respond differentially to familiar versus novel stimuli after familiarization has been found by Pancratz and Cohen (1970), Cohen et al. (1971), and Weizmann et al. (1971). The implications of these sex differences to differences in memory processes are unclear. It is unlikely that the young female is incapable of storing visual information since females are equally capable of performing at other learning tasks and demonstrating other behaviors that require storage of stimulus information. A study reported by Cohen (1973) suggests that sex differences might be due to the fact that males and females are processing and storing different kinds of information about repeatedly presented stimuli. Males appear to be more likely to store information about the various components of a repeatedly presented stimulus, for example, its color or form. Information such as this determines the length of time an infant will continue to fixate a stimulus. When a comparator mechanism (see the following discussion of models of habituation) determines that incoming information matches stored information, fixation ceases. The lack of habituation shown by female infants, according to Cohen, might in part reflect their lesser tendency to store such specific stimulus information. Cohen further suggests that females, unlike males, are more likely to store information about the consequences of orienting, or the reinforcing value of visual orienting. Evidence for this hypothesis comes from data that show that female, but not male, infants will differentially increase or decrease their latencies in turning to look at a peripherally presented stimulus as a function of the complexity of immediately prior stimuli. That is, the more interesting a stimulus is on a given trial, the faster the female will orient on subsequent trials. Males showed similar decreasing latencies but the amount of decrease did not vary as a function of the nature of previously encountered stimuli.

Sex differences in the tendency to process visual information have also been reported by Watson (1969). In attempting to operantly condition visual orienting responses of 14-week-old infants to a specified location, Watson obtained a Sex × Modality of reinforcement interaction reflecting greater learning by boys with visual reinforcement and greater learning by females with auditory reinforcement. This tendency of males to be attuned more to visual information is consistent with results showing more response habituation in males to visual patterns. One might have expected, however, on the basis of Cohen's (1973) hypothesis, that females would have learned under the visual reinforcement in Watson's situation since storage of specific visual information about the reinforcer was not a necessary antecedent of learning. Whether or not Watson's results are at odds with Cohen's hypothesis is difficult to determine because of the many differences in procedures and response measures. In fact, generally, procedural variations among studies make it difficult to isolate the factors responsible for the contradictory data on sex differences reported in the literature. At this time one can only speculate regarding the extent to which these early sex differences reflect varying cognitive styles, state differences, or perhaps even discrepancies in rates of intellectual development.

3. FAST VERSUS SLOW HABITUATORS

Much has been made of the relationship between habituation rate or preferences for novelty and the cognitive ability of the infant (Lewis, 1971; McCall, 1972). For example, one could argue that if habituation reflects memory, then the rate at which the infant habituates should reflect the rate at which a model, schema, or engram of the repeated stimulus if formed. Similarly, the degree of preference for novelty should reflect the accuracy of the model and the ease with which the infant can discriminate it from novel stimuli. Furthermore, since memory is an essential component of much cognitive activity, the ability to habituate or show a novelty preference should be related to performance on other cognitive tasks as well.

Considerable evidence supports this view. As we have seen, older, presumably more cognitively advanced infants habituate more rapidly and prefer novel stimuli sooner than do younger ones (e.g., Lewis, 1971). Full-term infants prefer a novel stimulus more than premature infants do even when the two groups are equated for conceptional age (Sigman, 1973). When the differences between novel and familiar stimuli are subtle, normal infants show a greater novelty preference at an earlier age than do Down's Syndrome infants (Miranda & Fantz, 1974).

In a review of research on individual differences in response decrements (i.e., habituation) and early cognitive growth, Lewis (1971) reports evidence that response decrements are also related to Apgar score and medication at birth, CNS (central nervous system) dysfunction, and socioeconomic status of the father. Response decrements at 1 year were also predictive of discrimination learning and IQ at 44 months. Gelber (1972b) has also shown that for 4-month-old females the degree of habituation to a visual pattern predicts their performance on a subsequent two-choice discrimination problem. Taken together, all of this evidence suggests that tests of infant recognition memory may be tapping some basic cognitive operations.

As more and more investigators begin to look at individual differences in response decrements or habituation, the problems associated with how to decide when an infant habituates or how to separate infants into fast and slow habituators become increasingly important. These two problems are closely related since one cannot decide whether an infant habituates rapidly or slowly until he has defined the criterion for habituation, and which criterion he selects depends upon his assumptions regarding the nature of the habituation process.

These problems become critical when the initial response level to the stimuli differs between groups or individuals. For example, on the first trial, fixation times are frequently found to be greater for younger than older infants (e.g., Cohen, 1969). Consider the three hypothetical examples presented in Figure 5.3. Each set of curves represents the fixation times of younger (Group Y) and older (Group O) subjects when they are repeatedly shown the same visual stimulus. In all three examples Group Y looks 8 sec on the first trial, while Group O looks 4 sec.

One approach assumes habituation proceeds as in Figure 5.3a. When both groups decrease their responding by the same fixed amount (e.g., 3 sec) they have habituated equally. While this approach is usually not stated explicitly, it is assumed whenever the raw data are examined by a traditional Groups × Trials analysis of variance. If the two curves are parallel as in Figure 5.3a, habituation is assumed to be the same for the two groups; if the curves are not parallel, an interaction occurs, and in the case of Figures 5.3b and 5.3c, the younger group would be assumed to habituate more

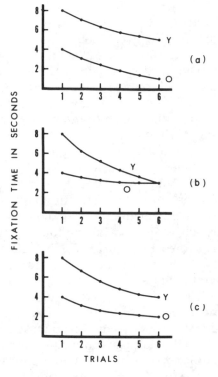

Figure 5.3   Hypothetical forward habituation curves illustrating the effects of different criterion measures of habituation for younger (Y) and older (O) groups of infants. In (a) habituation of the groups would be equal if the criterion were based upon the same decrease in absolute fixation time. In (b) habituation would be equal if the groups habituated to a common final asymptotic level. In (c) the groups would habituate equally if they had the same proportional decrease in fixation time.

rapidly than the older one. As attractive as this simple model of habituation may seem, it is intuitively unreasonable. If Group O's initial fixation time were 2 sec rather than 4 sec, it would be impossible for them to decrease their response by 3 sec. A more reasonable assumption would be that the response level decreases to some asymptotic level at or above zero and then levels off.

The second commonly used approach is to arbitrarily pick some criterion value, such as a fixation time of 3 sec, and assume all infants have habituated when their response reaches that value. This approach assumes habituation proceeds as in Figure 5.3b, and using the 3-sec criterion, the older infants but not the younger ones would have habituated in Figures 5.3b and 5.3c. The approach makes some sense in that infants are not required to respond less than zero, but it includes the assumption that regardless of initial response level all infants will arrive at the same final level. Whether the assumption is true or false is open to empirical test. One disadvantage of the approach is that it can lead to a violation of the usual definition of habituation, a decrease in responding over trials.

If an infant's initial fixation time is equal to or less than the criterion value of 3 sec, one would be forced to assume habituation on a single trial even though the response may never decrease or may even increase on subsequent trials.

The third approach is represented in Figure 5.3c. Here infants are assumed to have habituated equally when their response decreases the same proportional amount. In the example presented in Figure 5.3c, both groups of infants decrease their fixation time to one-half their original level. Using this criterion, the older group would have habituated more than the younger group in Figure 5.3a, and the younger group would have habituated more than the older in 5.3b.

Use of a proportional criterion has several advantages. It is more consistent with the definition of rate of habituation, infants all have to decrease their responding somewhat, and they are allowed to reach their own asymptotic level. It has a disadvantage, if as is assumed in Figure 5.3b, infants tend to reduce their responses to some common final level regardless of how long they looked on the first trial.

The point of this discussion is not that any one approach is necessarily superior to any other. Rather it is that what one considers to be equal amounts or rates of habituation depends upon a number of assumptions, in fact depends upon one's model of the habituation process. The model will also influence how one interprets the data when a novel stimulus is introduced to test for recognition memory. Should the amount of recovery be based upon the difference between the infant's response to the novel stimulus and his final response to the familiar stimulus, upon how close his response is to some arbitrary level, or upon the proportional increase of his response? Again, different approaches can yield different results. Unfortunately, up to now, no one has presented a model explicit enough to permit unambiguous selection of one of these approaches. Until someone does, any attempt to compare the results of different experiments on rate of habituation or fast versus slow habituators, when each experiment uses a different criterion, will be a difficult, if not futile endeavor.

Nevertheless, some interesting results have come from attempts to separate infants into rapid and slow habituators. McCall and Kagan (1970) tested the hypothesis that, "If . . . the rate of habituation of attention to a repeatedly presented standard is an index of the acquisition of an engram for that stimulus, then infants that display rapid habituation should respond more positively to discrepancies than those who do not evidence habituation

[McCall, 1971, p. 121]." Four-month-old infants were shown the following sequence of standard (S) and discrepant (D) stimuli: SSSSSDSSSDSSSDSSS. On the basis of a proportional measure computed from trials 2 through 5, infants were classified as rapid or slow habituators. (Those who had consistent short looks and did not show much decline over trials were also included as a separate group in the analyses, but will not be discussed here.) Rapid habituators increased their response to the first discrepant stimulus, but slow habituators did not. This difference between the two groups was not surprising since the slow habituators never really habituated. They were looking much longer than the fast habituators on trials 4 and 5, and probably could not have increased their response to the discrepant stimulus no matter what was presented. This experiment illustrates the difficulty in interpreting recovery to a discrepant stimulus when the groups are at different levels at the end of habituation. A difference score measure would indicate little or no recovery for the slow group, but a proportional measure would indicate almost complete recovery.

A better procedure for assessing differences between rapid and slow habituators would be to continue presenting the standard stimulus until all infants reach the same criterion. In the study by McCall *et al.* (1973), all subjects were shown the same vertical or horizontal arrow until they looked 3 sec or less on two consecutive trials following the first five presentations. Various rotations of the arrow were then presented to determine the infants' response to discrepancy. Rapid habituators displayed an inverted-U curve as a function of the discrepancy while slow habituators responded most to the most discrepant stimulus. In a second similar experiment (McCall *et al.*, unpublished, 1974) the same results were obtained following a 5-sec retention interval. Following a 15-sec interval, however, it was the slow habituators who showed the inverted-U, while the rapid habituators had a U-shaped curve. Although the meaning of these results is unclear, apparently some differences between rapid and slow habituators still remain, even after they are habituated to a common criterion, at least as long as the discrepancy involves a rotation of the same stimulus elements.

A very different result is obtained when the discrepancy involves entirely new stimuli. DeLoache (1973) habituated 4-month-old infants to a stimulus consisting of four simple patterns, each of a different color and shape. Her criterion was a proportional measure, three consecutive looks equal to or less than one-half of the first three looks. An interesting finding was that the infants fell into two distinct groups: Fast Habituators, taking 8 trials or less to reach criterion, and Slow Habituators, taking 11 trials or more.

Reexamining DeLoache's data using backward habituation curves revealed that the basic assumption that fast habituators store information more rapidly than slow habituators may be in error. As can be seen in Figure 5.4, both groups actually habituated on a single trial. Furthermore, both showed the same peak in fixation just before they habituated. The main difference between the groups appears to be the greater number of trials it took the slow habituators to reach the beginning of the peak. The same general results were found in another study where checkerboard patterns were the stimuli. These results are presented in Figure 5.5. In both experiments, fast and slow habituators show the peak and then habituate rapidly.

Additional evidence from the checkerboard experiment suggests that information may be stored in memory during the period of the peak. Infants in the study were actually repeatedly shown either a 2×2, 8×8, or 24×24 checkerboard pattern. If the more complex checkerboard required more information processing, one would expect the duration and height of the peak to be greatest for those infants given the 24×24 pattern. As can be seen in Figure 5.6, this is precisely what happened. Infants in the 24×24 group initially fixated about the same amount as those in the other two groups, but then increased their responding much more than the other groups just prior to habituation.

One reasonable interpretation of the data from both experiments is that fast and slow habituators do not differ from one another in the time needed to process and store visual information, but that they do differ in the number of trials or fixations before they *begin* to process the information. Some infants come into the situation ready to go. They peak early and habituate almost immediately. Other infants take longer to get involved in the task. They may look without remembering for any number of trials. Once they do begin to store the information, however, they peak and habituate just as quickly as the fast habituators.

At this point in time, research is so meager on backward habituation that one does not even know if the difference between fast and slow habituators results from transient variations in state or from persistent individual differences. One of the first tasks now confronting researchers of infant habituation will be to conduct repeated testings of the same infants to see if the differences

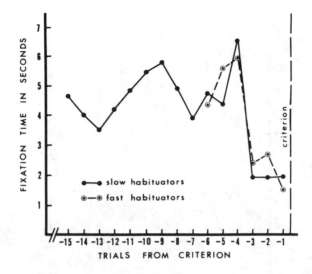

Figure 5.4 Backward habituation curves for fast and slow habituators from the colored shape experiment.

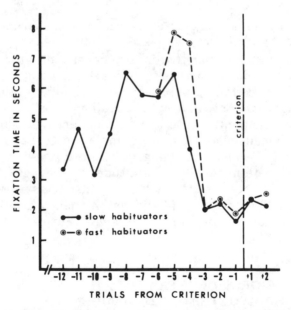

Figure 5.5 Backward habituation curves for fast and slow habituators from the checkerboard experiment.

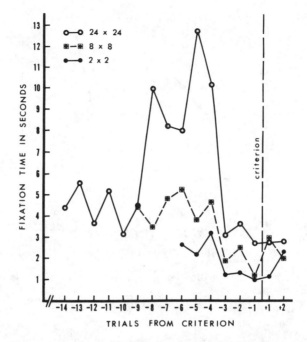

Figure 5.6   Separate backward habituation curves for infants receiving repeated presentations of either a 2 x 2, 8 x 8, or 24 x 24 checkerboard pattern.

between fast and slow habituators are consistent within the same individual over time and across stimulus dimensions.

One thing is certain. Simple models of infant attention and memory, which say only that with repeated exposures to the same stimulus the infants process and store an engram or schema of the stimulus, are inadequate. A more complete model is needed that explains what the infant is doing during the prepeak time, what initiates and determines the magnitude of the peak, and what causes him to decrease suddenly his response to asymptote on one or two trials. The adequacy of the few models which do exist to explain infant habituation and memory will be examined in the next section.

VI.   MODELS OF INFANT HABITUATION AND MEMORY

This section of the chapter will consider four conceptualizations of habituation that are frequently cited in the infant literature. One is a general model of habituation, the other three are based mainly on infant research. All four make certain common assumptions. First, they all assume that habituation or differential responding to novel and familiar stimuli implies some type of memory; second, that this memory is of long enough duration to persist across several trials; and third, that on any given trial, the organism compares his current input with the information that is stored. If there is a match, the organism will cease responding. If there is a mismatch, the response will continue. While the models all appear quite similar, as we shall see, there are also some significant differences between them.

A. Sokolov

Of the several models of habituation, the most widely cited is that of Sokolov (1963, 1969). His theory developed as a result of his research on the orienting reflex (OR) and its interrelationship with the adaptive and defensive reflexes. The OR consists of a complex set of physiological and behavioral responses that occur to changes in the environment. Physiological indices of the OR include a change of heart rate, galvanic skin response, or vasoconstriction and dilation. Orientation of the receptors toward the source of stimulation is the most common behavioral measure.

Sokolov's neurological model of habituation attempts to account for the fact that with repeated presentations of a nonsignal stimulus the OR to it wanes and gradually disappears (habituation), but that any change in the stimulus reactivates the OR. In simplified form, according to Sokolov, a trace or model of a repeated stimulus is formed in the nervous system. Each incoming stimulus is compared to the trace or neuronal model from past stimulation. If the input matches the model the OR is inhibited. The amount of inhibition varies with the strength or clarity of the neuronal model, thereby producing gradual response reductions or habituation as a concomitant of model or memory trace formation. Conversely, if an incoming stimulus fails to match the neuronal model, the OR is elicited, the magnitude of the reaction being a function of the degree of discrepancy between the model and the novel stimulus.

One chief limitation of Sokolov's model as it is applied to infant visual attention is that it predicts a gradual decrease in attention over trials as the incoming stimulus and neuronal model begin to match. As we have seen from backward habituation curves, infant attention may actually increase just before habituation occurs. The model also does not explain the behavior of those infants (e.g., Cohen, 1973) who look at a stimulus, look away, look, and look away again several times during the course of an experiment even though they never habituate.

Although Sokolov's model is couched in neurological terms, it has a strong cognitive flavor. An adaptation of Sokolov's model that is more explicitly cognitive and deals more directly with infant behavior has been offered by Lewis.

B. Lewis

Lewis (1971) conceptualizes habituation as a cognitive process by which the infant learns not to attend to irrelevant or unimportant information in his environment. The infant will maintain his attention to relevant environmental events, but if the event is unimportant, he will cease attending and turn to analyzing other events, potentially more important. Lewis provides evidence that response decrements are related to CNS functioning and are under cognitive control. He assumes that the rate of decrement reflects the growth of internal representations against which external events are compared, so that those infants who display more rapid decrements are those who build internal representations faster.

While Lewis recognizes the similarity between Sokolov's model and his own, he does take issue with a simple match–inattention, mismatch–attention explanation that assumes that sensory experiences are merely stored for later comparison. For Lewis, internal representations of external events are more than mirror images of sensory experience. With repeated exposures to the same object in a variety of different settings and from a variety of different angles, the organism constructs an internal representation that is a composite of his entire experience, an idealization transcending any number of specific sensations, allowing the object to maintain its invariance even when presented from a new angle or orientation.

Thus, according to Lewis, the organism plays a more active role in the processing and storing of information than one might assume from Sokolov. For Sokolov, any change in stimulation will produce recovery of the OR. For Lewis, not any change will be sufficient. The change must also be at least a partial violation of an existing idealization or schema.

One of the chief limitations of Lewis's model is its lack of specificity. Although he says the infant plays a more active role in deciding whether a stimulus is relevant or irrelevant, he does not indicate the rules by which that decision is made. Although he stresses the importance of organized units of perception or schemas rather than mere sense impressions, he does not tell us what constitutes a schema or how schemas are formed. He assumes that older or more cognitively advanced infants should habituate at a faster rate, but does not specify which measure of rate to use. In essence his predictions regarding habituation are much the same as those of Sokolov. Repeatedly present a relatively neutral stimulus and the infant should gradually reduce his response to it. Present a discrepancy, and recovery of the response should occur, with the recovery being greater the greater the discrepancy. Stated in this way, Lewis's model, like Sokolov's, does not explain the peak in the backward habituation curve. Nor does it explain the behavior of those infants who repeatedly look away from the stimulus but do not habituate. Nevertheless with his emphasis on the information-processing aspect of attention, Lewis has pointed out an important dimension in the study of infant memory.

C. McCall

McCall's model, like Lewis's, assumes that when an infant is repeatedly presented with the same stimulus, an engram or schema of the stimulus is stored. Following habituation, presentation of a discrepant stimulus will produce recovery of the response. Unlike Lewis, McCall assumes an optimal level of discrepancy, so that stimuli too similar to or too different from the familiarized standard will produce less recovery than a stimulus with an intermediate amount of discrepancy.

A description of the model and evidence for and against it were discussed earlier and so will not be covered in detail again here. However, one additional point should be made. In order to test the validity of the discrepancy hypothesis, McCall and his associates have concentrated upon the recovery or test phase of their experiments. But, predictions can be made regarding the course of habituation itself. If a highly discrepant stimulus is less preferred than a moderately discrepant stimulus, which in turn is preferred to the nondiscrepant standard, it would seem to follow that attention to the initial presentations of the standard should be very low since it is highly discrepant from existing engrams at this time. With repeated presentations, as a model of the standard is formed, the same stimulus should yield an increasing magnitude of responding, until an optimal discrepancy is reached. This should then be followed by response habituation as the degree of discrepancy continues to decrease between the model and additional presentations of the same stimulus. In other words, the discrepancy hypothesis would actually predict the peak found in backward habituation curves. To be sure, the rapid rate of habituation would not be predicted, but the increasing and then decreasing function would be. One reason McCall may not have emphasized the habituation phase of his experiments is that until recently he has been analyzing habituation only by typical forward group curves. Unpublished evidence from McCall's laboratory, however (personal communication), indicates that some of his infants do show the peak in responding before they habituate. Perhaps then, the discrepancy hypothesis will hold more reliably for the acquisition of an engram than for the response to a novel stimulus once the engram is fully formed.

D. Cohen

Cohen's (1973) model of infant visual attention is the most explicit one applied to infant habituation research. The model has been generated inductively from experimental findings and is not yet considered complete. Cohen makes the same fundamental assumption as the other models that attention will be a function of the comparison between incoming stimuli and some internal representation or memory. The model is presented schematically in Figure 5.7. While there are some similarities to the other models there are also a number of unique features dictated by empirical evidence from infant research. One of the most important is Cohen's postulation of two independent processes in infant visual attention: an Attention-Getting process that determines whether an infant will orient his head and eyes toward a visual pattern, and an Attention-Holding process that determines how long he will fixate after he has turned. These processes have been shown to be affected by different stimulus parameters. For example, Attention-Getting is more affected by size or movement, while Attention-Holding is more a function of the complexity or familiarity of the pattern (Cohen, 1969, 1973).

According to the model, both processes are involved in habituation—fixation time decreases over the course of an experiment, and eventually the orienting response to the pattern may also be inhibited. As Figure 5.7 shows, the Attention-Getting process is set in motion by any environmental event with sufficient brightness, size, movement, etc., to activate the Peripheral Perceiver. If not inhibited by the OR Inhibitor–Facilitator, an orienting response will then occur, followed by fixation of the stimulus. During fixation, two memory systems are engaged. An incoming stimulus is analyzed by the Perceptual Processor, a short-term or operative memory. On each trial this system builds up a representation of the stimulus. The Comparator–Decider compares the representation to the current stimulus. When they match, the subject stops fixating and turns away. Thus the Perceptual Processor initially determines how long the subject's fixation time will be on any given trial. Presumably, the more information in the pattern (i.e., the more complex it is) the longer it takes for the Perceptual Processor to develop an adequate representation, and hence the longer the fixation. As soon as the infant turns away, however, the short-term representation is displaced so that on the next trial the process must start over again.

The Long-Term Memory System also influences fixation time. On

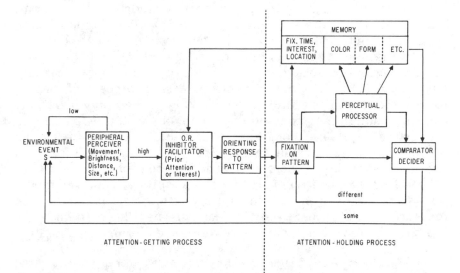

Figure 5.7 A schematic representation of Cohen's model of infant attention and habituation. [From Cohen, 1973.]

each trial some information about the stimulus goes from the Perceptual Processor into long-term memory where it is stored. We have reviewed evidence in this chapter suggesting that, up to 4 months of age, infants will break down compound stimuli into their constituent components, and that is indicated in the model by the separate boxes labeled "color, form, etc." As a representation of the repeated stimulus builds up over trials in this memory system, it is retained and becomes more accurate until it closely matches the incoming stimulus. In addition to comparing the current stimulus to the short-term representation in the Perceptual Processor, the Comparator–Decider compares it to the Long-Term Memory model. After a number of trials, the long-term memory becomes accurate enough for a match to be achieved, and the infant habituates.[2]

Thus Cohen's model hypothesizes that the length of a subject's fixation on any trial is a function of both short- and long-term memory systems. A match of the representation developed by either to the incoming stimulus will end the fixation. The short-term memory accounts for the infant's turning away from a stimulus when he is not habituating, and the long-term memory accounts for his turning away once he does habituate.

To complete the picture, changes as a function of trials also occur in the Attention-Getting process. Cohen suggests that in addition to storing information about the physical characteristics of the stimulus, infants also store something about their own reactions to it, such as how interesting the pattern was, how long they looked at it, as well as its location. This information goes to the OR Inhibitor–Facilitator and influences the subject's behavior on succeeding trials. Thus infants may increase or decrease their speed of turning toward the stimulus according to what they saw on previous trials. Cohen assumes that conditioning is involved. If the pattern is interesting or produces long fixations, the subject will increase his turning speed; if it is uninteresting or produces short fixations, his speed will slow down. There is evidence (Cohen, 1973; DeLoache *et al.*, 1972) that tends to support these assumptions. Thus, the model points out the danger of using total fixation time per trial as a measure of habituation. Does the decrease one is likely to find over trials result from an actual reduction in the duration of the infant's

---

[2] As originally presented, the model did not specify whether habituation would require several trials, reflecting a gradual increase in accuracy of the long-term memory, or would occur in one or two trials, reflecting the fact that some threshold in accuracy had been reached. Given the data from backward habituation curves, the latter alternative seems more reasonable.

looking at the stimulus, or from a reduction in his tendency to turn to look? Most evidence (e.g., Cohen, 1969, 1973) suggests it results from a reduction in the duration of each fixation, but without separate measures of Attention-Getting and Attention-Holding one cannot know for certain.

The specificity of Cohen's model represents both a major strength and a chief weakness. It does summarize coherently a great amount of data. Unlike the other models it provides an explanation for infants' turning away from a stimulus before they have habituated. It is also consistent with the rapid habituation found in backward habituation curves. By separating infant behavior into Attention-Getting and Attention-Holding processes it has led to a refinement in experimental procedure that has resulted in more precise measurements of infant attention and memory. However, in some respects it is not specific enough. Like other models, it does not specify how rate of habituation should be measured. Neither does it explain why infants increase their attention just prior to habituation. On the other hand, it may also be too specific. The model has been generated primarily from data on 4-month-old infants. It says nothing about developmental changes in attention, habituation, or memory. Neither it nor the other models presented in this chapter can explain why newborn infants habituate but 6- to 8-week-old infants do not, or why a 2-month-old may actually look longer at a familiar than at a novel stimulus.

The introduction of backward habituation curves may make all of these models obsolete. They have concentrated on what causes the infant to decrease his response. A more interesting question could be what causes him to increase his response. In fact, the data from backward habituation curves open up a whole new set of questions. Why do some infants take several trials before their peak appears, while for others the peak occurs almost immediately? Do age or population differences in habituation reflect differences in pre-peak behavior, in behavior during the peak, or in both? Is the onset of the peak actually the onset of long-term memory, or do infants retain information even on the pre-peak trials? On those early trials does the infant really store information in short-term memory, as Cohen proposes, or is he turning away from a stimulus because he is just tired of looking in that direction? In other words, is the information on these trials actually processed by the infant, or is it analogous to what frequently happens to most of us when, for example, we read a page from a book, stop to recall what we have read, and realize nothing has been retained.

All of these questions can be explored experimentally, and the answers can lead us a long way toward the understanding of infant habituation and memory. Even if the models in their present form do become obsolete, they have provided a valuable service. By generating interest in the phenomenon of infant habituation and by serving as the impetus for innumerable studies of infant attention, they have laid the foundation for future research and theorizing on infant recognition memory.

VII. SUMMARY AND CONCLUSIONS

In this chapter we have tried to show that much of infant behavior is dependent upon infant memory, but that the investigation of infant memory, particularly recognition memory, is best served at this time by concentrating on either of two experimental paradigms. In both, the infant is familiarized to one stimulus and then tested with one or more novel stimuli. One paradigm involves simultaneous pairing of two stimuli (the paired-comparison method), while the other involves successive exposures of a single stimulus (the habituation method). Each paradigm has its own specific methodological limitations, but evidence provided by both usually tends to agree.

Research on infant memory has tended to show that infants can recognize a pattern up to 2 weeks later, and that under certain specified conditions recognition can be interfered with. In general it has been found that the more novel a stimulus the more the infant will prefer it, but this conclusion must be qualified in at least two respects. There is evidence that at approximately 8 weeks of age infants may actually prefer familiar stimuli. Also, other evidence indicates that if the novel stimulus differs from the familiar one in arrangement or rotation of elements the most novel stimulus may not be the most preferred.

Age, sex, and other individual differences occur in habituation and preferences for novelty, and it has usually been assumed that the more advanced an infant is cognitively, the more marked his novelty preference or the more rapid his rate of habituation. However, no one has yet provided an adequate rationale for the use of any one particular measure of habituation rate, and different measures can lead to different conclusions regarding who is a fast and who is a slow habituator.

Several models of habituation have been evaluated in this chap-tor. While differences exist between them, both in content and in specificity, they all assume that while the infant is watching a stimulus, a representation or model of the stimulus is being built up and stored, so that later presentations of that or some other stimulus can be compared to the model.

Finally, recent evidence from backward habituation curves may mark a transition in the study of infant habituation and memory. Instead of indicating, as most investigators believed, that habituation involves a gradual decrease in responding, the data have shown that under certain conditions, at least, habituation may be all or none, occurring on a single trial, and that just preceding this sudden decrease the infant may exhibit an increase or peak in his response. Future research must determine the generality of this finding and whether or not the peak reflects the onset of long-term memory.

ACKNOWLEDGMENTS

We wish to offer special thanks to Judy DeLoache and Marian Sigman for their critical reading of the chapter and their many helpful suggestions for improving it.

REFERENCES

Berlyne, D. E. Motivational problems raised by exploratory and epistemic behavior. In S. Koch (Ed.), *Psychology: A study of a science.* Vol. 5. *The process areas, the person, and some applied fields: Their place in psychology and in science.* New York: McGraw-Hill, 1963. Pp. 284–364.

Bower, T. G. R. Discrimination of depth in premotor infants. *Psychonomic Science,* 1964, *1,* 368.

Bower, T. G. R. Heterogeneous summation in human infants. *Animal Behaviour,* 1966, *14,* 395–398.

Brown, A. L., & Scott, M. S. Recognition memory for pictures in preschool children. *Journal of Experimental Child Psychology,* 1971, *11,* 401–412.

Bruner, J. S. The course of cognitive growth. *American Psychologist,* 1964, *19,* 1–15.

Caron, R. F., & Caron, A. J. The effects of repeated exposure and stimulus complexity on visual fixation in infants. *Psychonomic Science,* 1968, *10,* 207–208.

Caron, R. F., & Caron, A. J. Degree of stimulus complexity and habituation of visual fixation in infants. *Psychonomic Science,* 1969, *14,* 78–79.

Caron, R. F., Caron, A. J., & Caldwell, R. C. Satiation of visual reinforcement in young infants. *Developmental Psychology,* 1971, *5,* 279–289.

Charlesworth, W. R. The role of surprise in cognitive development. In D. Elkind & J. H. Flavell (Eds.), *Studies in cognitive development: Essays in honor of Jean Piaget.* New York: Oxford Univ. Press, 1969. Pp. 257–314.

Cohen, L. B. Observing responses, visual preferences, and habituation to visual stimuli in infants. *Journal of Experimental Child Psychology,* 1969, *7,* 419–433. (a)

Cohen, L. B. Alternative measures of infant attention. Paper presented at the meeting of the Society for Research in Child Development, Santa Monica, March 1969. (b)

Cohen, L. B. Attention-getting and attention-holding processes of infant visual preferences. *Child Development,* 1972, *43,* 869–879.

Cohen, L. B. A two process model of infant visual attention. *Merrill-Palmer Quarterly,* 1973, *19,* 157–180.

Cohen, L. B., Gelber, E. R., & Lazar, M. A. Infant habituation and generalization to repeated visual stimulation. *Journal of Experimental Child Psychology,* 1971, *11,* 379–389.

Collard, R. B., & Rydberg, J. E. Generalization of habituation to properties of objects in human infants. *Proceedings,* 80th Annual Convention, American Psychological Association, 1972.

Cornell, E. H. Infants' discrimination of faces following redundant presentations. Unpublished doctoral dissertation. Case Western Reserve Univ., Cleveland, Ohio, 1973.

Cornell, E. H., & Strauss, M. S. Infants' responsiveness to compounds of habituated visual stimuli. *Developmental Psychology,* 1973, *9,* 73–78.

Corsini, D. A. Memory: Interaction of stimulus and organismic factors. Paper presented at the meeting of the Society for Research in Child Development, Minneapolis, Minnesota, April 1971.

DeLoache, J. Individual differences in infant visual memory. Unpublished doctoral dissertation, Univ. of Illinois, Champaign, Illinois, 1973.

DeLoache, J., Wetherford, M., & Cohen, L. B. The effects of motivation and conditioned head turning on infant attention to patterns of varying complexity. Paper presented at the meeting of the Midwestern Psychological Association, Cleveland, Ohio, 1972.

Dember, W. N., & Earl, R. W. Analysis of exploratory, manipulatory, and curiosity behaviors. *Psychological Review,* 1957, *64,* 91–96.

Fagan, J. F. Memory in the infant. *Journal of Experimental Child Psychology,* 1970, *9,* 217–226.

Fagan, J. F. Infants' recognition memory for a series of visual stimuli. *Journal of Experimental Child Psychology,* 1971, *11,* 244–250.

Fagan, J. F. Infants' recognition memory for faces. *Journal of Experimental Child Psychology,* 1972, *14,* 453–476.

Fagan, J. F. Infants' delayed recognition memory and forgetting. *Journal of Experimental Child Psychology,* 1973, *16,* 424–450.

Fagan, J. F. Infant recognition memory: The effects of length of familiarization and type of discrimination task. *Child Development,* 1974, *45,* 351–356.

Fagan, J. F., Fantz, R. L., & Miranda, S. B. Infants' attention to novel stimuli as a function of postnatal and conceptional age. Paper presented at meeting of the Society for Research in Child Development, Minneapolis, Minnesota, April 1971.

Fantz, R. L. Visual experience in infants: Decreased attention to familiar patterns relative to novel ones. *Science,* 1964, *146,* 668–670.

Fitzgerald, H. E., Lintz, L. M., Brackbill, Y., & Adams, G. Time perception and conditioning of an autonomic response in young infants. *Perceptual and Motor Skills,* 1967, *24,* 479–486.

Friedman, S. Habituation and recovery of visual response in the alert human newborn. *Journal of Experimental Child Psychology,* 1972, *13,* 339–349. (a)

Friedman, S. Newborn visual attention to repeated exposure of redundant vs. "novel" targets. *Perception and Psychophysics*, 1972, *12*, 291–294. (b)

Friedman, S., & Carpenter, G. C. Visual response decrement as a function of age in human newborn. *Child Development*, 1971, *42*, 1967–1973.

Friedman, S., Carpenter, G. C., & Nagy, A. N. Decrement and recovery of response to visual stimuli in the newborn human. *Proceedings, 78th Annual Convention, American Psychological Association*, 1970, *5*, 273–274.

Friedman, S., Nagy, A. N., & Carpenter, G. C. Newborn attention: Differential response decrement to visual stimuli. *Journal of Experimental Child Psychology*, 1970, *10*, 44–51.

Gelber, E. R. The effect of time and intervening items on the recovery of an habituated response. Unpublished master's thesis, Univ. of Illinois, Champaign, Illinois, 1972. (a)

Gelber, E. R. Habituation, discrimination learning, and visual information processing in infants. Unpublished doctoral dissertation, Univ. of Illinois, Champaign, Illinois, 1972. (b)

Glanzer, M., & Clark, W. H. Accuracy of perceptual recall: An analysis of organization. *Journal of Verbal Learning and Verbal Behavior*, 1962, *1*, 289–299.

Greenberg, D. J., & Weizmann, F. The measurement of visual attention in infants: A comparison of two methodologies. *Journal of Experimental Child Psychology*, 1971, *11*, 234–243.

Greenberg, D. J., Uzgiris, I. C., & Hunt, J. McV. Attentional preference and experience: III. Visual familiarity and looking time. *Journal of Genetic Psychology*, 1970, *117*, 123–135.

Horowitz, F., Paden, L., Bhana, W., & Self, P. An "Infant Control" procedure for studying infant visual fixations. *Developmental Psychology*, 1972, *7*, 90.

Hunt, J. McV. Intrinsic motivation and its role in psychological development. *Nebraska Symposium on Motivation*, 1965, *14*, 189–282.

Jeffrey, W. E., & Cohen, L. B. Habituation in the human infant. In H. Reese (Ed.), *Advances in child development and behavior*. Vol. 6. New York: Academic Press, 1971, 63–97.

Lewis, M. Individual differences in the measurement of early cognitive growth. In J. Hellmuth (Ed.), *Exceptional infant*. Vol. 2. *Studies in abnormalities*. New York: Brunner/Mazel, 1971. Pp. 172–210.

Martin, R. M. Long-term effects of stimulus familiarization. Paper presented at the meeting of the Society for Research in Child Development, Philadelphia, Pennsylvania, March 1973.

McCall, R. B. Attention in the infant: Avenue to the study of cognitive development. In D. Walcher, & D. Peters (Eds.), *Early childhood: The development of self-regulatory mechanisms*. New York: Academic Press, 1971. Pp. 107–137.

McCall, R. B. Habituation and the response to discrepancy: Implications for memory, retrieval and processing perceptual information. Paper presented at the meeting of the American Psychological Association, Honolulu, Hawaii, September 1972.

McCall, R. B., Hogarty, P. S., Hamilton, J. S., & Vincent, J. H. Habituation rate and the infant's response to visual discrepancies. *Child Development*, 1973, *44*, 280–287.

McCall, R. B., & Kagan, J. Stimulus-schema discrepancy and attention in the infant. *Journal of Experimental Child Psychology*, 1967, *5*, 381–390.

McCall, R. B., & Kagan, J. Individual differences in the infant's distribution of attention to stimulus discrepancy. *Developmental Psychology*, 1970, *2*, 90–98.

McCall, R. B., & Melson, W. H. Attention in infants as a function of magnitude of discrepancy and habituation rate. *Psychonomic Science*, 1969, *17*, 317–319.

McCall, R. B., Wycoff, H. E., Hamilton, J. S., & Hogarty, P. S. The infant's fixation to discrepancies from a decaying perceptual memory engram. Unpublished paper, 1974.

McClelland, D. C., & Clark, R. A. Antecedent conditions for affective arousal. In D. C. McClelland, J. W. Atkinson, R. A. Clark, & E. L. Lowell (Eds.), *The achievement motive*. New York: Appleton, 1953.

McGurk, H. The role of object orientation in infant perception. *Journal of Experimental Child Psychology*, 1970, *9*, 363–373.

McKenzie, B., & Day, R. H. Operant learning of visual pattern discrimination in young infants. *Journal of Experimental Child Psychology*, 1971, *11*, 45–53. (a)

McKenzie, B., & Day, R. H. Orientation discrimination in infants: A comparison of visual fixation and operant training methods. *Journal of Experimental Child Psychology*, 1971, *11*, 366–375. (b)

Miranda, S. B., & Fantz, R. L. Recognition memory in Down's Syndrome and normal infants. *Child Development*, 1974, *45*, 651–660.

Nickerson, R. S. A note on long-term recognition memory for pictorial materials. *Psychonomic Science*, 1968, *11*, 58.

Norman, D. A. (Ed.) *Models of human memory*. New York: Academic Press, 1970.

Paivio, A. Mental imagery in associative learning and memory. *Psychological Review*, 1969, *76*, 241–263.

Pancratz, C. N., & Cohen, L. B. Recovery of habituation in infants. *Journal of Experimental Child Psychology*, 1970, *9*, 208–216.

Parry, M. H. Infants' responses to novelty in familiar and unfamiliar settings. *Child Development*, 1972, *43*, 233–237.

Piaget, J. *The origins of intelligence in children*. New York: International Universities Press, 1952.

Piaget, J., & Inhelder, B. *Memory and intelligence*. New York: Basic Books, 1973.

Reese, H. W., & Lipsitt, L. P. *Experimental child psychology*. New York: Academic Press, 1970.

Reitman, W. What does it take to remember? In D. A. Norman (Ed.), *Models of human memory*. New York: Academic Press, 1970. Pp. 469–509.

Saayman, G., Ames, E. W., & Moffett, A. R. Response to novelty as an indicator of visual discrimination in the human infant. *Journal of Experimental Child Psychology*, 1964, *1*, 189–198.

Sigman, M. Visual preferences of premature and full-term infants. Paper presented at meeting of the Society for Research in Child Development, Philadelphia, Pennsylvania, March 1973.

Sokolov, E. N. *Perception and the conditioned reflex*. New York: Macmillan, 1963.

Sokolov, E. N. The modeling properties of the nervous system. In M. Coles & I. Maltzman (Eds.), *A handbook of contemporary Soviet psychology*. New York: Basic Books, 1969. Pp. 671–704.

Thomas, H. Discrepancy hypotheses: Methodological and theoretical considerations. *Psychological Review*, 1971, *78*, 249–259.

Watson, J. S. Memory and "contingency analysis" in infant learning. *Merrill-Palmer Quarterly*, 1967, *13*, 55–76.

Watson, J. S. Operant conditioning of visual fixation in infants under visual and auditory reinforcement. *Developmental Psychology*, 1969, *1*, 508–516.

Weizmann, F., Cohen, L. B., & Pratt, J. Novelty, familiarity, and the development of infant attention. *Developmental Psychology*, 1971, *4*, 149–154.

Welch, M. J. Infants' visual attention to varying degrees of novelty. Unpublished doctoral dissertation, Case Western Reserve Univ., Cleveland, Ohio, 1973.

✕ Wetherford, M. J., & Cohen, L. B. Developmental changes in infant visual preferences for novelty and familiarity. *Child Development*, 1973, *44*, 416–424.

Zeaman, D., & House, B. J. The role of attention in retardate discrimination learning. In N. R. Ellis (Ed.), *Handbook of mental deficiency*. New York: McGraw-Hill, 1963. Pp. 159–223.

Author Index

Sprague, J. M., 95, *130,* 160, 161, 162, *246*
Stark, L., 41, 42, 46, *74,* 143, 171, *244*
Stechler, G., 180, *246, 276, 345*
Steele, B., 40, 43, 44, 45, *66,* 175, 177, *237*
Steinman, R. M., 169, *246*
Steinsiek, K. J., 27, *70,* 104, 109, *128*
Stern, E., 177, *244, 246*
Stewart, D. L., 94, *130*
Stiles, W. S., 153, 174, *246*
Stirnimann, F., 276, 299, *345*
Stone, E., 63, *74*
Strauss, M. S., 374, 375, *400*
Streiff, E. B., 167, 169, *246*
Stromeyer, C. F., III., 147, *246*
Sturr, J. F., 146, *243*
Suitt, C. D., 27, 31, 35, *69,* 104, *127,* 297, *343*
Sutherland, N. S., 138, *246*
Sutton, P., 147, *236*
Sutton, S., 26, 30, *70*
Sweet, J. A., 84, *125*

T

Tauber, E., 44, 48, *74*
Taylor, D. M., *246*
Taylor, J. H., 98, 120, *130,* 147, *244*
Thach, W. T., Jr., 169, *238*
Thatcher, R. W., 100, *128*
Thibos, L. N., 147, *239*
Thines, G., 136, *243*
Thomas, H., 176, 193, *246,* 378, *402*
Thomas, J., 99, *131*
Thompson, R. F., 100, *131*
Tinbergen, N., 137, *246*
Todd, A., 2, *74,* 178, *246*
Todd, T., 2, *74,* 178, *246*
Tordoir, W., 23, 26, 27, *73*
Treisman, A. M., 140, *247*
Tresselt, M. E., 146, 154, *243*
Trevarthen, C., 39, 63, *74,* 139, 158, 160, *242, 247*
Trevarthen, C. B., 234, *247*
Trincker, D., 26, *74*
Trincker, I., 26, *74*
Tronick, E., 39, 40, *75,* 175, 179, 180, 229, *247*
Tsuchida, Y., 18, 19, *71*

Tursky, B., 39, *74*
Twarowski, C. J., 178, *243*

U

Udelf, M. S., 44, 45, *68,* 78, *127,* 251, 343
Uhr, L., 138, *247*
Umezaki, H., 23, 25, 30, 31, 32, 34, *75*
Uttley, A. M., 138, *247*
Uzgiris, I. C., 380, *401*

V

Vallecalle, E., 99, *131*
Van der Tweel, L. H., 109, *131*
Vanzini, P., 99, *131*
Vanzulli, A., 23, 24, 25, 28, 29, 31, *75*
Verduyn Lunel, H. F. E., 109, *131*
Verzeano, M., 99, *131*
Vincent, E., 63, *73*
Vincent, J. H., 377, *401*
Vinh-Bang., 141, *244*
Vitova, Z., 23, 29, 32, 34, *75*
von Noorden, G. K., 146, 147, *247*
von Senden, M., 148, 149, *247*
Vossler, C., 138, *247*

W

Walk, R. D., 92, 93, 94, *129, 131*
Wallace, J. G., 148, *239*
Walls, G. L., 3, *75,* 150, *247*
Walsh, F., 42, 44, 47, *75*
Walters, C. P., 93, *131*
Walton, D., 7, 8, 9, *75*
Warkentin, J., 94, *131*
Watanabe, K., 24, 25, 29, 32, 34, *75*
Watanabe, S., 99, 100, *126*
Watson, J. S., 356, 383, *402*
Weale, R. A., 151, 153, *245, 247*
Weber, R. B., 168, 186, *247*
Weinmann, H., 104, *131*
Weiskrantz, L., 158, 160, 206, *241*
Weisstein, N., *247*
Weitzman, E., 42, 43, *69*
Weizmann, F., 292, *343,* 365, 366, 380, 381, *401, 403*
Welch, M. J., 374, 377, *403*
Weled, B., 25, *69*
Wenner, W. H., 177, *244, 246*

Subject Index